FOR REFERENCE

Do Not Take From This Room

D1737678

Alternative Healing in American History

Alternative Healing in American History

An Encyclopedia from Acupuncture to Yoga

MICHAEL SHALLY-JENSEN

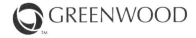
GREENWOOD

An Imprint of ABC-CLIO, LLC

Santa Barbara, California • Denver, Colorado

Copyright © 2019 by ABC-CLIO, LLC

Library of Congress Cataloging-in-Publication Data

Names: Shally-Jensen, Michael, author.
Title: Alternative healing in American history : an encyclopedia from acupuncture to yoga / Michael Shally-Jensen.
Description: Santa Barbara, California : Greenwood, [2019] | Includes bibliographical references and index.
Identifiers: LCCN 2019008161 (print) | LCCN 2019008711 (ebook) | ISBN 9781440860348 (eBook) | ISBN 9781440860331 (hardcopy : alk. paper)
Subjects: | MESH: Complementary Therapies—history | United States | Encyclopedia
Classification: LCC RM700 (ebook) | LCC RM700 (print) | NLM WB 13 | DDC 615.8/2—dc23
LC record available at https://lccn.loc.gov/2019008161

ISBN: 978-1-4408-6033-1 (print)
        978-1-4408-6034-8 (ebook)

23 22 21 20 19   1 2 3 4 5

This book is also available as an eBook.

Greenwood
An Imprint of ABC-CLIO, LLC

ABC-CLIO, LLC
147 Castilian Drive
Santa Barbara, California 93117
www.abc-clio.com

This book is printed on acid-free paper ∞

Manufactured in the United States of America

Contents

Alphabetical List of Entries

Introduction

If you walk into your local coffee shop, food market, library, or campus center, chances are that you'll encounter ads for a variety of complementary and alternative health products and services. Acupuncture, tai chi classes, breathing and meditation exercises, naturopathic clinics, detox diets, Ayurvedic consultations, and various mental health approaches are just a few of the many options one can choose from for one's health maintenance needs. You are also likely to find, in the pharmacy or the pharmacy section of any supermarket, shelf after shelf of dietary supplements along with essential oils, nature-based lotions and toothpastes, and, nearby, numerous herbal teas, and the like. In fact, if you are like many other Americans, you will have already sampled one or more of the broad selection of options available, even if it was only to have had a little "soothing" Ayurvedic tea, or placed a pretty "healing" crystal on your nightstand, or explored visualization exercises to get at the connection between the mind and the body. Perhaps, even, your physician has recommended that you try fish oil or some other supplement or that you see a chiropractor or massage therapist for a particular ailment. Similarly, if you've visited a bookstore or magazine stand, you will have noticed whole sections devoted to health and wellness, most featuring works on "self-help" or the programs of various health "gurus." If you've had occasion to visit a large hospital recently, you may have discovered that it has a "wellness center" or signs indicating the presence of different "integrative therapeutics" such as Reiki, biofeedback, or somatic methods ("bodywork"). Such is the state of complementary and alternative medicine (CAM) today that virtually everyone knows at least something about it, and more and more businesses and organizations are making its products and services accessible to the public.

Complementary health approaches include an array of ideas and practices with a history of use outside of conventional Western medicine (or *biomedicine*, as it is often called). People use complementary health approaches to improve general health and well-being, to relieve symptoms associated with chronic diseases, or to lessen the side effects of conventional medicine. Most people in the United States use such approaches as an auxiliary to conventional medical care rather than as a replacement for it. Nevertheless, usage occurs on a sliding scale, as it were: some CAM purists avoid standard biomedicine to an extreme degree, while, at the opposite end, many people rely on biomedicine as their primary health resource and are mere dabblers in alternative approaches.

Outlines of Current Use

The latest data from the National Center for Complementary and Integrative Health (2018) concerning CAM usage are not as comprehensive as in previous years, but one can look at them in connection with earlier reports to get a picture of what has been happening (see also National Center for Health Statistics 2015, for data from 2012). As of 2012, and most likely today, the most commonly used complementary health approach is the taking of dietary supplements, such as fish oil, ginseng, and glucosamine: nearly 18 percent of adult Americans took (nonvitamin, nonmineral) supplements in 2012. (Vitamins and minerals, which are in even wider circulation, are not considered part of CAM by NCCIH.) Another popular modality is yoga, whose use has continued to increase over the years and now is enjoyed by 14.3 percent of adults, especially by women (19.8 percent of women versus 8.6 percent of men). Almost on par with yoga is meditation, with 14.2 percent of adults making use of this approach in 2017. The use of chiropractic care was the fourth most commonly used approach in 2017, with 10.3 percent of American adults taking advantage of it—again representing a solid increase from previous years. Other moderately popular approaches used in recent years include deep-breathing exercises, whether alone or in combination with another activity; and tai chi and qigong, which have shown a slow but steady rise. Approaches with lower but by no means insignificant rates of prevalence include homeopathic treatment, acupuncture, and naturopathy along with Ayurveda, biofeedback, guided imagery (visualization), and energy healing therapy such as Reiki. Some observers have commented that, in light of earlier surveys, these statistics probably greatly underestimate the percentage of people who have explored CAM approaches at one point or another and that the real figure is likely to exceed one-third of the U.S. population.

From whence did all these healing riches come? What forces brought them to the American medical marketplace, and when? Who makes use of them and why? How do they stand in relation to the medical establishment? Are they really useful or are they closer to a cultural fad of some kind? These are some of the questions that we explore in the present book. We examine the rise and fall and, in many cases, rise again of over a hundred different alternative healing strategies, ranging from Colonial-era witchcraft treatments and humorism (see below) to modern-day technologies. Although the bulk of the topics covered fall squarely within the alternative medicine camp, the line between mainstream and alternative/complementary has not always been sharply drawn; and for that reason we include some subjects that are now or may once have been considered ordinary, or orthodox, but over time have experienced their own cultural downturns or upturns. Therefore, we throw a wider net than might otherwise be expected in a book about "alternative" healing. We include mostly alternative approaches but also some key orthodox ones to help shed light on the broader picture.

We should begin, though, with a little background.

Development of Alternative Medicine

Before the last decades of the 19th century, when the germ theory first arose and became established, orthodox medicine was based on the humoral theory, an idea that had been around for centuries. The humoral theory held that four internal fluids, or humors, made up the human constitution: blood, phlegm, yellow bile (associated with the gall bladder), and black bile (associated with the liver). It was necessary to keep these humors in balance in order to maintain one's health; otherwise, illness could result. When someone did become sick, it was the physician's job to restore balance among the humors. This objective was commonly achieved through two simple yet dramatic procedures: bleeding the patient by lancing a vein, and purging the patient by administering a medication such as calomel, which often caused explosive vomiting and diarrhea.

Elaborate treatises were written on the humors and the whys and wherefores of the balancing act performed by doctors, but there was no concrete evidence for the workings of these fluids inside the body, and few homegrown doctors (or patients) bothered themselves with the details. What mattered most was that humoral medicine had been around for a long time, serving patient populations throughout the Western world. When doctors ordered patients to be bled and purged, they could feel that something was being done to "cure" the illness at hand. Blood and puke, after all, were clear signs that bodily fluids were on the move.

Both these procedures, unfortunately, severely depleted the energy resources of the patient and undoubtedly did more harm than good. Patients most often recovered on their own (or did not), depending on the type of illness they had and various other factors—most of which had nothing to do with the state of their humors. Such slow, painful illness experiences and recuperations, moreover, had little to recommend them: most people looked forward to a doctor's visit with about as much enthusiasm as they did a visit to the dentist, at a time when dentistry itself was quite distressful and anything but painless. For this reason, some enterprising men (and, eventually, women) in the 19th century undertook to develop alternatives to regular medicine. Not that they saw their systems as mere alternatives, however; for many, in fact, these systems were considered *better* than the conventional medicine of the time. Why not pursue something that promised to revolutionize health care?

One such fellow was Samuel Thomson, a self-trained New Hampshire physician who in the early part of the century began to promote the use of botanical medicines and other treatments for common ailments. Thomson had watched his mother suffer for weeks while she was bled and purged by local doctors, only to see her die of "galloping consumption" (severe tuberculosis) in the end. As a consequence, he came to regard conventional medicine as a loathsome business. He developed an alternative system based on maintaining bodily heat and ensuring good digestion. Thomsonian therapy consisted of ingesting spicy cayenne peppers and other vegetable matter and substituting the plant lobelia—known as puke weed—for toxic calomel as a means of cleansing the system. The system also entailed the use of blankets and steam to sustain body temperature. Thomson's goal was to make "every man his own physician," and he did so by actively marketing his products and methods to the masses. For a few decades before Thomson's death in 1843, his alternative form of healing was immensely popular in many parts of the United States.

Another early adopter of alternative thinking in medicine was Samuel Hahnemann, a German physician who favored herbal cures and invented the system called *homeopathy*. Like Thomson, Hahnemann thought the practice of bleeding and purging crude and ineffective. An observant practitioner as well as a medicinal tinkerer, he was led to conclude that he could cure a sick patient by supplying him or her with a tiny dose of a botanical or other substance that caused, in a healthy person, symptoms like those exhibited by the patient. For example, a bark powder that produced a fever or increased the pulse rate in a healthy person could be used to relieve the same fever or high pulse rate in a sick person. The idea was that a treatment regimen using minute amounts of a compound or highly diluted solutions worked to replace the patient's more pronounced symptoms with milder ones, thereby giving the patient's body a better chance to recover. Hahnemann's philosophy was "like cures like" (hence, the name *homeopathy*), and for a few decades between the 1840s and the late 1860s, homeopathy enjoyed great popularity, even drawing many "regular" doctors to its side. The American Medical Association, founded in 1847, resisted the pressure, however, and declared homeopathy to be a false system (even while it continued to endorse the humoral approach).

Of course, there had always been informal folk healers, "root doctors," bonesetters, tooth-pullers, preacher-counselors, and midwives working among the people, back when the nation was overwhelmingly rural. Indeed, many American families relied on their own limited medical knowledge and resources in treating themselves, drawing on remedies handed down through the generations along with farmers' almanacs and their knowledge of domesticated animals. They were fortunate, more or less, if the nearest local or itinerate doctor had a little training at a private medical school and a brief period of apprenticeship before going out on his own to explore the ways of disease. To be seriously ill, then, was not an experience for the faint of heart; one method after another might be tried while the patient remained bedridden or, in some cases, had to continue functioning in the household despite being ill. Death was a commonplace occurrence.

In the cities, things were a little different. There, an even greater variety of medical approaches was available. One of the most popular mid-19th-century competitors to Thomsonism and homeopathy, for example, was hydropathy, or *the water cure*. American hydropaths had been inspired by the success of water-treatment institutions in Europe. Similar in some respects to later "spas" and mineral-water resorts, but differing markedly from them as well, these hydropathic institutions employed all manner of cold baths and bracing water flows to establish health by contact with water and exposure to nature. Sitting for an hour or more in an open-air room on a cold day while wrapped in cold, wet sheets was one of the more highly touted "cures." Needless to say, the people who benefited most from the rigors of such treatment were the walking well, not the truly sick. Hydropathy appealed, as did the spas of the latter part of the century, primarily to educated city folk who needed a change of scene and/or a radical "fix" of some kind in their health status (physical or otherwise). Many of the fans of hydropathy also followed the health regimen promoted by Sylvester Graham, who argued for the importance of whole-grain breads, meatless dishes, temperance in drink and sex, nature walks, and other lifestyle changes. Graham was, arguably, the original diet and fitness guy—though one of a decidedly prudish sort.

Emerging in the second half of the 19th century were a number of alternative approaches linked loosely to the great popular phenomenon of mesmerism, or "animal magnetism," which had arrived on the scene in Europe—via Franz Mesmer—over 100 years earlier but lingered on in one form or another well after its creator's death in 1815. Thus, Christian Science, for example, founded in the United States by Mary Baker Eddy in the 1860s, preached healing through prayer, and prayer alone. Drawing on the notion of mesmerization, where ideas or experiences could seemingly be planted in the head, Eddy and the Christian Scientists argued that disease did not exist except as a construct in the mind; therefore, treatment of the sick consisted of changing their state of mind through prayerful action and the cultivation of faith. Christian Science was never a mass religious movement or a popular approach to health and wellness, but it caught on in some circles and continues to have a presence today. Far more successful as a popular culture phenomenon was a different sort of faith-based activity called *spiritualism*, which concerned itself with contacting the dead through spirit mediums and bringing consolation to the living. Spiritualism thrived in the post–Civil War era—so many dead soldiers waiting to be heard from—and enjoyed a modest renaissance after World War I.

Both osteopathy and chiropractic, created in the later decades of the 19th century, likewise shared a connection to mesmerism/animal magnetism through the idiom of magnetic healing, which the founder of each of these new healing methods practiced before hitting upon his own system of alternative therapy. Andrew Taylor Still, osteopathy's founder, had used magnetism to remove obstructions to the flow of body fluids before discovering that it was more effective to employ hands-on manipulation, particularly of the vertebrae and large bones, as a way of realigning any disarticulated regions and bringing health and healing to the patient. Still founded the American School of Osteopathy, in Kirksville, Missouri, in 1892—but it wouldn't be until the next century that osteopathy achieved broad success, in part by allowing its basic premise, or medical viewpoint, to evolve. Meanwhile, another former magnetic healer, Daniel David Palmer, founded the method of chiropractic manipulation around the same time, in Davenport, Iowa. In chiropractic's case, too, the original idea began as a vague understanding of fluidic blockages and then shifted to a concept of misaligned spinal parts and other problems involving pinched nerves. Chiropractic, likewise, would build up its reputation and gain broader appeal only in the 20th century, again by adapting to circumstances.

There are far too many developments such as the ones noted above, from both distant and more recent decades, to describe in an introduction such as this; we must allow these few early examples to serve as indicators of how the field of alternative medicine got off the ground and began its evolution—in many different directions over time. The reader is referred to separate introductions preceding each of the five sections of this book for historical background information, and to the entries themselves for more detailed information on the history, development, and uses of the various practices making up the field of complementary and alternative medicine.

Intercultural Sources

A word should be said here, though, about some medical traditions from cultures outside of North America that came to have an influence there. These traditions differ from the classic Western approach and yet share some surprising similarities with it.

In China and India, as well as in pre-modern Europe, the human body was traditionally viewed as a kind of microcosm of the universe. Physicians in these cultures held that the cosmos and the corporal substance of the body, along with certain aspects of the body's arrangement, had much in common—indeed, they were essentially the same. It was believed that the actions of the human body mimicked, in many ways, those of the cosmological world. The body was affected by the movements of heavenly forces. Chinese traditional medicine, Indian Ayurvedic medicine, medieval astrology and alchemy, and even some aspects of Native American traditional medicine all share this view. Chinese medicine, for example, gives primacy to the five main elements of the natural world: wood, water, fire, earth, and metal. There are also five planets, five directions (including the "center"), five tastes, fives smells, and five main organs: the heart, the liver, the spleen, the lungs, and the kidneys. Each of these components aligns with the others to compose a grand system of metaphysics, health, and wellness. Similarly, from the Indian subcontinent, Ayurveda features five elements (air, water, fire, earth, and ether), the five senses, and other fundamental connections while also giving primacy to the three *doshas*, or bodily humors (called, in this case, *vata, pitta,* and *kapha*).

These linkages between the composition of the body and the operations of the external world have long defined the way healers in these medical traditions approach health and illness. In each case, Indian, Chinese, and early European, practitioners treat disease as an imbalance of fluids or energies within the body that echo disturbances occurring in the relationship between the patient and his or her social and metaphysical environment. Native American traditional medicine, as well, shares some of these same traits. The goal of the healer in each case is to reestablish equilibrium by addressing both the personal and cosmological signs and symptoms involved, usually through a combination of approaches—material/

medicinal, behavioral/dietary, and spiritual. It is a regimen that demands attention to the subtleties of health and illness and, often, an ongoing effort by patients to maintain the proper balance.

Each of these ancient traditions has had a modest presence in Western culture since the mid-19th century. However, they became especially popular in the second half of the 20th century as part of the New Age movement and other developments. In the present work, we consider two of them—Chinese and Native American traditional medicine—in the context of their "pre-1900" existence, with comments provided about their "rebirth" in later decades. Ayurvedic medicine, on the other hand, is positioned as part of the 1960s–1970s New Age movement, because it tended to be less well known in the West until that time.

Mental Health

A separate overview should also be provided here regarding mental health and illness, because this subject has followed a somewhat different trajectory over the years and tells a slightly different story. Both mainstream and alternative approaches have played a part in that story, even though the line between them, again, is rather fuzzy in some instances.

As with "organic" illness, in the Colonial era mental illness was thought to result from both supernatural and natural causes. Protestant ministers and ordinary town folk were likely to blame mental and emotional troubles on "demons" inhabiting a person; the opportunity was thought to be given them by lapses of personal faith and poor moral judgment. Folk healers and midwives were sometimes accused of being sorceresses themselves, given that their trade required them to traffic in alchemical potions and the mysteries of the body. Meanwhile, doctors tended to attribute mental disturbances to the same four bodily humors that affected physical health and worked to restore balance as a means of treating patients. (Preacher-physicians, one supposes, took both approaches, moral and humoral.)

With the Enlightenment of the 18th century, mental illness—"madness" or insanity—came to be regarded as a problem with the individual's faculty of reason; in other words, illness was rooted in an inability to think logically and coherently, particularly in moral matters. One possible solution at the time was moral education, and for this reason various mental asylums were created to impart moral knowledge to patient populations instead of simply locking them up as hopeless "lunatics." One of the nation's founding fathers, Benjamin Rush of Philadelphia, was one of the first people to look at the mentally ill "compassionately" in this way.

Doctors working in psychiatric asylums in the 19th century had no standards of diagnosis and employed a variety of labels for different categories of illness, chief among them mania (hyperactivity and wild thoughts), melancholia (sadness or depression), dementia (incoherent or inconsistent thinking), and idiocy (gross mental/behavioral lapses). Various labels arose and fell over time, however, depending on the symptoms counted as definitive and the latest understanding about the sources of illness. In 1869, for example, a neurologist in New York,

George M. Beard, brought attention to a condition he called *neurasthenia*; it consisted of such symptoms as headaches, insomnia, exhaustion, and a general nervousness that Beard said stemmed from the stresses of modern living, particularly life in the cities. The diagnosis didn't last long, though, as other physicians began to find fault with it.

Mental conditions, then, seemed such vexing things from the modern scientific standpoint. *Hysteria*, for example, was another problematic label, being assigned mostly to women and seemingly brought on in odd circumstances reminiscent of mesmerism. One of the tools for exploring hysteria was hypnosis, which also served as a temporary treatment, of sorts. Hypnosis and the condition it was meant to address served, in fact, to reveal enough about the human mind to cause one neurologist from Vienna, Sigmund Freud, to shift his focus from organic medicine to the study of the psyche. Freudian psychoanalysis soon emerged as the latest and greatest explanation for mental illness—if not for the most serious of conditions, then at least for the many troublesome neuroses (disorders affecting only part of the personality) that people can and did experience. Especially in the United States, psychoanalysis came to dominate the psychiatric field for more than a half century in the 1900s; its central point of focus was psychic conflict caused by childhood sexual drives and the effect of those conflicts on the development of the person, or self. Nevertheless, after decades in the driver's seat, orthodox psychoanalysis began to lose ground to other competing approaches.

Behaviorism, humanistic psychiatry, sociological and clinical studies of sex, and similar challenges emerged in the 1950s. And, in the 1960s, an antipsychiatry movement, led by Thomas Szasz and R. D. Laing, promoted a broader conception of human "normalcy" and attacked what the movement's advocates called *the myth of mental illness*. By then, mental health was already starting to be understood as deeply enmeshed in social and cultural attitudes, not just in family dynamics during a child's developmental years. Although, ultimately, the antipsychiatry movement went too far in pursuing its new, alternative vision, it left a lasting mark on the field and lay behind later developments such as the recovery movement of the 1990s and, more recently, the notion of neurodiversity (an expanded concept of normality).

In the past few decades, many such alternative approaches have become marginalized in the psychiatric establishment by the paradigm of biomedicine, which has successfully demonstrated the power of drugs to control mental illnesses—not, however, with uniformly positive results. Drug therapy has experienced many of the same ups and downs as other approaches to mental health; it is not a straight evolutionary path. More recently, across the whole of the mental health field, and even in some circles within mainstream psychiatry, a recognition has arisen regarding the power of traditional approaches to the mind–body connection and the satisfactions that can be had by those who learn how to take advantage of that connection. Currently, then, while biological psychiatry holds center court, patients are likely to engage in various other, alternative pursuits as well. The present is indeed the era of "integrative" medicine, where patients act in conjunction with physicians to find the best solution for themselves and their general health and well-being.

Michael Shally-Jensen

Further Reading

Bivins, Roberta. 2007. *Alternative Medicine? A History.* New York: Oxford University Press.

Marchant, Jo. 2016. *Cure: A Journey into the Science of Mind over Body.* New York: Crown Publishers.

National Center for Complementary and Integrative Health and National Center for Health Statistics. 2018. "2017 National Health Interview Survey." https://nccih.nih.gov/research/statistics/NHIS

National Center for Health Statistics. 2015. "Trends in the Use of Complementary Health Approaches among Adults: United States, 2002-2012." https://www.cdc.gov/nchs/data/nhsr/nhsr079.pdf

Porter, Roy. 2002. *Madness: A Brief History.* New York: Oxford University Press.

Pre-1900

INTRODUCTION

In the United States, as in most of the rest of the world before the modern era, methods of treating illness were long rooted in local custom and belief. Until the start of the 20th century, really, there was no firmly established class of professional physicians, or even a convincing scientific model of health and illness. The medicine practiced in one region or by one group could be quite different from the medicine practiced elsewhere. Moreover, a range of new systems created by innovators who promised cures, and, in many cases, produced satisfied customers, arose at different times and places over the course of the 19th century. Not all of these alternatives lasted. Meanwhile, the standard medical system that eventually came to dominate the scene was still a century away. The "regular" doctors who operated in the 1800s employed much the same methods as those used by their predecessors in the 1700s or even earlier.

Medical Mélange

Nineteenth-century "irregular" doctors, or those pursuing alternatives to what then passed as "conventional" medicine, advocated a wide variety of approaches. There were magnetic healers, hydrotherapists, sellers of electrical shock equipment, makers of sham medicines, and more. Patients were urged to seek fresh air away from the cities or to recreate at hot spas, if one could afford it. There were mesmerism and spiritualism to address emotional concerns; there were diets of whole grains and simple vegetables to improve digestion; and there were homeopathic remedies containing tinctures of substances that caused symptoms similar to those of the very disease one wished to cure. Some of the characters behind these varied methods might be referred to as quacks, whereas many of them were dead serious and staked their lives and careers on the truth of their approach.

In many communities, laypersons combined folk customs with information gathered from almanacs and popular reference works to treat injuries and disease. At the same time, regular doctors, so-called, were trained through a mix of informal teaching and practical apprenticeship. What medical schools existed in the mid-19th century were, as often as not, business enterprises organized for the profit of the professors who managed them. Students, typically from middle-class or working families, were asked to pay to attend lectures of doubtful value. Even after the founding of the American Medical Association (AMA) in 1847, formal medical education at hospital- or university-affiliated institutions could vary in structure and content, as there was no standardized curriculum. In schools for "irregulars," meanwhile, the curriculum was organized around a particular *kind* of medicine: homeopathy, hydrotherapy (water cure), chiropractic, and so on.

Few people living in the 19th century, whether laypersons or doctor-healers, agreed on what form medicine should have. Indeed, many people were skeptical of those who sought to fix medical practice within a single therapeutic mold. Calls by orthodox practitioners for order and uniformity were taken to be attempts to secure legitimacy for their own version of healing. Throughout much of the century, the varied approaches of different groups produced an odd assemblage of therapeutic know-how and medical understanding. Training differed for urban doctors, rural doctors, homeopaths, allopaths (or what we now might call mainstream physicians), eclectics, herbalists, and a host of others. Those treating patients of different social classes, different ethnicities, and so on were often expected to adjust their practice to the realities of the situation; local traditions, social expectations, and cultural norms were hard to overcome.

Regular physicians, or those who came closest to having a medical education in the modern sense, relied heavily on bloodletting and on purgatives and emetics. They used calomel, for example, a toxic mercury-based compound, to induce vomiting. Bloodletting was intended to drain the body of unwanted "bile" and restore balance to one's natural "humors," or fluids and vapors. The basis of the medical approach was rather speculative, as there was as yet no understanding of germ theory and no thorough, science-based comprehension of anatomy and physiology. The "cause" of an illness might as often be ascribed to god (or one's offenses against him) as not. In the case of mental illness, in fact, the patient was usually thought to have strayed morally and therefore required a strong dose of moral and religious teaching to turn his life around. Only occasionally did such "therapy" produce long-term benefits, though it was certainly preferable to previous forms of mental health treatment involving imprisonment inside grim "lunatic asylums" or "madhouses."

In many cities and towns, regular practitioners were predominant. As the century progressed, however, they found themselves competing with homeopaths, herbalists, patent medicine salespersons (i.e., those promoting cheap nostrums), faith healers, and all variety of others. Self-taught itinerants offered their services as fever doctors, bonesetters, and dentists. Midwives provided birthing services, where they weren't pushed out by male physicians. Patients in the 19th-century United States had the advantage of choice when it came to maintaining their health, even though what they had to choose from often worked on the basis of wishful thinking and natural recovery over time.

Folk healers in rural areas already depended largely on plant-based treatments—solutions, ointments, burnings (inhalations), poultices, and so on—along with other folk remedies. This explains why the Thomsonian system of botanical treatment, developed by Samuel Thomson (1769–1843) as an alternative to regular medicine, became one the most successful "schools" of medicine in large areas of New England, the South, and the Midwest. Thomsonism, which involved the use of herbs, spices, laxatives, and steam baths, was really the first "trending" form of medicine on the continent, the popular "alternative" of the day. Thomson reminded all who would hear him that only pain and suffering resulted from the bleeding, blistering, and purging of regular medicine. He and other irregular healers believed in their right to practice and in the public's right to choose how and by whom they were treated.

People who feared that regular medicine was too harsh but weren't sold on the benefits of herbs, cathartics, and steam treatments might instead turn to another, equally mild form of practice: homeopathy. A European import, homeopathic medicine appealed to people on the basis of its unusual rationale—that is, that tiny amounts of potentially *damaging* substances could help build up the constitution. Homeopathy also attracted merchants because of the ease of transporting small vials of medicine—in an era of lax regulatory controls over such items.

Meanwhile, another group of practitioners—eclectics, as they were known—went one step further and used botanicals, purgatives, folk remedies, homeopathy, and whatever else was available. Eclectics were reviled by regular doctors nearly as much as irregulars were.

Broad claims were made, too, by the inventors of patent medicines. These were sold through touring medicine shows in rural areas and towns alike. They sold well in these venues, and they also were sold through advertising and, later, via mail order. Indeed, if patent medicines did not actually launch the advertising business in the United States, they certainly pushed it to the next level. What they might have lacked in substance, it seems, had to be made up for by their creators in the form of populist, no-holds-barred advertisements. These ads were usually as florid as the circuslike pitches made by salesmen at medicine shows. A person could, it was proclaimed, heal virtually any condition by swallowing some "amazing" cure-all or taking a few incredible "liver pills," say, which in truth contained indeterminate ingredients and were of dubious manufacture.

Then there was phrenology, which wasn't exactly a type of medicine but rather a way to "read" the characters of different people and understand what might be going on with them. It accomplished this task through an examination of the skull, with special attention being paid to its bumps, their size and location. Personality, health, career, and social prospects might be outlined by such an exam. Phrenology enjoyed great popularity in the 1870s, and professional phrenologists and courses in phrenology became widely available in the cities. It was, however, ultimately a passing fad.

Doctors' Progress

Regular doctors viewed the various irregular systems with skepticism. They considered irregular medicine as a baseless mix of common substances and sometimes dangerous methods foisted upon the public as a cheap alternative to the real thing. Physicians were, for the most part, "family" or "community" practitioners who engaged in general medicine; very few of them specialized in surgery, neurology, or other areas. As such, they typically lived in the communities where they practiced, making house calls or treating patients in their offices located at their home in town. Often they and their patients were members of the same church or club. The doctor would preside at significant family moments like births and deaths. It was his role to comfort the family during an illness, and he might spend many hours inside a patient's home during the course of it.

These doctors were working in an era of uncertainty regarding medical procedures and outcomes. Because of the sketchy nature of medical knowledge, and the fact that doctors depended on their patients for a living, regulars tended to practice in ways that were familiar to their patients. In many ways, in fact, their knowledge was not much more sophisticated than that of their patients. Most doctors employed bleeding, cupping, purging, and other relatively harsh measures to treat their patients. Calomel was just one of a host of violent purgatives employed to cleanse the intestines. Incised veins were allowed to release a pint or more of blood at a time. Given the association of illness with moral failing, the cruelty of the medical method can be viewed as being part of the treatment process. It worked almost like a confessional: one admits a problem, suffers for his or her sins, and then comes out of it—hopefully—renewed and reinvigorated.

This type of "heroic" medicine, as it is sometimes called, began to change near the end of the century. By the 1890s doctors had come to understand the role of viruses and bacteria in causing disease. They learned the significance of personal contact and insects in the spread of infectious disease. They knew how to wash their hands before surgery and how to reduce infection through sanitation. They started to grasp more thoroughly how organs functioned. Even while cures remained elusive, advances were made in the theory, classification, and diagnosis of disease.

By the turn of the century, therefore, there was a movement to reform medical education. Calls for standardizing the training of physicians and controlling entry into the profession through licensure won favor. Medical education was to be grounded in laboratory science and clinical training, the reformers made clear. Medical practice itself started to become more uniform, more rigorous, more standardized.

Battles between the American Medical Association and proponents of alternative therapies had occurred earlier in the 19th century. Now they became even more serious. Chiropractic, for example, was the subject of a sustained campaign by physicians to discredit it—partly because it enjoyed significant success and doctors were losing patients to it. What was particularly unfortunate about this conflict was that musculoskeletal discomfort, especially back pain, was an area that regular medicine had largely disregarded. Chiropractors, along with osteopaths, developed methods to address it. Indeed, they and the other irregulars did not necessarily think of their type of medicine as "alternative" but merely as *not* regular medicine. Irregulars speculated on the cause of disease and presented believable theories, however unorthodox. They promised their patients/clients a direct path to wellness. Their ideas helped patients to make sense of sometimes confusing and often vague symptoms. Although their methods were somewhat hit or miss, often enough they got things right. They helped people gain a sense of control over their illness and feel that they were getting better instead of worse.

Other Traditions

We also look here at a couple of non-Western medical traditions that played a role in the development of modern complementary and alternative medicine in North America. Native American remedies, for one, had been relied on for millennia before the arrival of Europeans. They continued to do service as part of the Western materia medica in the New World. Botanical medicines used by U.S. physicians were most often based on indigenous plants, and Native American preparations, not their European counterparts. In addition, the connection with Native Americans was exploited on the basis of their having ancient and exotic wisdom unfamiliar to whites. Especially in patent medicines and medicine shows, Native American–themed products and entertainments became big attractions, even though they were typically "made up" examples. A somewhat truer use of Native American medicines and practices occurred a century later, in the New Age movement of the 1970s. In the latter case, the intent was to reveal the "natural healer" within all of us, and to explore new, "deeper" meanings of health and well-being.

Another ancient tradition of medicine that made inroads in the West was Chinese traditional medicine. Here, again, Chinese communities in North America had long relied on this system before Euro-Americans discovered its value as a complementary or alternative form of medicine. The holistic health ideology that emerged in the 1960s and 1970s fostered an interest in the classical traditions of the Far East. Acupuncture, in particular, seemed to embody the esoteric—and spiritual—nature of Chinese medicine, and it seemed to work in many cases. In the section that follows, we consider Chinese traditional medicine and philosophy as a whole, and look at acupuncture, along with its distant cousins Tai Chi and Qigong, in later sections.

A third important non-Western system, Ayurveda, is explored only in a later section, reflecting the fact that it did not have a strong presence in the United States until sometime in the 1970s and 1980s, when the South Asian Indian population began to grow significantly and the New Age/holistic health movement was in full swing.

Further Reading

Janik, Erika. 2014. *Marketplace of the Marvelous: The Strange Origins of Modern Medicine.* Boston: Beacon Press.
Shorter, Edward. 2003. *A History of Psychiatry: From the Era of the Asylum to the Age of Prozac.* New York: Wiley.
Starr, Paul. 2017. *The Social Transformation of American Medicine.* 2nd ed. New York: Basic Books.
Whorton, James C. 2002. *Nature Cures: The History of Alternative Medicine in America.* New York: Oxford University Press.

BLOODLETTING AND LEECHING

Bloodletting, or the practice of draining a certain amount of the patient's blood, has existed for thousands of years. It is, in fact, one of the oldest medical practices. Historians believe that it dates back at least to ancient Egypt, from whence it migrated to Greece. By the time of the Middle Ages in Europe, bloodletting was the preferred treatment for most ailments. The practice began to die out only in the second half of the 19th century, when the germ theory displaced the long-standing humoral theory of illness (according to which sickness results from an imbalance of bodily "humors," or fluids). When modern medications like vaccines and penicillin became easily available, bloodletting died out almost entirely. Modern doctors, however, have found that bloodletting is still very useful, albeit in limited settings.

Traditional Practice

Bloodletting treatments were common in ancient Greece by the third century BCE, when the physician Erasistratus commented that all illness was caused by an excess of blood, or *phlethoras*. Erasistratus's work was based on the fifth-century BCE writings of Hippocrates. The latter believed that the body was controlled by four humors: blood, phlegm, yellow bile, and black bile. When these four humors were

---

How Bloodletting May Have Killed George Washington

On two cold, rainy days in December 1799, George Washington rode out to see to his plantation. After the second day, however, Washington awoke early in the morning and summoned aides and doctors, extremely ill. Modern experts believe that he most likely had strep throat. Today, this is an easy infection to treat with antibiotics; in 1799, no such medication existed. The general was treated by bloodletting; he died later that same day.

Washington is far from the only person to have been bled as they were on their sickbeds; King Charles II of England suffered a stroke in February 1665 and died four days later. During that time, he endured many different treatments, including cupping and bloodletting.

In France in 1778, Marie-Antoinette was in labor with a crowd observing, hoping to see the birth of the next dauphin. At one point, Marie-Antoinette fainted. Her surgeon quickly applied his lancet, and she revived; it's worth noting, however, that the accounts of the time also note that the windows were simultaneously opened to let in some fresh air.

George Washington is perhaps the most famous person to have directly died due to bloodletting, although that summation may not be entirely fair. Modern physicians believe the swelling in the former president's throat was extreme and that the amount of blood drained was an attempt to clear that swelling. Still, losing roughly half his blood in just a few hours was clearly the ultimate cause of death.

in balance, the body was healthy. When they were out of balance, the individual would become ill. The nature of the person's illness would show which humor was out of balance; someone with melancholia, for example, would have too much black bile. Black bile was associated with cold and dry elements, so the physician would treat the patient with warm, wet herbs or foods.

Erasistratus recommended reducing the plethoras in many different ways, including sweating, limiting food intake, and vomiting. It was the Roman-era physician Galen of Pergamum who, in the second century CE, studied Hippocrates and then wrote and advocated for the use of bloodletting in many different circumstances to relieve imbalances of the humors. At the time a lively debate broke out between those siding with Galen and those preferring Erasistratus's method and explanation.

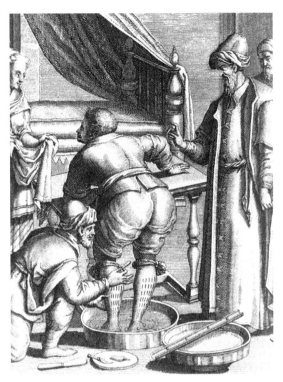

A bloodletting procedure as published in *Lugduni Batavorum*, 1718. One man is making incisions with a lancet on the backs of the legs of a man standing in a tub of water while a woman stands to the left with a towel. Other instruments and another tub are on the floor. The physician stands to the right. (National Library of Medicine)

Many cultures have a medical history that involves the imbalance of different bodily energies or elements. Ayurvedic medicine, for example, focuses on the three doshas; and the Chinese Wu Xing, or five elements, are the foundation of Chinese medicine. Greek humors, however, are considered very different from these other systems because they focus on specific bodily fluids instead of energy flows.

Bloodletting as a medical treatment seems to have spread with the Roman Empire, becoming popular in Europe and the Islamic world. Some medical histories believe that bloodletting was compared to menstrual bleeding: doctors thought that the monthly bleeding that women endured was to purge their body of old blood that had been used up. Special tools were developed to nick veins and arteries. In the ancient world, tools were as simple as a sharpened piece of wood or a small metal knife. Later on, lancets were developed that made more precise punctures. A specific amount of blood would be drawn off, relieving the patient's illness.

In some situations, leeches were considered simpler to use than the other tools available. A certain number of leeches would be applied to the body, and when they dropped off, the bleeding was complete. Some healers did not believe that the procedure was complete until the patient came close to fainting.

Barbers and Business

Until the mid-1100s, bloodletting treatments were often performed by monks or priests, who generally stood in for doctors during the period. The Church was horrified by the practice, however, and forbade religious authorities from using bloodletting in 1163.

By that time, barbers had begun to arise in cities and villages, offering haircuts and shaves; with their familiarity with sharp blades and skin surfaces, they were the natural replacements for those who favored bloodletting for their ailments. Barbers could also be found who offered cupping, tooth extractions, and even amputations when necessary. Barber-surgeons would hang blood-stained towels outside their businesses to let the public know that they were available; indeed, this is the origin of the modern white-and-red striped barber pole.

Bloodletting continued to be a regular medical practice throughout the 19th century, with physicians using more and more specialized tools to draw their patient's blood with as little scarring and damage to the skin and vessels as possible. Surgical techniques and overall anatomical knowledge had greatly increased since the early Greek work of Hippocrates, but the knowledge of how actually to cure disease would continue to elude doctors for decades to come. Knowledge of germs and the development antibiotics were still a long way off, and until those medical developments unfolded, doctors were generally unable to do much to treat their patients. Bloodletting at least offered a placebo effect, and doctors often felt better doing something rather than nothing at all.

Modern Bloodletting

In the world of modern medicine, the practice of deliberately removing blood is called phlebotomy. If you have ever been to the doctor and had your blood drawn for testing, you've seen a phlebotomist. There are also a few modern illnesses that benefit from phlebotomy—the modern version of bloodletting. These diseases all require the reduction of red blood cells. For example, hemochromatosis is a disease in which the red blood cells carry too much iron, causing severe damage to organs if untreated. Some versions of porphyria, the condition believed to have affected King George III of England, are best treated by phlebotomy. There is also a disease of the blood marrow called polycythemia vera, in which the marrow makes too many red blood cells. Again, removing blood in a controlled fashion can keep patients healthy. Phlebotomy may also be a successful treatment for fluid overload in chronic heart failure, and may reduce overall blood pressure in severe situations. The uses of bloodletting, in other words, are somewhat fluid.

Modern phlebotomy looks different from old fashioned bloodletting, though similarities are certainly present. When ancient and medieval physicians practiced bloodletting, they used a metal tool and let the blood drain into a bowl. Nowadays, we use very small needles and tubing, then allow the blood to drain off into a sterile plastic bag. In both situations, doctors are precise about how much blood they draw off. The main difference may be that in modern phlebotomy, the puncture that is left from the needle is so small that bleeding is easily stanched. Other tools, such as blood pressure and heart monitors, can also be used if necessary to make sure that a patient's vital signs are strong and steady while blood is being drawn.

Leeches and Severed Limbs

Leeches have also seen a resurgence in modern surgical techniques. When limbs have been amputated and reattached, doctors have frequently struggled to reconnect all the tiny blood vessels between the amputated limb and the rest of the body. Blood would often pool in the reattached body part and cause it to need to be removed again, this time permanently.

When the body's arteries have been reconnected and the limb reattached, leeches can be used like external veins. They draw off the blood that would otherwise accumulate. Over time, the body will regrow small veins, allowing the blood to circulate properly; then, leeches are no longer needed.

The reason leeches work so well in this situation is that they are designed to suck blood slowly and steadily; doctors say that if you draw blood too quickly after a surgical reattachment, you might as well not have bothered to reattach the limb. There are other options that doctors can use, but they are fairly gruesome: in the case of a finger, for instance, doctors can remove the fingernail and then scrape the raw nail bed so that it continues to slowly bleed. Most patients prefer the leeches. Leeches are also a cheap treatment, medically speaking, costing around $7 per leech.

While we often think of bloodletting as an ancient practice that has no relevance to modern life, it is easy to see how the treatment has evolved into a currently used medical practice that helps us stay healthy. We now have better treatments for conditions like epilepsy, depression, and bacterial illnesses, but we also use phlebotomy to safely draw blood for testing, and to treat certain medical conditions for which we do not have a better, safer treatment.

Kay Tilden Frost

See also: Acupuncture; Alternative Diagnostics; Chinese Traditional Medicine; Cupping; Purgatives and Emetics

Further Reading

Cohen, Jennie. 2018. "A Brief History of Bloodletting," *History*, October 15.
Greenstone, Gerry. 2018. "The History of Bloodletting," *BC Medical Journal*. October 15. https://www.bcmj.org/premise/history-bloodletting
McCann, Henry. 2014. *Pricking the Vessels: Bloodletting Therapy in Chinese Medicine.* London: Singing Dragon.

CHINESE TRADITIONAL MEDICINE

Traditional Chinese medicine is a diagnostic and therapeutic system based on two central philosophical principles: (1) yin and yang, or the interaction of opposites; and (2) the five elements of wood, fire, earth, metal, and water. Other factors are also important in this complex cultural system. The traditional Chinese approach was developed in ancient times and encompasses a variety of therapeutic techniques, ranging from acupuncture and herbal medicines to movement (e.g., Tai Chi) and diet.

In looking at Chinese traditional medicine, it is useful to set out some of the basic philosophical themes underlying the subject.

Astrology and the Body

Throughout much of Chinese history, court astronomers observed the sky carefully and recorded what they saw. They assumed that the position of the sun in relation to the stars and planets affected the fortunes of individuals and could be used to determine the auspiciousness (or inauspiciousness) of certain days for carrying out particular actions. Astrologers thus might give advice on the best day to launch a war or the worst day to stage a wedding. If the advice was wrong, it sometimes meant death or imprisonment for the practitioner. Most of the time, however, the astrological signs were simply reinterpreted to "prove" the outcome as correct. Astrology was also applied to illness and the body to identify the external forces that could be at work and the best way to address them. The body was thought to be a kind of mini-cosmos, with the same forces and alignments shaping it that shaped the heavens.

Alchemy and Yin-Yang

The ancient science of alchemy drew on the materials and methods of medicine, chemistry, and metallurgy to bring about natural reactions. These reactions typically involved two contrasting substances, corresponded to the interplay of *yin* and *yang*, the complementary opposites in the cosmos. Yin, the feminine (passive) principle, and yang, the masculine (active) principle, interacted to produce all phenomena. The chemical and other reactions designed by alchemists were aimed at exploring yin-yang interactions and revealing the Dao (Tao), or the cosmic unity that pervaded all.

The connection of alchemy with medicine in China gave the latter some of its metaphysical force. The most potent alchemical elixirs were thought, for example, to confer immortality, while the lesser ones could cure an illness, particularly if one also meditated on the Dao. As with astrology, therefore, alchemy was a science that concerned the link between large forces of the universe and the smaller, visible forces that one could manipulate for good or evil.

Medicine

Traditional Chinese medicine has lasted through the ages and is now part of contemporary alternative and complementary health care. The knowledge compiled in roughly 10,000 early medical treatises is tied together through a complex theory of body processes, health, and illness. Diagnosis in the classic Chinese system consists of four main methods: (1) observation (i.e., examination of the skin, eyes, tongue), (2) sensing (listening and smelling), (3) pulse taking, and (4) questioning the patient (along with his or her family members). All were important, but appearance, breath, and, especially, the pulse were key. Lengthy works were written about the latter, and Westerners still have great difficulty "reading" the pulse in accordance with the Chinese system.

Central to the system, again, are yin and yang. Health is the balance of these vital forces, not only inside the body but also in the body's interactions with the mind, the emotions, and the environment. A proper diagnosis and therapeutic plan considers every aspect of that complex relationship. All parts of the body interact, because they are connected by the circulation of vital forces. Thus, even a rash or wound is treated as a problem involving the entire body, not just as a localized impairment.

The Chinese system of medicine contains resources that make surgery seem inappropriate. Medicines derived from plants, animals, or minerals can produce mild effects on the system to adjust most imbalances, in combination with dietary regulation, massage, breathing exercises, and other measures. Under the well-known treatment of acupuncture, slender needles are inserted at key points along circulation pathways to correct any imbalances. Modern research indicates that acupuncture may possibly affect the nervous system and also trigger the production of pain-reducing substances called endorphins in the brain. Acupuncture is widely used by traditional practitioners as a first-line treatment for a range of disorders, among them minor muscular and neurological complaints. It is also used in modern settings to treat pain, stress, smoking, and other conditions.

Chinese herbal medicine includes the use of a variety of vegetable products, some of which have found their way into modern orthodox medicine. The modern drug known as ephedrine (used for low blood pressure, asthma, and other conditions) was first isolated from the herb *má huáng* in China over 2,000 years ago. In general, treatment in the Chinese system is based on the identification of particular *patterns* based on the information gathered from the patient. Unlike Western medicine, which seeks a lasting "cure," or at least a decisive change, Chinese medicine seeks to restore a healthy balance between imposing forces (or energies) for the benefit of the patient.

Five Elements

The five elements too are an integral part of Chinese culture. Five-element theory is central not only to medicine but also to such Chinese disciplines as feng shui (siting or positioning), the martial arts, and cosmology. Serving as a comprehensive template, the five elements represent all natural phenomena as ordered into five master groups or patterns. Each of the five groups—wood, fire, earth, metal, and water—include categories or qualities such as season, direction, climate, stage of growth and development, internal organ, body tissue, emotion, aspect of the soul, taste, color, sound, and so on. The whole system provides a master blueprint for how nature interacts with the body and how the different dimensions of life and being impact each other. Key medical associations include liver–wood, heart–fire, spleen–earth, lung–metal, and kidney–water, but there are many others. The five elements show how the structures and systems of the body are interconnected and how a healer might treat a patient's condition by addressing imbalances using countervailing elements.

Tai Chi, Qigong, and Feng Shui

Movement, positioning, and the control of natural energies are also key elements of traditional Chinese medicine and philosophy. These principles are embodied, for example, in the therapeutic techniques known as Tai Chi and Qigong and in the art of siting, or physical arrangement, known as Feng Shui. All are based on the idea of a flow of opposite yet complementary yin and yang fluids. These fluids correspond to the configuration of the land as well as the various circulatory pathways in the body, and therefore it is beneficial to conform one's motions, thoughts, and actions to their shape and direction.

Tai Chi, which has links to the martial arts, is a system of movements and postures designed to enhance mental and physical health. It is influenced by Confucian and Buddhist philosophy. A series of gentle and graceful movements is accented by moments when a particular posture is held for a short period of time, thus operating as both a physical stimulus and an effort at balance. Qigong (chee-gong) likewise employs gentle, focused exercises for mind and body to restore or increase the flow of qi (life energy), either for the general maintenance of health or to aid in the healing process. Qigong uses both movement and meditation, motion and relaxation. An external practitioner may also be utilized to direct qi energy onto the patient by means of hand manipulations or breath.

Feng shui (fung-shwā) specialists, like healers, are concerned with dynamic balance. Whether depending on intuitive judgment or manipulating a traditional compass device, these experts look for points of harmony between high and low, watercourse and landform, at which to locate a house or a tomb, or to situate a person for optimal health. Correctly orienting oneself with respect to natural surroundings is part of the Chinese art of healthy living.

Michael Shally-Jensen

See also: Acupuncture; Astrology; Folk Medicine; Herbal Remedies; Macrobiotics; Meditation and Mindfulness; Mind–Body Medicine; Tai Chi and Qigong

Further Reading

Kaptchuk, Ted J. 2000. *The Web That Has No Weaver: Understanding Chinese Medicine.* New York: McGraw-Hill.

Lloyd, G. E. R., and Nathan Sivin. 2002. *The Way of the World: Science and Medicine in Early China and Greece.* New Haven, CT: Yale University Press.

Maciocia, Giovanni. 2015. *The Foundations of Chinese Medicine.* 3rd ed. Edinburgh: Elsevier.

FOLK MEDICINE

Although most practices belonging to folk medicine, or "prescientific" medicine, are rooted in cultural traditions and social customs, many of them have been found to work reasonably well by the folks who use them. The cultural origins of folk practices, in other words, sometimes obscure their empirical worth in the eyes of outside observers. Folk medicine often deals with the emotional needs of the patient as well as the physical matter at hand. A curative ritual of some kind—not just medication alone—is sometimes involved in the healing process.

Thoroughly Unmodern Medicine

In the colonial era, few men or women practicing medicine had obtained a university degree or received formal training. Most were midwives, nurses, or folk healers who based their actions largely on a set of beliefs inherited from premodern Europe. This included the doctrine of the four humors, or bodily fluids: yellow bile (or choler), blood, black bile (or melancholy), and phlegm. The idea was that one's health and temperament depended on the balance of these four humors inside the body. Every person was thought to have his or her own unique blend of humors; therefore, medical practice was individualized to the patient and aimed at restoring equilibrium. (Or so went the theory; in actuality, a standard grab bag of remedies was often relied on, albeit adjusted to the situation.)

Astrology, too, was a popular medical resource in the 17th and 18th centuries. Astrological readings were used for the diagnosis of illness or disease as well as for choosing among treatments. Nicholas Culpeper's *Astrological Judgment of Diseases* (1655), for example, was distributed widely in the colonies and reprinted for many decades. (His astrologically informed *Complete Herbal* remains in print in several editions.) Popular almanacs, likewise, included medical information that linked, for example, preferred bloodletting sites on the body to the positions of the sun and the moon. Both astrology and alchemy were taught in U.S. colleges into the mid-1700s, when Enlightenment values pushed them aside. At the "folk" level, however, astrology continued to have a presence.

Witchcraft and magic also were elements of early medical practice. Religious traditions that held witches responsible for causing illness and death, among other troubles, were pervasive throughout much of the colonial period and beyond. Midwives were both a source of medical knowledge and a threat to male cultural domination; as such, they were sometimes labeled as witches and sentenced to death for their alleged crimes against humanity. Women, more broadly, could build up an understanding of basic medical matters on the basis of their role in the family, but to become a village healer was a different situation altogether, for to do so, again, challenged male authority. The exclusion of women from the healing arts became particularly strong when the medical profession began to organize itself nationally (and internationally) in the mid-19th century.

Medical care also came in the form of herbal remedies. Some healers—herbalists—specialized in this field, drawing on tradition along with developing their own botanical preparations. Undoubtedly, the most prominent herbalist in the early 19th century was Samuel Thomson (1769–1843), a self-taught medical promoter whose motto was "Every man his own physician." Thomson detested "regular" or "learned" doctors with their vile mineral medicines (like calomel) and arch theories and practices. In their place he proposed citizen curers who took care of their own and their families' medical needs by means of herbs, enemas, and steam. Among the various herbal powders, tinctures, syrups, and infusions that Thomson included in his pharmacopoeia, the one that took center stage was lobelia, used as a purgative. Thomson's therapeutics were aimed at restoring *body heat* through the use of plant remedies and steam vapor baths. The first step was to employ emetics and enemas to purge the body and prepare it for the return of its natural heat. Cayenne pepper enemas were recommended, along with libations of lobelia, turpentine, horseradish, and other substances. Thomson's patented "kits" for home use became immensely popular as a way to treat illnesses without the benefit—or expense—of a regular doctor. Subsequent stages of treatment involved steam inhalation and/or hot baths followed by warm blankets to build up internal temperature. Ultimately, although Thomsonianism was perhaps useful in addressing mild fevers, it was anything but helpful for a variety of other ailments. Its chief effect was to have left a strong sense in the patient that powerful measures had been undertaken on his or her behalf. The Thomson system faded away almost as quickly as it arose after peaking in the 1830s.

Another popular system emerging in the 19th century was homeopathy, a European import. Homeopaths served a more upscale clientele in the cities in addition to selected populations in the hinterlands. Unlike botanic medicine, homeopathy was based on the use of minuscule doses of drugs that were meant to produce symptoms of the very disease with which one was trying to dispense. Thus, for example, practitioners used a faint trace of onion powder for treating hay fever and watery eyes or a vanishingly small amount of a strychnine (poison) dilute to treat disordered bowels. Besides its unique, counterintuitive system, homeopathy had going for it the fact that many *regular* medical doctors took it up—to the dismay of their more orthodox colleagues. It could not necessarily be practiced by a run-of-the-mill herbalist or folk healer. In fact, by the late 1800s there were several homeopathic schools and hospitals in the United States, along with a number of professional societies and medical journals.

Other medical sects from roughly the same era included hydropaths, who advocated water cures, cold and hot baths, and wet sheets; chiropractors, who concentrated on manipulation of the spine to address specific diseases or conditions; magnetic healers, who sought to control human electromagnetic impulses or forces to cure illnesses; and eclectics, who combined therapies from several different traditions. There were also a few early diet and exercise proponents (such as Sylvester Graham) along with a host of traveling medicine shows whose focus was the hawking of patent medicines that contained more promise than substance.

Regional Specialties

As a result of geographic or social isolation, peoples of various ethnic groups and rural locales in the United States long retained their own systems of folk medicine. In Appalachia, for example, a combination of rustic wisdom and simple practicality produced a folk system based on regional medicinal herbs, a try-and-try-again treatment philosophy, and the use of moonshine whiskey as both an analgesic and general tonic. Remedies for arthritis included the drinking of a cocktail made of vinegar, honey, and moonshine. Burns were treated as they were in many other rural areas in the country: by the application of a poultice made of goose grease. The common cold could be treated with quinine or moonshine—or both.

In northern New England, particularly in Vermont, folk medicine was based partly on foods. Honey, cider, vinegar, lemon juice, castor oil, and corn oil were all substances commonly used in the treatment of diseases. Hay fever, for example, was dealt with by the chewing of a honeycomb during the main allergy-producing months. A mixture of apple cider vinegar, honey, and water, taken regularly, was used for the treatment of arthritis. A potassium-bearing food such as acorn squash, along with clover honey, was recommended for the common cold. Oil and seaweed were prescribed for a thyroid condition.

The Pennsylvania Germans, also known as the Pennsylvania Dutch (from the German *Deutsch,* meaning "German"), adopted various Native American plants and remedies into their folk system. Tobacco, for example, was chewed for toothaches, sassafras and other bitter herbs were drunk to "purify" the blood, and peppermint was consumed to help reduce a fever. The Pennsylvania Dutch also were fond of bloodletting as a means of clearing out impurities and restoring equilibrium to the body. Not too far away, in various Shaker villages of the northeast, a vast number of herbs were produced both for domestic medicinal use and for sale to outside patent medicine manufacturers.

In African American communities, particularly in the south, "root doctors" prescribed a combination of herbal treatments and spiritual rites to chase out bad influences and restore health to patients. In many cases African Americans had no choice but to rely on traditional methods, as mainstream methods were not available to them. The local environment supplied the materia medica, including Spanish moss (to lower blood pressure), sassafras tea and similar drinks (for fatigue or worms), and local and more exotic, imported oils (for aches and pains). Charms and amulets played their part, as did spiritual beliefs and stories about encounters with demons and other such threats.

In San Francisco's Chinatown, and in other, smaller Chinatowns in New York and Chicago, traditional Chinese medicine was the norm. The Chinese community drew on such concepts as chi and yin and yang. Chi is the life force that flows through the body, particularly along pathways known as meridians. Acupuncturists using needles and moxibustionists using burning substances tapped into this energy field to ensure its proper functioning. Similarly, healers specializing in Chinese botanicals would seek to adjust the balance of yin (the feminine, passive element) and yang (the male, active element) inside the body by making special preparations for patients.

Members of the Latin American community relied on a a system based on "hot" and "cold" properties. As with the humoral system, the body was believed to fluctuate between "hot" and "cold." Medicines, too, exhibited one of these qualities or the other—if only symbolically. The system assigned "hot" medicines to "cold" illnesses and "cold" medicines to "hot" illnesses. Arthritis and the common cold, for example, were both considered "cold" diseases, for which a "hot" medicine like alcohol might be prescribed. Diarrhea, on the other hand, was a "hot" condition, for which a "cold" therapeutic agent like whole milk might be prescribed.

Although a number of the various folk traditions can still be found today, by the turn of the 20th century many of them had gone into decline, spurned by patients and families drawn to advances in medical science and the ever-growing professional medical marketplace. Laboratories began to synthesize the active ingredients in plants and could, moreover, produce standardized dosages in sterilized containers to satisfy the increasing demand. In addition, improved surgical procedures, radiological advances, and discoveries like antibiotics positioned modern medicine to take over and soon far exceed folk medicine as a resource of first, and last, resort. People came to expect fast and dramatic results as opposed to the somewhat slower, less definitive outcomes of ye olden times. Nevertheless, with the "back to the land" movement in the 1970s, folk medicine began to make a comeback. It got an additional boost from the New Age movement in the 1980s. Nowadays, complementary and alternative medicine, with its roots in folk traditions, is a major industry.

Michael Shally-Jensen

See also: Astrology; Bloodletting and Leeching; Chinese Traditional Medicine; Faith Healing and Prayer; Herbal Remedies; Homeopathy; Hydrotherapy; Medicine Shows; Purgatives and Emetics; Voodoo and Santería; Witch Trials and Exorcisms

Further Reading

DeStefano, Anthony. 2001. *Latino Folk Healing.* New York: Ballantine.
Janik, Erika. 2014. *Marketplace of the Marvelous: The Strange Origins of Modern Medicine.* Boston: Beacon Press.
Jarvis, D. C. 1985. *Folk Medicine.* New York: Fawcett.
Mitchem, Stephanie. 2007. *African American Folk Healing.* New York: NYU Press.
Wallnofer, Heinrich, and Anna von Rottauscher. 1975. *Chinese Folk Medicine.* London: White Lion.

HOMEOPATHY

Homeopathy is an alternative/complementary method of therapy based on the idea that the best way to address a medical condition is to introduce small doses of drugs or other agents to reproduce the symptoms of the malady one is seeking to cure or prevent. In homeopathic therapy, for example, arsenic, which ordinarily produces vomiting (or death) when swallowed, is diluted to an extreme degree and then consumed as a treatment for . . . vomiting. Although treatments are often tailored to an individual's own "chemistry" and needs, the basic premise is that "like cures like."

In fact, homeopathic medicines today are often prepared in such a way as to leave virtually no detectible active ingredients in place, or else they likely would have a hard time being marketed in today's regulated environment. In a typical preparation, a diluted form of an ingredient is dropped on a sugar pill and allowed to evaporate, leaving barely a trace of the original substance. Homeopathic remedies are derived from substances that come from plants, minerals, or animals, such as red onion, arnica (mountain herb), crushed whole bees, white arsenic, poison ivy, belladonna (deadly nightshade), stinging nettle, and snake venom. Some supporters call it "nanomedicine" because of the tiny dosages.

History and Theory

The person primarily credited with advancing the theory that "like cures like" is the German doctor Samuel Hahnemann (1755–1843). After practicing medicine for a number of years, Hahnemann began studying chemistry and pharmacology and looking into what he would eventually call "homeopathy." At the time, medical treatment consisted largely of bleedings, purges, baths, and peculiar diets. Medicines, such as they were, were anything but uniform from one apothecary to the next, and they were often mixed in with other substances or combined with other drugs. One drug used then was cinchona, a South American tree bark from which quinine is derived and known to be effective in treating persons with malaria. Hahnemann undertook to test the drug by administering it in small doses to a healthy person; the subject soon developed symptoms of malaria. When the treatment was stopped the patient "recovered." From there, Hahnemann went on to test numerous other drugs on himself, laying the foundations for homeopathy. He published his findings in 1796 as *A New Principle for Ascertaining the Curative Power of Drugs*.

The key to Hahnemann's technique was the "minuscule dosage rule." The homeopathic physician (or homeopath), he observed, should use the least amount of the prescribed substance needed to produce the reaction expected. Selecting the correct drug and the proper dosage was the essence of Hahnemann's homeopathy. He believed that the closer a drug's action matched the symptoms of the condition or illness being treated, the less one needed to apply to ensure that the body had been stimulated to heal itself.

Proof of Hahnemann's theories seemed to come during a cholera epidemic that swept Europe in 1831 and then spread to the United States. Thousands of people lay suffering and dying, and Hahnemann took the opportunity to prescribe homeopathic drugs that for the most part functioned better than existing treatments (which were ineffective, in any case). Regular physicians, whom Hahnemann labeled "allopaths" (because their remedies produced effects *different* from those caused by the disease itself) considered the new science nonsense, even dangerous. But patients disagreed and flocked to it, demanding home homeopathic kits containing ingredients and lists of symptoms, illnesses, and suggested dosages.

Subsequent Developments

As homeopathy increased in popularity, a variety of professional societies, journals, and clinics were established in a number of countries. One such organization was the American Institute of Homeopathy, founded in 1844. By the turn of the 20th century, there were twenty-two schools of homeopathy in the United States along with a monument in Washington, DC, honoring Samuel Hahnemann. In Germany, meanwhile, a new generation was making refinements to homeopathic science. Hugo Schulz and Rudolph Arndt, for example, developed more precise protocols for achieving results based on dosage amounts ranging from the infinitesimal to the more substantial. In the 1920s Karl Kotschau drew on the existing homeopathic practice of taking detailed patient histories to make doses more specific to individual cases. Indeed, what helped make homeopathy so popular in its early years was the attention paid to patients by practitioners, the availability of practitioners (licensing requirements were minimal or nonexistent), the accessibility of the underlying concepts, and the fact that homeopathic therapy did *not* involve the likes of cold baths, bleedings, hot poultices, purgatives, emetics, and other harsh measures.

Inevitably, though, time seems to have caught up with homeopathy. As advances in orthodox medicine increased in the 20th century, homeopathy began to lose its popularity, and homeopathic practitioners found it harder to apply their trade in the professionalized medical arena. Schools began to close, and professional societies and journals were shut down. The theory of minute dosages was maligned as unscientific and wrongheaded, as were Hahnemann's and his followers' ideas about illnesses and their sources. By midcentury the American Medical Society held that homeopathy was of interest only as a historical development situated somewhere between modern science and primitive medicine.

In Europe, on the other hand, homeopathy hung on, to a degree, and in India it continued to expand from its 19th-century colonial origins there, generally in combination with traditional Ayurvedic practices as well as with Western science. A pragmatic attitude underlay medical practice in India, as summarized by the Sanskrit verse lines, "That alone is the right medicine which can remove disease; He alone is the true physician who can restore health" (quoted in Bivins 2007, 156). There was none of the taint of the "unscientific" in the case of Indian homeopathy; if anything, the method was associated with modern medical knowledge and practice and brought a degree of prestige to its practitioners, even as it continued to be "vernacularized" through local applications. Some observers noted that Hahnemann himself had examined medical traditions in India in the course of developing homeopathy, thus demonstrating the latter's kinship with Ayurveda. Moreover, folk healers in India, like homeopaths, were often loath to apply severe remedies that seemed to physically (or mentally) harm the patient, as in the case of (early) Western medicine; homeopathy was regarded as more humane. Finally, there is something "exotic," perhaps even "karmic," about the concept, promoted by leading homeopaths, that a lack of active ingredients in homeopathic medications is not an issue because the surrounding water molecules "remember" or encode the shape of the active substance molecules and thereby deliver the essence of the original to the consumer. Whether this is nanomedicine or, as homeopathy's critics maintain, an elaborate, unscientific rationale is ultimately in the eyes of the patient.

Back in the United States

In the 1970s homeopathy was reintroduced to U.S. consumers via India. It was a time when young Americans actively sought out elements of Eastern traditions to expand their awareness and enrich their lives. Thus, homeopathy was part of a broader importation of alternative systems of medicine, including acupuncture, herbal medicine, and Ayurvedic therapies. All were considered attractive because they featured natural components and holistic philosophies. They also did *not* represent standardized Western medicine, as epitomized by large pharmaceutical corporations, medical insurance companies, and big, impersonal hospitals and clinics. These are all factors that continue to keep homeopathic medicines on the shelves of "natural" food and health stores and in home medicine cabinets today.

Nevertheless, homeopathy is a somewhat controversial topic from the point of view of mainstream medical research. Several of the key concepts of homeopathy are incompatible with basic understandings of chemistry and physics. It is not possible, for example, to explain in regular medical terms how a remedy containing little or no active ingredient can have any effect. Moreover, research into the matter is difficult because, obviously, one cannot identify the presence of an ultradiluted or "vanished" ingredient in order to test for its effects and any claims made on a label.

At the same time, while most homeopathic remedies are highly diluted, some of them may *not* be; they might contain measurable amounts of active ingredients. Thus, like any drug or dietary supplement that contains chemical ingredients, these homeopathic products may cause side effects or drug interactions. One should be sure to discuss the issue with one's care provider.

Homeopathic remedies are regulated as drugs under the Federal Food, Drug and Cosmetic Act (FDCA). However, under current agency policy, the FDA does not evaluate the remedies for safety or effectiveness. Only when a homeopathic remedy claims to treat a serious condition such as arrhythmia must it be sold by prescription. Most often, homeopathic remedies are used for minor health problems, such as colds and headaches, which generally go away on their own; these remedies can be sold without a prescription.

Michael Shally-Jensen

See also: Aromatherapy and Essential Oils; Ayurvedic Medicine; Folk Medicine; Herbal Remedies; Naturopathic Medicine

Further Reading

Bivins, Roberta. 2007. *Alternative Medicine? A History.* New York: Oxford University Press.

Singh, Simon, and Edzard Ernst. 2008. *Trick or Treatment: The Undeniable Facts about Alternative Medicine.* New York: W. W. Norton.

U.S. National Institutes of Health, National Center for Complementary and Integrative Health. 2015. "Homeopathy." https://nccih.nih.gov/health/homeopathy

Whorton, James C. 2002. *Nature Cures: The History of Alternative Medicine in America.* New York: Oxford University Press.

HYDROTHERAPY

Also known as the "water cure," hydrotherapy is to be distinguished from "spa therapy," mainly on the basis of the temperature of the water used (cold versus hot or warm) and the water's mineral content (none versus some). Hydrotherapy, at least in its original form, relied on cold water not necessarily drawn from a mineral spring to treat a variety of physical and emotional stresses and strains. The liquid was both applied externally and drunk in large quantities by the patient. For a couple of decades in the mid-19th century, hydrotherapy was considered quite the medical revolution—at least as a major new *alternative* medicine.

The People's Panacea

Popular spa destinations had been around in Europe for over a century by the time that hydrotherapy, with its unusual methods, first emerged in the 1830s. At places such as Baden-Baden, Germany, and Bath, England, a well-off clientele with complaints of gout, rheumatism, or bladder stones, for example, would converge to take advantage of the warm springs there and drink down the fresh mineral water. Water, however, was never the sole remedy used at these centers; rather, the usual premodern medical arsenal, including bleeding and purging, was present as well. Moreover, matters of health were never the only thing that clients had in mind at these resorts. They also came for the entertainments: dancing, dining, gambling, drinking, and romancing. These trips were costly affairs and could be indulged in only by elites or upcoming professionals.

In contrast, hydrotherapy originated with an Austrian peasant named Vincent Priessnitz (1799–1851). Priessnitz had had some success as a youth applying cold compresses to his own sprains and bruises and dipping affected body parts in local watering holes; he also experimented on farm animals and family members. By 1826 he was seeing patients at his Grafenberg Water Cure, and by the end of the decade he was well known and doing a lively business. Visitors were instructed in a series of demanding cold-water activities, from soaking and showering to wrapping (in wet sheets) and sweating (in wet blankets). Drinking substantial amounts of water and undergoing cold-water enemas were also part of the healing process. Priessnitz theorized that, internally, added water helped to break up disease-causing matter and bring it to the surface, where, with the proper external treatment, it could then pass through the skin and be washed away. As with a few other 19th-century cures, the method was designed to bring about a "crisis" in the patient, whereby severe shivering and sweating were viewed as signs that the treatment was working. In most cases, rashes, blisters, sores, and diarrhea were regarded as positive signs, as well. Consuming 10 to 12 glasses of water per day kept the bladder active—and yet some followers felt that that number was too low and aimed instead to drink 30 or more.

By the 1840s hydrotherapy (or, as it was commonly then called, hydropathy) had spread to other areas in Europe and to the United States. Many of the older spa centers adopted it to cash in on a good thing and stay relevant in a changing health market. Old-school doctoring was facing increased pressure from a number of new, alternative methods, including mesmerism, magnetism, homeopathy, herbalism, chiropractic, and hydrotherapy. These were developing as accessible, "middle-class" treatments that seemed to work quite as well as the standard medical treatments of the time and yet were more available and affordable. U.S. spas centering on mineral springs, such as the one at Saratoga Springs, New York, were being modeled both on their older European cousins and, in part at least, on Priessnitz's Grafenberg center. In Brattleboro, Vermont, a hydropathic institute opened in the early 1840s and soon became a major operation. It featured some two hundred rooms for residents and was equipped to handle a wide variety of medical conditions, including rheumatism, neuralgia, throat and lung diseases, scrofula, fatigue, asthma, dyspepsia, and gout.

What made the growing popularity of the water cure particularly surprising is that it emerged at a time when most Americans were not accustomed to bathing regularly. Days, weeks, even months would pass before ordinary citizens thought it time to bathe or shower. Some even worried that a weekly wash (or less) might have a deleterious effect. When it came to alternative therapies, on the other hand, people seemed more than willing to explore. The magazine *Water-Cure Journal*, which began publication in the early 1840s, acquired a sizable readership and lasted until 1897—although its best years were in the middle decades. It was taken over early in its history by the Fowler brothers, Orson and Lorenzo, known for their popularization of the equally new field of phrenology, or skull reading.

Hydrotherapy, Holism, and Health

As hydropathy/hydrotherapy developed, some of its followers began to see it as part of a larger trend toward holistic health and self-improvement that included vegetarianism, temperance (avoidance of alcohol or caffeine), hygiene, phrenology, and even women's health—a virtually taboo subject in the Victorian era. One emerging feminist, Mary Gove Nichols (1810–1884), made use of hydrotherapy during her pregnancy and touted it as a means of achieving pain-free—or nearly pain-free—birth. Nichols also promoted the use of douching to maintain vaginal health. The program of walking outdoors, as illustrated by Catharine Beecher's account, was likewise a fairly new phenomenon, especially for women. Indeed, as more and more women became acquainted with the water cure, it became clear that it was having an effect, even, on their dress. A garment known as the "wet dress," a loose-fitting gown with wide sleeves and a skirt falling over pantaloons, was designed to permit ladies to move comfortably while soaking. In time, the "wet dress" came to be adopted by the likes of Amelia Bloomer and others in the dress reform movement, giving women everywhere the opportunity to forgo corsets and other encumbrances associated with traditional women's wear. Articles and ads in the *Water-Cure Journal* were central to this transformation.

Other social reform movement that flourished in association with hydrotherapy were antigambling campaigns, public hygiene or sanitation campaigns, mental hygiene or psychic health programs (pouring water on the head was one technique), the parks and recreation movement, and even some art movements like the Hudson River School of painters, whose members were fond of depicting waterfalls, rivers, lakes, and great cloud formations in their works. It was as though society had discovered an entire water world lying beneath (or sitting atop) the regular world. In the 1850s there were nearly 50 water-cure institutes in the United States, and by the end of the century the total (including both defunct and existing ones) had reached almost 200. Most of them were located in the northeast—New York, Pennsylvania, Massachusetts, and New Jersey. This probably had to do with the fact that much of the appeal of "the cure" was that it took place in scenic rural areas situated outside the big urban centers. Taking a shower, therefore, also meant smelling the roses, or, in other words, getting a break from one's daily routine.

A *Water-Cure for Ladies* came out in 1844 and a *Water-Cure Encyclopedia* in 1851. Meanwhile, U.S. medical journals did everything they could to discourage the flood of interest in hydropathy. Regular physicians considered the whole business quackery, even though many of their own kind ended up abandoning normal medicine in favor of the new water cure and allied measures. In cartoons published in widely read newspapers and magazine, hydropathy patients were variously shown exploding from having imbibed too much or being wrung out like a wet rag after a treatment. The alternative healing field as a whole suffered a drop in public interest after the Civil War, as people came to question the notion of perfecting the human species through novel health measures.

Standard medicine, with its "regular" doctors, enjoyed a wave of popularity in the postwar years, despite its rather dismal record during the preceding conflict. At least, by then, medicine had going for it the germ theory, which not only helped doctors advance their claim to being experts but also led to the recognition of bathing and general hygiene as socially valuable. Such recognition, combined with the increased availability of home plumbing systems, cut into the perception of the water cure was somehow unique or special. It was, after all, really just the introduction of a healthful medium generally. The people that it "cured" at far-off hydro-centers were primarily sufferers of comparatively mild conditions who may well have got better on their own after a few weeks or months. The more seriously ill type of patient could hardly be expected to travel overland and then undergo repeated chillings and sweatings in an aqueous environment without facing serious harm. No, the rigorous methods of the water cure favored those who could endure and even come out the better for it. Hydropathy was for hardy souls. Today, hydropathy/hydrotherapy survives mainly in the of form steam rooms, hot tubs (or Jacuzzis), foot baths, athletic cold compresses, and the daily shower.

Michael Shally-Jensen

See also: Bottled Water; Cupping; Magnet Therapy; Mind–Body Medicine; Neurasthenia, or Nervous Exhaustion; Purgatives and Emetics; Sanatoriums; Spas and Mineral Waters; Sweat Lodges and Saunas

Further Reading

Cayleff, Susan. 1987. *Wash and Be Healed: The Water-Cure Movement and Women's Health.* Philadelphia: Temple University Press.
Janik, Erika. 2014. *Marketplace of the Marvelous: The Strange Origins of Modern Medicine.* Boston: Beacon Press.
Silver-Isenstadt, Jean L. 2002. *Shameless: The Visionary Life of Mary Gove Nichols.* Baltimore: Johns Hopkins University Press.
Whorton, James C. 2002. *Nature Cures: The History of Alternative Medicine in America.* New York: Oxford University Press.

HYSTERIA

The infliction known as hysteria is such an odd beast that no one has quite known what to do with it or how to treat it over its long history. It has taken so many shapes and forms over the centuries, depending on how it is conceived and dealt with, that one probably shouldn't even think of it as a solitary "it"; perhaps it is better thought of as a "they."

Historically speaking, hysteria represents a psychoneurosis characterized by complaints of physical illness or incapacity but without any identifiable organic disease lying behind it. People who have suffered from classical hysteria have been found to be emotionally disordered and to present a variety of troubling symptoms—blindness, for example, or paralysis, insomnia, or deafness. The hysterical patient of lore, in other words, exhibited a physiological malfunction without having any of the usual material causes present to account for his or her symptoms. In addition, there was often (but not always) a degree of fear or panic on the part of the patient together with, somewhat bizarrely, attention-seeking behavior—that is, a tendency to dwell on one's symptoms and seek to express them, sometimes quite dramatically, in front of others. Such overdramatization often came with a lack of self-criticism, or even self-awareness. The hysteric's basic emotions were so strong that she or he behaved in uncontrolled ways, like gasping for air or fainting. Yet the hysteric was, at the same time, highly suggestible (i.e., susceptible to suggestion by others). Hysterics could be readily hypnotized, for example—far more easily than most people. In short, hysteria is and always has been something of a mystery, both alluring and strange. Complementary and alternative approaches have been tried against it, as have any number of "regular" medical approaches.

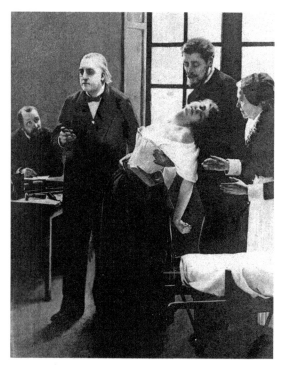

Jean-Martin Charcot demonstrating hypnosis on a "hysterical" female patient, who is supported by another doctor, at the Salpêtrière Hospital School in Paris. (National Library of Medicine)

Today, the term *hysteria* is no longer used by clinicians. The symptoms associated with the condition have been assigned to other psychiatric categories, such as somatic symptom disorder (conversion disorder) and histrionic personality disorder. The term does, of course, continue to be used in the popular culture—for example, when talking about a performer's "hysterical fans" or an individual's becoming "hysterical" during an argument. For present purposes, however, we are interested primarily in the medical condition—and its unusual "disappearance" in the modern age.

History of Hysteria

Long considered a disease specific to women, hysteria was attributed by the Greek physician Hippocrates to the movement of the uterus (*hysteron*) from its normal position to other areas of the body. Galen, of the second century CE, felt that possibly menstrual blood was involved, but more likely the cause was the retention of the "female seed." Hippocrates recommended marriage as a cure and Galen, sexual intercourse. Centuries later physicians were still speculating about the womb as a source of hysteria.

The so-called mass hysteria sometimes associated with the Salem witchcraft trials of 1692–1693 was of a unique nature. There, three teenage girls fell ill, and, encouraged by the adults around them, leveled accusations of witchcraft against a number of village residents, claiming to have witnessed their evil "specters" flying about and behaving badly. Other citizens joined in. Were not the accusers true religious "seers," people asked? Or were they perhaps just anxious youngsters making much ado about nothing? This was a major controversy in the small community, and its echoes lingered long after the fact. The Salem variety of hysteria, however, was less a matter of clinical illness than one of the "extraordinary popular delusions and the madness of crowds," as one famous book title (from 1841) put it. The "cause" of the community's craziness was not organic or psychological but rather sociocultural, having to do with magical beliefs and local social tensions.

One common symptom of classical hysteria is a sense of constriction in the throat, which early writers felt must be caused by the uterus becoming lodged in that area. Later, when the "wandering womb" theory of hysteria was finally abandoned, it was replaced by the idea that "noxious vapors" rose up from the womb and suffused the brain—hence the phrase "attack of the vapors" in reference to a woman who became emotionally indisposed. The first medical writer to recognize that men, too, could suffer from the condition was the 17th-century English physician Thomas Sydenham, who took careful case notes regarding hysteria patients. As Sydenham noted with respect to the gender differences, he observed, "women, except for those who lead a hardy and robust life, are rarely quite free from it [i.e., hysteria]; those men who lead a sedentary or studious life are subject to the same complaint; in their case, it is indeed called hypochondria [i.e., the persistent belief that one is sick], but this disease is as like hysteria as one egg is like another. Men are less subject to it than women because of their more robust habit of body" (quoted in Pearce 2016).

Sydenham, moreover, believed that hysterical symptoms could mimic virtually any known medical condition. His preferred remedy was bloodletting and purging followed by a round of medicinal substances: steel filings, wormwood extract, castor oil, and laudanum (an opium tincture).

Investigation into the possible neurological roots of hysteria was first undertaken by the French physician and anatomist J.-M. Charcot (1825–1893). Initially, Charcot believed that hysteria was caused by some as yet undetected disruption of the nervous system, but through his rigorous clinical studies, he showed that hysterical symptoms could be removed through hypnosis and could often be initiated by suggestion. This tended to indicate a psychological cause, or perhaps a psychosomatic (mental and material) basis for the condition. Charcot demonstrated that in some cases a patient's hysterical symptoms did not "make sense" physiologically—they might not conform to known nerve pathways, for example. The patient's mind, therefore, had to be involved in the makeup of the disease.

The founder of psychoanalysis, Sigmund Freud (1856–1939), observed Charcot's use of hypnosis in connection with hysteria and was struck by the malleability of his patients. Freud and his own early collaborator, Joseph Breuer, further explored the use of hypnosis but ultimately turned to something new in the world of medical science: free association as a means for getting at patients' subconscious thoughts. In 1895, Freud and Breuer published *Studies in Hysteria,* concluding that hysterical symptoms resulted from the repression by the mind of some emotionally unsettling experience. The two clinicians theorized that in order to treat hysteria, the physician should encourage the patient to express his or her suppressed emotions via a kind of forced mental "crisis," or catharsis. It was through the writings of Freud and his followers that a consensus eventually developed regarding the psychological origins of hysteria—or, arguably, the psychosexual origins, because the blocked experiences at issue were frequently found to involve sexual themes. The Freudians also reaffirmed that men as well as women could be affected by the condition, even though some old-school physicians at the time continued to insist that hysteria could only be caused by uterine problems.

In World War I, severe neurotic reactions among combat troops were called "shell shock" and were originally thought to be caused by microscopic brain lesions resulting from the concussive blasts of exploded ordnance. Later, it was hypothesized that many of these reactions were hysterical in nature—that is, they arose from the soldier's sense of conflict over his strong desire to flee from the battle, on the one hand, and his duty to stay and fight bravely, on the other. When a soldier developed hysterical paralysis of the leg, for example, he obviously could neither run nor perform his duties but was frozen in place. He would then be removed from the battlefield and given a brief period of rest. Military commanders nevertheless expected that the soldier would return to the battlefront. The cause of his condition, they thought, was simply a lack of fortitude. Manly combat would restore it. As a result, many shell-shock victims died "doubly"—both mentally and in actuality after their return.

By the time of World War II, the term "shell shock" would be replaced with "combat fatigue." Treatment then consisted of a combination of rest, drugs, and occupational therapy. The results were not overwhelmingly positive, however. In subsequent conflicts, the diagnosis of posttraumatic stress disorder and/or traumatic brain injury would be applied, along with, occasionally, selected psychosomatic conditions. The word *hysteria* dropped out from the lexicon.

Postmodern Developments

In psychiatric circles, and in the culture at large, psychoanalysis held sway for more than half a century as the dominant method of treatment for psychological disorders. By the last quarter of the 20th century, however, the Freudians' emphasis on repressed sexual drives as the cause of hysteria and related disorders was beginning to lose out to other perspectives. Researchers were beginning to explore the roles of nonsexual anxiety and depression in the genesis of hysterical symptoms. Certain common stressors, that is, might manifest themselves as physical illnesses or psychosomatic conditions. The "hysteric" might be suggestible precisely because he or she was looking for a solution to his or her conflict. Thus, newer forms of therapy, such as cognitive behavioral therapy, avoided delving deeply into psychosexual matters and instead explored with the patient ways to reduce stress, cope with physical symptoms, manage emotional issues, reduce one's preoccupation with the condition, and generally improve one's quality of life. This, in most cases, remains the goal today.

Hysteria, which always had to do with the "social construction of illness" (i.e., how an illness is defined by its sociocultural setting) as well as with the "presentation of self" in society (how one manifests oneself socially), experienced a dramatic rise beginning in the late 1700s and an equally dramatic fall sometime around the mid-1900s. It can be seen, like melancholia, neurasthenia ("nervous anxiety"), and, in our own time, eating disorders, as a historically specific form of disease. As the public shed the repressive Victorian—and pre-Victorian—culture and became more sophisticated about medical symptoms, cases of classical hysteria started to wane, both in number and in scale. The more "florid" types of hysteria that seemed to express the style of the era became increasingly rare. In addition, psychological science contributed to the dissipation of the disease by advancing clinical analysis and symptom classification. By the 1960s, the diagnosis of hysteria was thought to be medically inappropriate, as newer "somatoform" disorders and various personality disturbances came to take its place.

Michael Shally-Jensen

See also: Anxiety and Its Treatment; Breathwork; Deep Brain Stimulation; Electroconvulsive Therapy; Hydrotherapy; Mesmerism and Hypnotherapy; Neurasthenia, or Nervous Exhaustion; Neurodiversity; Psychoanalysis; Witch Trials and Exorcisms

Further Reading

Hustvedt, Siri. 2010. *The Shaking Woman; or, A History of My Nerves.* New York: Henry Holt.
Micale, Mark S. 2008. *Hysterical Men: The Hidden History of Male Nervous Illness.* Cambridge, MA: Harvard University Press.
Pearce, J. M. S. 2016. "Sydenham on Hysteria." *European Neurology* 76 (3–4): 175–81. Available at http://www.karger.com/Article/FullText/450605 (Visited 5 May 2017).
Sabine, Arnaud. 2015. *On Hysteria: The Invention of a Medical Category between 1670 and 1820.* Chicago: University of Chicago Press.

MEDICINE SHOWS

The traveling medicine show was a popular form of entertainment and hucksterism that flourished in the 19th-century United States. It combined free amusement with the sale of well-hyped "nostrums," or medicines whose ingredients were kept secret and whose effectiveness went unproved. Drawing on the circus format, and employing profit-minded carnival barkers who often called themselves "doctors," the medicine show was a lively affair that attracted big crowds in rural areas and large towns alike. These itinerant events were always publicized in advance with handbills, posters, newspaper ads, and painted signs or billboards.

Historically, the peddler of cheap "miracle medicines" represents a figure situated somewhere between the classic charlatan who exploited fairgoers in early modern Europe and the contemporary television ad spokesperson who promotes health and wellness products while wearing a physician's white coat—as the words "Not a Doctor" appear in fine print below. Many of the techniques of modern high-pressure salesmanship were pioneered in the medicine show.

Itinerate Showmanship

Medicine show pitchmen often wore frock coats, top hats, fancy vests, and polished leather boots or shoes. In this way, they sought to impress their audiences with their sophistication, wealth, and worldly experience. Following an introductory piece of entertainment—an animal act, some comedy or ventriloquism, a little song and dance, perhaps—the showman would step up onto a raised platform and begin delivering his grandiloquent "lecture" on the marvels of the cure he held in his hand. It might be an herbal tonic used as a cathartic, an oil rub or liniment for pain, a salve for cuts or bruises, a cure for catarrh (excessive mucus), a corn remedy for bowel problems, a scalp preparation for baldness, or a "medicated"—that is, aromatic—soap. Snake oil was, at first, a particularly popular item. Allegedly derived from rattlesnake venom, or from some other frightful serpent, it was prized for its powerful effect on the user, even if entirely imaginary. Later, of course, "snake oil" became a slang term for fraud and flim-flam.

The medicine shows followed the season from north to south and east to west, traveling in horse-drawn wagons or trains and playing in grange halls and country opera houses during the winter months, and at fairgrounds or town commons during the summer. The roster of performances could be quite extensive, depending on the size of the show. There might be displays of marksmanship mixed in with blackface minstrel entertainments; magic and acrobatics combined with strongman exhibitions; or a dog and pony show followed by a tomahawk-throwing contest. The performers often worked on a small stage and sometimes came out among the audience; the stage typically featured a backdrop of painted scenes together with a smattering of props. At key moments, the "doctor" or "professor" would emerge from behind the curtain to promote his fabulous cure-alls to the excited group of onlookers.

Central to the pitchman's art was his knowledge of popular psychology and his skill at public oratory. He would use folksy expressions to gain the confidence of his listeners, change pace to maintain their attention, use sympathy and fear-mongering to remind people of the human condition, and rattle off a string of Latin (or Latin-like) medical terms to legitimate his claims. Frequently, a demonstration of the cure was presented to the group, such as using ear drops on someone with a hearing problem and then surreptitiously inserting a finger inside the ear to "pop" it in order to get a rise from the patient. Shills, or actors who were in on the trick, were often used in these ploys. "Testimonials," too, might be delivered by a paid informant planted in the audience and brought onto the stage. Such sales spiels, when successful, would be followed by a clamor to purchase the medicine. If need be, another shill could lead the charge.

Women also ran or participated in medicine shows. One such person, Princess Lotus Blossom, a Minnesota entrepreneur (Violet McNeal), marketed Vital Sparks, which she sold as a restorer of male virility; it was, in fact, a kind of tart candy in "buckshot" form that crackled when chewed. (McNeal said that it came from rare Asian turtles.) Another pitchwoman, Madame DuBois, had a brass band and worked together with her husband, Dr. Andre Dupre. The pair's specialty was tooth-pulling, which was a popular medicine show sideline and served a practical purpose at a time when professional dentistry was still in its infancy.

Native American characters often appeared on stage, both to provide "exotic" entertainment and to call attention to the indigenous medical knowledge that frequently was said to lie behind a product. In fact, because early Anglo-American herbal remedies were based primarily on English botanicals rather than on common North American species, there was some resistance at first among customers and sellers to take advantage of native plants. Yet, as the market for such remedies ripened over time—partly through the work of medicine shows—various "Indian-branded" patent medicines and manufacturing companies became hugely popular. One of the largest and most successful of these was the Kickapoo Indian Medicine Company, founded in 1881—in Connecticut. One of the first nationwide marketing organizations, the Kickapoo company sent out annually up to 75 traveling troupes of Indian "warriors," dancers, and musicians to sell its pharmaceuticals, among them the bestselling "Sagwa" tonic, whose name was made up. The potion was intended as a "blood, liver, and stomach renovator" and contained a mixture of herbs, roots, bark, gum, buffalo tallow, and alcohol.

Signs of Decline

Essentially a 19th-century phenomenon, and relying on the scarcity of knowledge at the time and people's limited access to goods, the medicine show thrived for decades. On the wane in the early 20th century, the shows nevertheless persisted, albeit with trucks instead of wagons and radio ads augmenting the traditional printed announcement. As early as the 1910s, rural areas had started to become less isolated and people began to discover alternative forms of diversion, including circuses, carnivals, Wild West shows, minstrel shows, and vaudeville. Eventually, radio programs and the silent screen drew increased attention among the populace. Audiences became less tolerant of the florid language of the medicine man's pitch and the deceptive practices that went with it. Moreover, regulations started to be put in place to restrict commercial activities in local communities, and governments demanded increased fees from show producers to offset the costs involved and generate revenue. The medicine show could not long hold its own under such circumstances.

The 20th century also saw an expansion of science-based remedies and a growth in the physician population, thus allowing citizens to access the healing arts more easily. Drugstores, even chain drugstores, began to crop up to replace the wagon-borne apothecaries of old. Improved over-the-counter medicines, conforming to new, stricter federal guidelines, started to replace the dubious patent medicines that had been the basis of the medicine show. For these and other reasons, the curtain came down on the great American medicine show sometime around the end of the Depression. By the 1940s, it was already largely a thing of the past.

In more recent times, the medicine show might be compared to the "New Age" fairs and expositions that took place in the 1970s and 1980s. At such events, vendors offered items like healing magnets and crystals, aromatherapy materials, homemade herbal compounds, taped audiovisual materials, fortune-telling services, past-lives encounters, extraterrestrial explorations, and many other unconventional items for a new generation of consumers. Even today, this type of small-scale public vending continues at the local level, while at the retail level (stores and online) many different types of health and wellness merchandise, from the mundane to the exotic, continue to be marketed vigorously, occasionally displaying echoes of the fancy salesmanship that preceded it in the medicine show era. The weight-loss industry, for example, is known for its sometimes overblown rhetoric and questionable promises. Each little pop-up ad promoting a "miracle" diet substance or quick "hard-core abs" owes a debt to the medicine show. The more things change, it seems, the more they stay the same.

Michael Shally-Jensen

See also: Diet Pills and Metabolism Boosters; Folk Medicine; Homeopathy; Infomercials and Wellness Promotion; Mesmerism and Hypnotherapy; Patent Medicines; Phrenology

Further Reading

Anderson, Ann. 2000. *Snake Oil, Hustlers, and Hambones: The American Medicine Show.* Jefferson, NC: McFarland.
Armstrong, David, and Elizabeth Metzger Armstrong. 1991. *The Great American Medicine Show.* New York: Simon and Schuster.
McNamara, Brooks. 1995. *Step Right Up.* Rev. ed. Jackson: University Press of Mississippi.

MESMERISM AND HYPNOTHERAPY

The theory and method known as mesmerism was named after its French inventor, Franz Anton Mesmer (1734–1815). Although it was later derided as a pseudoscience, mesmerism was a great sensation when it first arrived on the scene. It helped pave the way for the study of the unconscious (or subconscious) and the practice of hypnosis. Mesmerism contributed, therefore, to the rise of modern psychiatry.

Mesmer and Mesmerism

Franz Mesmer was born in the small village of Iznang, near Lake Constance, inside the Austrian Empire. He studied theology and philosophy before switching to law and moving to Vienna; subsequently, he turned to medicine. His doctoral dissertation, completed in 1766, was on the influence of planets on human disease. Mesmer believed that the movements of the planets, and of the moon, set up gravitational forces that affected not only the earth's surface but also the human body. In particular, Mesmer thought, the nervous "fluid" running through the body ebbed and waned according to celestial motions. Mesmer held, moreover, that disruptions to this fluidic system caused or affected the courses of human diseases. In 1774 he treated a 27-year-old woman suffering from recurring attacks of hysteria.

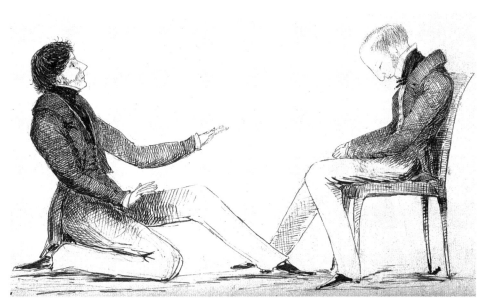

A practitioner of mesmerism performs therapy on a male patient, early 19th century. Mesmerism drew on the idea of a universal magnetic force that could be used for spiritual healing. (Wellcome Library)

Noting the periodic nature of her symptoms, Mesmer thought to apply magnets to the woman's body, theorizing that in doing so he might control the "tides" or rhythms driving her illness. Passing the magnets over the patient's stomach and legs caused her to become visibly excited and proclaim she was experiencing a powerful energy flowing inside her. After the initial experiment, Mesmer repeated the process to quell her seizures, eventually bringing her condition under control and pronouncing her cured. Two years later Mesmer moved to Paris to set up a practice, which brought him both fame and notoriety.

As he developed his method, Mesmer also modified his theory. Instead of seeing the planets as playing the central role in the movement of the magnetic ether, he came to view the fluid as universally present and as something that could be transferred from one person (or object) to the next. He called this subtle substance "animal magnetism," because it animated its subjects and was magnetic in nature. In Mesmer's eyes, his new discovery was a major achievement in world science, and the cure based on it—a nonmedical one—was no less significant. It seemed effectively to heal a variety of illnesses, especially those of a mental or psychosomatic character, such as melancholia, hysteria, vapors (fainting), dyspepsia, seizures, and fevers. It also avoided the pain and suffering caused by conventional medical treatments and drug therapy, both of which were, in the late 1700s, quite primitive. Animal magnetism was thought by Mesmer to be on par with gravity, magnetism, and electricity as a fundamental force in the universe.

A corollary to Mesmer's new theory was that the healing process, by its very nature, led to a "crisis" in the patient, whereby she or he would become agitated and sometimes tremble, faint, or enter into a trancelike state before recovering. To some critics, this made mesmerism suspect and mysterious. To Mesmer, however, it was proof that animal magnetism was real: the "crisis" could be explained as the body struggling to reestablish its fluidic balance. Some observers both past and present, including the medical historian James C. Whorton, have described the therapeutic crisis associated with mesmerism—particularly in the case of female patients—as veering dangerously close to orgasm. In the healing sessions, the master or a younger male associate would sit before a seated patient and clamp her knees between his own while touching and stroking her body and looking directly into her eyes in order to stir up her animal magnetism. More so than male patients, female patients experienced the classic mesmeric "crisis" in these situations. Accounts of patients' reactions at the time include mention of "flushed" faces, "ardent" eyes, shortened respiration, "tremors" in the limbs, "spasms" of the body, and a relaxed moment of "languor and quiescence" at the end (quoted terms from Whorton 2002, 107). Such provocative descriptions do indeed suggest heightened sexual arousal, if not outright orgasm, on the part of women patients.

In Paris, Mesmer and his practice were all the rage, particularly among the aristocracy. So sensational was the public response that in 1784, French authorities demanded a scientific review of the matter. A team was assembled that included such eminent figures as the chemist Antoine Lavoisier and the U.S. inventor and diplomat Benjamin Franklin. The group's investigation led them to conclude that animal magnetism was nothing but a figment of the imagination, and that mesmerism was no more than wishful thinking on the part of its adherents. The essence of this perspective is captured in the popular use of the word "mesmerize," which means to fascinate, enthrall, or spellbind. Mesmer himself was ultimately ruined by the scientists' finding and decided to relocate to Meersburg (southern Baden, Germany), where he lived in virtual isolation until his death in 1815. Today, few know that mesmerism is anything *but* a word in the English lexicon.

Hypnosis and Hypnotherapy

With the fall of classical mesmerism, Mesmer's followers began to explore one of the common side effects of the process, namely, the trancelike or "somnambulant" state that patients often experienced in the final stages of their "crisis." French mesmerists of the second generation generally abandoned the theory of animal magnetism in favor of the notion of psychic influence, or willpower, on the part of the practitioner vis-à-vis his subject. Bringing about sleep, or trance, instead of violent nervous crisis became the goal now. Such practicing "somnambulists," as they were called, seemed capable of bringing about healing through their force of will or by the power of suggestion. They found assurance in the fact that a patient who felt she was being aided by hypnotic treatments was likely to improve, because a good attitude can sometimes help in such situations. Although there were limits to what somnambulism—or what later came to be referred to as *hypnotism*—could achieve, as early as the 1830s physicians were using it to relieve symptoms of pain, even going so far in some cases as to employ it in place of anesthesia during surgery.

In the United States, a mix of old-line "magnetic" healers and newfangled "somnambulists" practiced side-by-side into the mid 1800s. Charles Poyen introduced magnetic healing to America in 1835, and helped popularize it by pairing it in his demonstrations with feats of clairvoyance. A hypnotized assistant, for example, would be asked by Poyen to "see" objects hidden inside other objects, or to intuit the thoughts of members of the audience. In reality, this was a demonstration of the power of suggestion, and the subtle art of mental manipulation. Indeed, a number of religious leaders in the country began to worry that such acts, allegedly based on the channeling of magnetic forces and the ability to tap into people's consciousnesses, were ungodly and should be condemned. Others worried that skilled practitioners, or those pretending to be practitioners, might undertake to seduce unsuspecting female patients. Despite such fears, however, numerous forms of treatment based on mesmerism/hypnotism developed in America: they ranged from "electrical psychology" and "mental electricity" to "phreno-magnetism" and "psycheism." All were based on a premise of "energy flow" between individuals, and all sought to exploit the link between mind and body to effect a sense of healing and/or improvement. Writers such as Edgar Allan Poe and Margaret Fuller drew on mesmerism and its variants in creating some of their notable literary works.

Back in France, the great neurologist Jean-Martin Charcot (1825–1893) pioneered in the clinical study of hysteria and hypnosis. Initially Charcot believed that hysteria was an inherited neurological disease, but in his mature years he came to regard it as a psychological disorder, or neurosis. One of the key characteristics of hysteria, Charcot determined, was susceptibility to suggestion by the person suffering from it. As the mesmerists had shown, excitability and trance (or somnambulance) seemed to go hand in hand. Charcot achieved fame with his dramatic clinical demonstrations in pursuit of understanding this strange connection. Patients were presented on a lighted stage while Charcot reviewed their case histories and illustrated their symptoms before the audience. His research revealed a clinical link not only between hysteria and the hypnotic state but also between hysteria and *trauma*. Patients, including male patients, who had suffered traumatic events in their pasts were seen to exhibit "hysteria" as a result. Moreover, their symptoms could be controlled, at least temporarily, by means of hypnosis. One of Charcot's most famous students, Sigmund Freud, became particularly fascinated by these developments.

Hypnotherapy, or the application of hypnosis to patients for therapeutic reasons, eventually came to be recognized as a standard medical and psychiatric tool. Physicians learned to hypnotize in order (1) to decrease or eliminate the perception of pain, (2) to allay common fears or anxieties, (3) to suppress psychological symptoms such as stress, (4) to help identify repressed thoughts or emotions and thus aid in the diagnosis and treatment of neuroses, and (5) to assist in the abatement of addictions such as smoking or Internet addiction. The American Medical

Association (AMA) approved hypnotherapy in 1958, followed by the American Psychological Association (1960) and the American Psychiatric Association (1961). Because of controversies regarding its use, however, the AMA withdrew its endorsement in 1987. The other two professional organizations continue to regard selected use of hypnosis by a trained professional in a therapeutic setting in a favorable light. And then, of course, there are the stage performers known as *mentalists* who continue to use hypnosis and clairvoyance to impress audiences around the globe.

Michael Shally-Jensen

See also: Hysteria; Magnet Therapy; Neurasthenia, or Nervous Exhaustion; Psychoanalysis; Reiki and Therapeutic Touch

Further Reading

Hughes, William. 2015. *That Devil's Trick: Hypnotism and the Victorian Popular Imagination.* Manchester: Manchester University Press.

Jackson, Stanley W. 1999. *Care of the Psyche: A History of Psychological Healing.* New Haven, CT: Yale University Press.

Mills, Bruce. 2005. *Poe, Fuller, and the Mesmeric Arts.* Columbia: University of Missouri Press.

Whorton, James C. 2002. *Nature Cures: The History of Alternative Medicine in America.* New York: Oxford University Press.

MORAL TREATMENT

The concept of moral treatment concerns not any specific *type* of therapeutic intervention but rather an entire *approach* to treating those suffering from mental illness. On the one hand, there was the medieval approach that saw the emotionally disturbed person as irreparably damaged. In this pretreatment age, people were considered to have become sick largely owing to "fate," "god's will," or possession by devils. For such people, there was little that could be done other than to lock them away in wretched asylums, under dungeonlike conditions—chains, whips, gruel, and all. These poor souls were basically *punished* for being who they were. "Madness," or "lunacy," as it was called, was both a sickness and a form of eternal damnation. No one among the ordinary citizenry much cared about how these "fools" and "idiots" were treated.

On the other hand, in the late-18th and early-19th centuries, there developed a somewhat more modern view that saw people suffering from mental illness not as harboring devils (though that idea would persist) or as permanently damaged, but rather as being afflicted with a kind of moral or civic depravity. They had not benefitted from or otherwise absorbed a proper moral upbringing. Such individuals came to be regarded, moreover, as imminently *curable*—at least within limits. Under this comparatively more modern, more humane view, it was incumbent on doctors and caretakers to treat patients respectfully, to a degree, to recognize their basic humanity, their circumstances, and their moral and ethical needs. Punishment was no longer the treatment of choice. Instead, care and understanding became the norm—at least for the first several decades of this period. The new form of treatment was called *moral treatment*, to distinguish it from the horrendous, amoral practices of the past.

A handful of key practitioners started the ball rolling in the direction of moral treatment. They do not represent a coherent group, and, often, the progress they made was counterbalanced by setbacks. Still, it is useful to look at their individual contributions.

Benjamin Rush

The U.S. physician and social and political reformer Benjamin Rush (1746–1813) was one of the most prominent figures of his day. Rush is sometimes called the father of American psychiatry for his pioneering contributions. Nevertheless, not all of his contributions were entirely humane, nor did they all withstand the test of time.

Born in Pennsylvania, Rush attended the College of New Jersey in Princeton and then served as an apprentice physician in Philadelphia. He obtained his doctorate in medicine from the University of Edinburgh (the top medical school at the time) in 1768. Returning to Philadelphia, he practiced medicine and taught chemistry and medicine, the latter at the University of Pennsylvania. During the Revolutionary War, Rush sided with the patriots and represented Pennsylvania in the Continental Congress in July 1776, becoming a signer of the Declaration of Independence. Between 1776 and 1778 Rush served as Continental physician general, overseeing medical care for George Washington's army.

Although he was involved in a number of social reform movements such as anti-slavery and anti-capital punishment, Rush's most lasting influence was as a physician. He explored new ways to identify and treat diseases, sometimes stirring debates among fellow physicians. During a yellow-fever epidemic in the Philadelphia area in the 1790s, Rush observed that mosquitos seemed to be more prevalent but nonetheless argued for bleeding and purging of the victims rather than addressing the matter of contact with insects. He applied the remedy to himself in 1793 and fell severely ill as a consequence. In the area of mental health, Rush was an innovator—first and foremost for recognizing mental illness for what it is. At Pennsylvania Hospital, where he opened a special wing for the mentally ill, he used "shock therapy" of cold and hot baths. Believing that mental illness was caused by disturbances in blood circulation, he also employed a large centrifugal spinning board to which patients were attached and rotated. In addition, Rush used a "tranquilizer chair" fitted with bodily restraints and a sensory-depriving head device to isolate patients and minimize any stimulation from the outside. Rush compiled his findings in *Medical Inquiries and Observations upon the Diseases of the Mind* (1812), the first book of its kind in the United States—and one of the first anywhere.

While his techniques did not always prove effective, and his methods could be a little crude, Rush at least had his patients' interests in mind. He questioned the use of dungeons and chains and approached sufferers, instead, as human beings. For these reasons and more, he stands as an early figure in the moral treatment movement.

Philippe Pinel and William Tuke

The French physician Philippe Pinel (1745–1826) was a major proponent of moral treatment. Both his father and grandfather had been physicians, and the young Philippe studied medicine at Montpellier and Toulouse before going on to Paris, in 1778, to specialize in psychiatry. In 1792 Pinel became chief physician at Bicêtre asylum for men, followed three years later by a similar assignment at the Salpêtrière hospital for women. His experiences demonstrated for him that the insane were not possessed by demons but instead suffered from psychological and social pressures, sometimes aggravated by physical ailments and/or hereditary conditions. As a result, he introduced new methods of treatment and generally broadened the medical profession's understanding of mental illness.

One of Pinel's first actions was to unchain the asylums' inhabitants and call a halt to bleeding, purging, cold baths, and other harsh practices. In their place he launched a therapeutic program that included warm baths, informative dialogues with the patients about their conditions, periods of practical work (occupational therapy), and occasional musical and other entertainments. Pinel also divided the asylums into sections based on the severity of patients' symptoms and worked, in all cases, to heal patients as best as could be managed.

He felt that it was important to hire former mental patients as staff in order to enhance understanding on the floor and avoid any problems concerning mistreatment. This had the salutary effect of making convalescing staff members responsible for their own recovery, even as they assisted others. (In this respect, Pinel was a founding figure in the *recovery movement*.) In general, Pinel fought to overcome the social biases and prejudices that surrounded mental illness, and for this reason he is remembered as a leader of moral treatment. His major published work, *Le Traité medico-philosophique sur l'aliénation mentale* (1801), was translated as *A Treatise on Insanity* (1806).

Around the same time that Pinel implemented his reforms, William Tuke (1732–1822), an English Quaker, founded a retreat in York for the care of the insane. Rejecting harsh medical intervention, Tuke emphasized the rural quiet of the retreat, where patients could engage in reading, light manual labor, and conversation. Serving no more than 30 patients at a time, the York Retreat was small enough to enable caretakers to focus on the individual needs of the residents. Tuke's son Samuel was also involved in the effort and wrote an 1813 book that promoted the principles of moral treatment. Critics, however, pointed out that the Tukes were keen to cultivate the religious, intellectual, and moral capacities of the individual in order to make him or her more tractable. The goal for the Tukes was not "recovery" in the modern sense but self-restraint and the cultivation of a favorable attitude toward learning and good manners.

Dorothea Dix

The American social reformer Dorothea Dix (1802–1887) was noted for her work to improve conditions for prisoners and treatments for the mentally ill. Born in Maine, Dix, by the age of 14, was teaching school in Worcester, Massachusetts. In 1821, she opened a school for girls in Boston and began writing children's books. In 1841, she started a Sunday school program in a house of correction outside of Cambridge, Massachusetts. Dismayed by the conditions she found there, especially by the mingling of violent criminals with the mentally ill as well as by the filthy, unheated cells, Dix undertook to survey Massachusetts prisons, almshouses, and insane asylums. Her findings, presented to the state legislature in 1843, led to major improvements at the Worcester state insane asylum and other such institutions.

On the basis of her success in Massachusetts, Dix launched a nationwide crusade, eventually visiting every state in the union east of the Rockies. She achieved some success in New York, New Jersey, Pennsylvania, and other states after documenting conditions in each of them. In 1848, Dix arrived in Washington, DC, aiming to win passage of a bill to provide public land for use in caring for those with mental disorders. A bill was ultimately approved by Congress but was vetoed by President Franklin Pierce in 1854, on grounds that such functions were more appropriately handled by the states. Dix was severely disappointed but continued her fact-finding and reform campaign both in the United States and in Europe. Between 1854 and 1856, she traveled to 14 countries, including Japan. After returning the United States, she got caught up in the Civil War. She was appointed superintendent of women nurses in the Union Army, the highest office held by a woman during the war.

After the war, Dix largely withdrew from public life. In all, she was responsible for the founding or improvement of 32 mental health institutions in a dozen states, Canada, Britain, Continental Europe, and Japan. In 1881, she chose to reside at the New Jersey State Hospital in Trenton, the first mental hospital built as a result of her efforts. Dix died there in July 1887.

Change and Demise

At their peak during the period between 1815 and 1845, early mental health "retreats" and/or specialized hospital wings serving up to 200 patients each—a quite manageable number—had success or recovery rates of around 80 percent, or so it has been reported. This is surely an admirable result, particularly as compared to what went before, when healing or recovery was not even thought possible. After the interregnum of the Civil War, mental hospitals continued to grow exponentially, both in number and in size—thanks, in part, to the work of Dorothea Dix. At the same time, it was this very expansion of asylums and asylum beds that ultimately led to the demise of the model of moral treatment. As patient populations grew and became more diverse, including more of the poor and of immigrants and social misfits, staffing requirements at these institutions exceeded their capacities, and standards of professionalism were lowered. Another notable figure in the history of mental health, Clifford Beers (1876–1943), wrote about his time in a mental ward during this period and claimed that his symptoms only got worse there. Practices in the wards became strict and streamlined, so that by the 1920s many patients were once again being "warehoused" in large, impersonal institutions and received little in the way of individualized care. It would take another revolution, that of the depopulation of the big state mental health institutions and a shift toward community-based plans beginning in the 1960s, before a new version of mental health treatment would emerge in the form of the recovery movement.

Michael Shally-Jensen

See also: Behavioral Theories and Therapies; Electroconvulsive Therapy; Lobotomy and Other "Psychosurgeries"; Mental Hospitals; Milieu Therapy and Therapeutic Community; Recovery Movement

Further Reading

Davidson, Larry, Jaak Rakfeldt, and John Strauss. 2010. *The Roots of the Recovery Movement in Psychiatry.* Hoboken, NJ: Wiley-Blackwell.

McKown, Robin. [1961] 2016. *Pioneers in Mental Health.* N.p.: Palala Press.

Shorter, Edward. 1997. *A History of Psychiatry.* New York: John Wiley and Sons.

Skull, Andrew. 2016. *Madness in Civilization: A Cultural History of Insanity.* Princeton, NJ: Princeton University Press.

NATIVE AMERICAN TRADITIONAL MEDICINE

Most of the healing practices used by American Indian peoples today and in the past are considered traditional or "indigenous." Some of these practices, nevertheless, have evolved over time or been passed between tribes in the course of Native peoples' long history in North America.

At the time of the first encounters between whites and Indians, the European arrivals had only the scantiest of "folk knowledge" regarding medical matters; many of them, therefore, were impressed with the apparent effectiveness of the various Indian practices and remedies. Ever since, it has been an up-and-down, love-hate relationship, with interest (among whites) in Native healing surging and waning depending on the times.

Herbals, History, and Healing

As with indigenous systems everywhere, the healing practices of Native Americans varied greatly with locale. There was not, and never has been, a single "Indian medicine"—although in recent decades a convergence, of sorts, has occurred with the increased market availability of remedies and the greater ease of access enjoyed by consumers. In the past, though, what a healer in one tribe did to address a particular medical condition might be looked askance at by a healer in another

Native American Medicine and the "Spiritual Indian" Trope

From the *X-Files* episode "The Blessing Way" to the Disney movie *Pocahontas*, Native Americans have struggled with what is referred to as "positive discrimination." While the tropes and stereotypes held around the particular group of people might overall be positive, the discrimination still limits how individuals can be perceived.

While Native Americans have faced a number of stereotypical presentations, from Tonto to the Noble Savage, the "Spiritual Indian" is a particularly egregious example. The idea is that since Native Americans are somehow closer to nature than Europeans, they are more magical and "in touch" with the world around them. When Native Americans get to see themselves in media at all, it's nearly always as the fierce warrior who is noble despite being uncivilized or as the medicine man who is somehow outside the conflicts happening around him.

With the ability for advocates to connect and create larger platforms on social media, many Native Americans are working together to make sure that more positive and diverse representations of Native Americans are visible in the entertainment world. For example, Sydney Freeland's movie *Drunktown's Finest* premiered at Sundance in 2014, and Rebecca Roanhorse's urban fantasy novel *Trail of Lightning* released in 2018. These examples tell indigenous stories from the point of view of indigenous characters, instead of the white people around them.

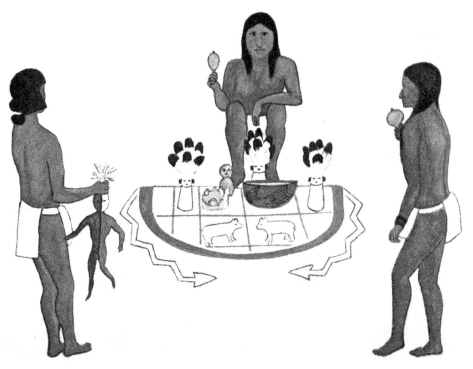

Illustration from a San Juan Pueblo tale about "Pah-tay and the Wind-Witch," showing medicine men with rattles, a kachina doll, and other objects. Illustration by Fred Kabotie (Hopi). (DeHuff, Elizabeth Willis. *Taytay's Tales Collected and Retold*, 1922)

tribe. For example, some tribes, along with the incoming European colonists, used bloodletting as a therapeutic procedure. The Algonkian tribes of the northeast, however, regarded bleeding as a detestable practice and felt that it weakened rather than healed those subjected to it.

Still, the healing systems of the colonists and the Native Americans shared a number of similarities. Belief in supernatural forces and the use of ritual and/or prayer pervaded each. White people brought from Europe the "doctrine of signatures," or the principle that herbs resembling different parts of the human body might be used by healers to treat ailments of those body parts. (Although traceable to ancient Greece, the doctrine of signatures in colonial times was justified by the argument that God would have wanted to reveal to humans what plants could be used for.) Most tribal healers employed the same or a similar system, looking to qualities such as shape, color, taste, and function to guide them in identifying remedies. Thus, members of the Meskwaki (Fox) tribe used the milky juice of the jack-in-the-pulpit plant (*Arum maculatum*) as a snakebite remedy, in part because it both looked like venom and had a sting to it (causing, in some cases, an allergic reaction); plus, the plant bore a resemblance to a snake's head.

A number of Indian remedies were clearly an improvement over European methods. Unfamiliar with the natural world in North America, and moreover seeing it as "a hideous and desolate wilderness" (William Bradford, 1620), Europeans preferred to import their herbal medicines from their homeland. In doing so they missed a variety of useful Native American preparations, such as one made from the foxglove herb and used as a remedy for dropsy (edema), or fluid in the legs caused by heart failure. Only in the 1780s would William Withering in England discover the same application from a folk healer's cure. Today, foxglove extract, known as digitalis, is used as a cardiac drug for the moderation of the heart rate.

As functional as the Native pharmacopoeia may have been, indigenous peoples were ill prepared for the spread of white people's diseases among their ranks. Although they had herbal and other treatments for such conditions as dropsy, scurvy (decoctions from the annedda, or Canadian spruce, tree), malaria (quinine, from the bark of the cinchona tree), they had nothing to deal with the ravages of smallpox, tuberculosis, venereal disease, and flu epidemics. They could nevertheless successfully reset broken bones, address various skin conditions, handle common stomach ailments and fevers, and, of course, delivery babies and ensure the health of mother and child.

Illnesses of the mental or psychosomatic variety, along with a wide variety of other, less specific conditions, were generally managed by shamanistic techniques. This would entail, for example, the burning of substances to be blown over, and sometimes inhaled by, the patient; chanting, drumming, and dancing around the patient; "sweating" the patient inside a sweat lodge; uttering special incantations; employing charms and amulets imbued with special powers; and magically "extracting" any foreign bodies or evil spirits from the patient's body. Such a regimen inevitably proved helpful enough in a sufficient number of cases as to become highly valued as both a practical solution and a time-honored tradition.

One practical problem for Native healers was that the natural resources upon which they drew were subject to fluctuations caused by drought, floods, fires, seasonal irregularities, and invasions of insects. This sometimes made access to medical supplies difficult or impossible. Another, graver issue was the effect of displacement by Europeans. As whites moved westward and forced Native Americans into settlements in unfamiliar territory, indigenous traditions suffered due to the alien flora and fauna in the new region and the general breakdown of social mores.

New World, New Age

As noted, Natives were considered by most white settlers as both ignorant savages and symbols of hardiness and vigor (the Noble Savage). They were thought not to suffer as many physical ills as whites. One Native practice that was found to be particularly conducive to good health was the sweat lodge, similar to a Finnish sauna. A hut was constructed out of branches and covered with hide. Inside were heated rocks and embers. The individual would sit in the structure until it became intolerable, at which point he would exit and douse himself in water or collapse in a snowbank. The idea was to purge oneself of impurities, either material or spiritual. Some colonists later took up this practice, although it became a popular trend among non-Indian Americans only in the 1970s and 1980s, when alternative health measures were being actively explored.

The medicines passed down from Native peoples to Euro-American settlers were arguably more effective than many of the Western remedies. Instead of eye of newt, oil of scorpion, and blood of serpent, for example, Indian tradition suggested sassafras (a general medicant), puke weed (a purgative), ginseng (an energy drink, with other applications), tobacco (a soothing social drug), and many other utile items. Most of these were brought back by traders to Europe, where they became popular. Tobacco, for instance, was used for over 350 years as a treatment for coughs and congestion of the lungs, before it was found to be a cancer-causing agent and generally unhealthful. (Native Americans preferred tobacco for ceremonial purposes, whereas Euro-Americans used it more frequently in leisure settings.)

Beginning in the 19th century, as U.S. folk medicine practitioners took to the road to sell their wares, Indian medicines started to be widely recognized as attractive to consumers. White purveyors of "patent medicines," which could be made up of virtually anything that the makers could get their hands on, traveled about as "Indian doctors"—that is, as persons claiming to have lived with a tribe and absorbed their "ancient methods" for the benefit of the rest of humanity. "Miracle potions" and "amazing elixirs," most of them having little or nothing to do with Native American cultures, were sold at a steady pace to buyers looking for a cure-all. Some of these medicines had vaguely Indian names, like Kickapoo Indian Oil, Seminole Cough Balsam, Comanche Blood Strength-O, Ka-Ton-Ka, and Sagwa (the latter two completely made up). At popular "medicine shows" people would gather to learn about the latest treatments and be entertained by pseudo-Native "characters" and other nonsensical personas and performances. The shows were at once enjoyable and rather dangerous, given the quality of the various "snake oil" remedies that were on offer.

Although much of Native American traditional medicine is forgotten today or ignored by the general populace, it still forms a part of the folk culture at some reservations and has a strong following among those open to alternative and complementary medicine. Sometime around the 1970s, particularly within U.S. hippie culture, Indian medicine took on a positive aura after more than a century of decline. Particularly popular was the hallucinogenic peyote plant, used more as a recreational drug than as a medicine. Then, in the 1980s, Native American healthways took on a slightly different cast as an integral part of New Age culture and the holistic health movement. The full range of medicinal practice was pursued, from herbal remedies to chanting, sweat lodges, and spiritual journeys (vision quests). Young White Anglo-Saxon Protestants (WASPs) took on Indian names (or Indian-sounding names) and, to a greater or lesser extent, abandoned their old WASP ways. Although many in the U.S. establishment questioned this cultural shift and lampooned it in the press, it served the signal purpose of raising awareness about Native American social and cultural life generally and Native health and wellness topics specifically. Native activists, too, raised questions about the appropriation of their culture by New Age seekers.

The combined U.S. Pharmacopoeia-National Formulary, an official compendium of recognized drugs in the country, has at one time or another listed some 200 American Indian herbals. Besides those mentioned already, commonly used Native medicinals include witch hazel (for skin conditions), mayapple (for warts), sarsaparilla (for anemia and other conditions), goldenseal (for muscle spasms and other ailments), and, from South America, ipecac (purgative). The continuing popularity of herbal remedies in the United States is, in a way, a tribute to American Indian cultural ingenuity.

Michael Shally-Jensen

See also: Herbal Remedies; Medicine Shows; Naturopathic Medicine; Paleo Diet; Psychedelic Drugs; Shamanism and Neo-Shamanism; Sweat Lodges and Saunas

Further Reading

Calabrese, Joseph D. 2013. *A Different Medicine: Postcolonial Healing in the Native American Church.* New York: Oxford University Press.

Cohen, Kenneth. 2003. *Honoring the Medicine: The Essential Guide to Native American Healing.* New York: Ballantine.

Lyon, William S. 1996. *Encyclopedia of Native American Healing.* Santa Barbara, CA: ABC-CLIO.

Vogel, Virgil J. 1990. *American Indian Medicine.* Norman: University of Oklahoma Press.

NEURASTHENIA, OR NERVOUS EXHAUSTION

Neurasthenia is a catch-all term for a variety of subjective complaints, including jitteriness, listlessness, lethargy, divided attention, lack of motivation, and feelings of weariness or weakness. Or, as *Merriam-Webster's Medical Dictionary* defines it, neurasthenia is "a condition that is characterized especially by physical and mental exhaustion usually with accompanying symptoms (as headaches, insomnia, and irritability); is believed to result from psychological factors (as depression or emotional stress or conflict); and is sometimes considered similar to or identical with chronic fatigue syndrome." The condition had a long and rich history before it ever was mentioned in the same breath with chronic fatigue syndrome, however—even though the comparison is an apt one. While no longer used as a diagnosis in American psychiatry today, neurasthenia continues to be recognized in Europe, Latin America, Asia, and elsewhere. Ironically, when it first came to notice in North America in the mid-1800s, it was considered an especially American disease, something associated with the unique stresses of modern American life.

"Neurasthenia Americana"

Neurasthenia, or nervous exhaustion, began to gain attention in the U.S. medical community in the years before the Civil War. In 1844, Joel Shew, a doctor and leading advocate of hydropathy, or the "water cure," suggested that the cause of virtually all disease was overwrought nerves. The idea was that a mechanical weakness in the nervous system—a disruption of the "nerve fluid"—caused imbalances elsewhere, leading to organic decline and, in some cases, psychological symptoms. Other physicians, too, started noticing more patients complaining about things like fatigue, headache, heart palpitations, high blood pressure, neuralgia (nerve pain), and depression. Often, the person complaining worked in a "professional" occupation—that is, business, finance, law, or medicine itself. There was no deep understanding or general consensus among medical practitioners of the time as to what lay behind the rise in complaints. Nor was any single cure advised; rather, a variety of therapies were initially proposed: hydrotherapy (cold water), mesmerism/magnetism, mineral water, spas, homeopathy, and so on.

After the war, a neurologist from New York, George Beard, began lecturing and publishing on the topic of neurasthenia. Although Beard's first works came out in the late 1860s, he wrote his most famous account, *American Nervousness: Its Causes and Consequences,* in 1881. In it, Beard argued that "nervousness" was especially prevalent in the northern and eastern sections of the United States and, in his view, was attributable chiefly to the development of "modern civilization." He pointed to a number of technological advances as contributing to the rise of the new disorder (steam power, the newspaper and magazine industry, the telegraph, and modern science) along with a variety of social factors such as the constant presence of death and bereavement (especially in the wake of the Civil War), business and family concerns, the stresses of birth (including the loss of the offspring), the consumption of stimulants and drugs, and the increasing involvement of women in society. Women, it should be noted, were believed to suffer from neurasthenia twice as often as men did.

In Beard's view, each person was assumed to have a set amount of "nerve force," or nervous energy, available to him or her. As the supply of nerve force dwindled in the face of heavy societal demands, or when one's nervous energy was not expended on worthy activities but was instead wasted on frivolities, nervous discord, or neurasthenia, resulted. Thus, activities like learning, productive work, spiritual pursuits, and the arts were beneficial uses of one's energies, whereas activities like gambling, drinking, and sexual debauchery were considered senseless drains of nervous force. Yet even refined or sophisticated members of society could be taxed, or stressed, by an overabundance of cultural activities; similarly, members of the lower orders of society could sometimes succumb to neurasthenia through the wasteful expenditure of their internal resources. The illness could be a sign of either moral development and sensitivity or moral depravity and decadence.

Symptoms might begin with little more than a mild case of "dyspepsia" (indigestion) or occasional insomnia but could go on to include asthma, hypochondria, skin rashes, hot and cold flashes, hysteria, mental collapse, and even insanity. In between, complaints such as a disinclination to engage in mental labor and a sense of being in an unsettled state were common.

Ironically, instead of regarding neurasthenia as a dreadful scourge, Beard considered it the natural effect of having developed a "superior" civilization; he therefore expected it to persist in parts of the United States and Europe as social evolution continued to unfold. Beard recommended a set of mild treatments to deal with most cases of the illness: fresh air, sunlight, water, rest, and light amusements. Phosphorous and arsenic (both known as toxins today) could also be introduced to help fortify the nerves. In more serious cases, a stronger form of treatment might be needed, namely, electrification of the body by means of copper leads. Intended to recharge the nervous system, the remedy was, in fact, an early form of electroconvulsive therapy, or "shock therapy." Sufferers could even purchase a variety of home electrical devices, such as an electric belt (the "Heidelberg") for men that delivered a charge to the groin.

From "Nerves" to Stress, Anxiety, and Fatigue

Although neurasthenia was one of the most common diagnoses made in the late-19th and early-20th centuries—one book about it was called *The Nervous Housewife* (Myerson, 1920)—it eventually began to fade as a medical term, replaced by diagnoses based on more specific sets of symptoms. By the mid-20th century, experts were talking more about *stress*, *anxiety*, and *fatigue* as debilitating conditions than they were about general "nervousness" or "nervous exhaustion." In *Identity and the Life Cycle* (1959), Erik Erikson described internal conflicts that can be sources of stress and anxiety. He said that the central internal conflicts typically revolve around issues of (1) autonomy versus dependence, (2) intimacy versus isolation, and (3) cooperation versus competition. Some people are better able than others to handle these kinds of dilemmas. For many, though, they experience a kind of existential angst when facing important decisions. They become anxious, exhibiting such signs as increased heart rate, elevated blood pressure, greater skin sensitivity, and heightened levels of adrenaline. Anxiety is a normal human response except when it overwhelms the person and makes him or her unable to act. Then it is potentially a medical condition, and the person is advised to seek help from a medical professional or mental health practitioner.

Stress operates in much the same way, with individuals reacting differently to stressful situations and being able to handle them or not depending on their unique makeup as a person as well as other factors. A particular stressor need not be present for the stress to be experienced, for the individual can think about or worry over the stressor at any time (including during sleep). The body's system for handling stress is designed to remain in a "ready" status most of the time, coming into play in difficult situations. When, however, people suffer from an overactive stress response that makes them react strongly to even minor provocations, they most likely are in need of assistance from a health care professional.

Another condition serving to replace neurasthenia in American medicine is chronic fatigue syndrome. Normal fatigue is a temporary state of physical, psychological, or emotional tiredness that can affect one's level of productivity. People suffering from fatigue report being overtired, overworked, feeling rundown, lifeless, and depleted of energy. Chronic fatigue syndrome (CFS), on the other hand, is a more serious condition marked by a state of exhaustion that lasts longer and is more profound than everyday fatigue and can result in diminished physical, mental, and emotional functioning. As with anxiety and stress-related disorders, the individual exhibiting signs of CFS should seek medical assistance.

The treatments for these three conditions vary. Generally speaking, however, for milder cases of stress and anxiety, relaxation techniques, such as meditation or progressive muscle relaxation, may be employed, perhaps aided by calming aural and aromatic stimuli. Education about the conditions is another standard element of most therapeutic regimens. Participants learn how to identify their personal sources of stress or anxiety, how to recognize the physiological and psychological signs of the conditions (including by means of biofeedback), and how to avoid or control their states of illness, to the extent that such is possible.

These and other strategies are often part of a cognitive-behavioral approach to therapy, which also can be used to control chronic fatigue syndrome. Under this approach, individuals are taught to monitor and change tendentious thoughts, to reorganize their activities and behaviors in such a way as to minimize illness reactions, and to make changes like prioritizing and managing their daily workloads and generally adopting a healthy lifestyle. In addition, an antianxiety (anxiolytic) drug may be prescribed in many cases. Alternatively, sufferers may choose to try acupuncture or bodywork (massage, etc.). Exercise, too, has proved beneficial. Chronic fatigue syndrome is perhaps the most difficult of the three to treat, as its causes are not well understood and no standard drug therapy has been developed for it.

In any case, we have come a long way from the neurasthenia of days past. Are we, however, perhaps missing a diagnosis that other cultures find to be legitimate?

Does neurasthenia no longer apply to contemporary U.S. life? Is the concept of the "nervous breakdown" so unscientific as to require banishment? A number of other cultures don't think so.

Michael Shally-Jensen

See also: Anxiety and Its Treatment; Homeopathy; Hydrotherapy; Hysteria; Mesmerism and Hypnotherapy; Spas and Mineral Waters; Stress and Stress Management

Further Reading

Gosling, Francis G. 1987. *Before Freud: Neurasthenia and the American Medical Community.* Urbana: University of Illinois Press.

Lutz, Tom. 2004. *American Nervousness, 1903: An Anecdotal History.* Ithaca, NY: Cornell University Press.

Myerson, Abraham. 1920. *The Nervous Housewife.* Boston: Little, Brown.

Ross, Zachary, and Amanda Glessman. 2004. *Women on the Verge: Neurasthenia in Late Nineteenth-Century American Art.* Stanford, CA: Stanford University Museum of Art.

Shorter, Edward. 2013. *How Everyone Became Depressed: The Rise and Fall of the Nervous Breakdown.* New York: Oxford University Press.

PATENT MEDICINES

Also known as proprietary medicines or "nostrums," patent medicines are medicinal products that at one time were sold directly to customers without any need for a doctor's prescription. They typically contained a "secret" ingredient known only to the manufacturer and were promoted in advertisements as "miracle" drugs that could cure a wide variety of ailments. Today, the Federal Food and Drug Administration (FDA) prohibits the manufacture and sale of medicines with undisclosed contents; all medicines must be labeled clearly as to ingredients and any restrictions on usage. They must also be free of harmful substances. In the 19th century, however, patent medicines based on dubious formulas were hugely popular and gave rise to an entire industry specializing in such over-the-counter products for consumers. Those same consumers, nevertheless, could not count on the purity or safety of the medicines they were buying. That would have required government regulation, which took hold only in the early decades of the 20th century.

The Trade in Medical Nostrums

Although some of the top patent medicine makers were physicians, or used the name of a physician on their labels, it was not at all necessary to have a medical background, or even a background in basic chemistry, to manufacture these medicines. All that was needed was the mixing of a variety of ingredients—the more exotic the better!—along with, usually, a good dose of alcohol to help the medicine go down and keep the customer happy. It is for this reason that promoters of such merchandise came to be known as "snake oil salesmen" or "toadstool millionaires"—the epithets referencing two favorite ingredients in the trade. Later on, of course, the phrase "snake oil" became a synonym for fraud.

Another key element in the proprietary medicine business was the creation of a distinctive bottle and brand name, together with some irresistible advertising copy. In fact, the name "patent medicine" is something of a misnomer. Most often, manufacturers would obtain a trademark registration for a brand name and the product's packaging (the bottle design functioning as a kind of "logo"), and would also claim copyright ownership with respect to the marketing copy employed. Very rarely did they seek a patent for the medicine itself, because doing so would require them to disclose the contents of a remedy and risk having it reproduced by competitors. Instead, they *talked* a lot about how unique and effective their products were—with very little to back up their claims.

Manufacturers used a variety of novel methods to attract consumers and get them to stop relying on old-fashioned home remedies. They created mixtures that were more pleasing to the senses and easier to take than, say, traditional calomel or cod liver oil. They might add cinnamon or mint to an elixir to make it more palatable. They innovated by making medicines in pill form, sometimes coating them with sugar to lessen any bitterness. They added aromas to lotions and ointments to make them smell better and seem more effective to users. And, again, they included substantial amounts of distilled spirits, and even small doses of narcotics like cocaine and opium, in order to cover symptoms of pain and reduce anxiety in their customers-patients. So successful were proprietary medicine makers in changing consumers' tastes and expectations, in fact, that "regular" doctors and pharmacists eventually had to follow suit in order to appease their own clientele and stay competitive in the marketplace.

Sold frequently through traveling medicine shows, as well as marketed nationwide via mail-order pioneers such as Sears, Roebuck and Montgomery Ward, patent medicines opened up a whole new category of medical consumption, namely, the casual buyer. Very early on, it seems, the industry learned how to *make* consumers out of the walking well or the near well; that is, they successfully convinced healthy or marginally ill individuals to try the new "wonder drugs" to see if they didn't bring (a sense of) relief or simply make one feel better. The more extensively and effectively a remedy was advertised, the more likely it was to achieve strong sales. The key for manufacturers was to reach ever wider audiences for their products and at the same time obtain repeat sales, thereby "validating" the extravagant claims made for their medicines.

Drawing on stereotypical images of American Indian healers (e.g., "Sagwa" Indian tonic from the Kickapoo Medicine Company), respectable family doctors (Dr. Keeley's "Gold Cure"), Quaker sensibility (Dr. Flint's "Quaker Bitters"), legendary characters (Hamlin's "Wizard Oil" liniment), or sage grandmothers (Lydia Pinkham's "Vegetable Compound"), nostrum makers demonstrated great skill in the art of marketing. They often included in their presentations testimonials by satisfied patients-customers; such statements were generally either made up or paid for, although some were genuine. In the medicine shows, elaborate narratives based on a particular brand's founding image or signature "theme" were often acted out on stage before a live audience. Manufacturers were able to do what they did, moreover, with little or no interference from government overseers. It was up to the customer to decide whether a product was safe and effective and lived up to its advertising. This model still applies in various areas of alternative medicine, such as the dietary supplement industry (which is largely free of FDA scrutiny). It is one that has served the industry well—and most customers seem not to object too strongly, because it gives them a continuing array of product choices.

Early remedies were marketed for the curing of "consumption" (tuberculosis), liver and bladder problems, ague (fever), dyspepsia (indigestion), piles (hemorrhoids), diarrhea, muscle pain, toothaches, foot ailments, nasal and cough problems, disorders of the nerves, skin conditions, "wind" (flatulence), grippe (influenza), worms, jaundice, dysentery, dropsy (fluid buildup), scrofula, spasms, dizzy spells, "brain exhaustion," biliousness (gas and/or gall bladder issues), catarrh (excess mucus), "languid" blood, "female complaints," "loss of manhood," inflammatory diseases, diseases of the lung and throat (e.g., asthma), kidney diseases, and so on ad infinitum. They contained ingredients such as corn oil, arsenic, mercury, sarsaparilla, celery, calomel, dandelion, root extract, catsup, beet, radon, cannabis, ginger, mineral oil, pepper, turpentine, camphor, and a host of others, along with the aforementioned narcotic substances and spirits.

The Marquee Comes Down

As the 19th century drew to its end, both the AMA and state legislative bodies began to push for reform of the patent medicine industry. One concern was the quality of the products themselves, made in far-flung factories with little or no quality control measures in place. Such medicinal items were subject to adulteration or contamination, not to mention fraudulent advertising as manufacturers tried to make the most of the goods they sold. Catsup and alcohol did not a healthy remedy make, and moreover there was no proof whatsoever that any such remedies addressed the conditions they claimed to address. Thus, cities and states began to pass laws establishing (minimal) standards for the manufacture and sale of food and drugs. The American Pharmaceutical Association developed a National Formulary to specify drug ingredients. Newspaper and magazine publishers denounced the practice by proprietary medicine companies of threatening to pull advertising accounts if a publication printed news that was unfavorable to the industry. More important, still, was a series of scathing stories in Collier's magazine between 1905 and 1907 by the muckraking journalist Samuel Hopkins Adams.

Called "The Great American Fraud" (and later published in book form under the same name), Adams's series exposed the chicanery engaged in by those in the patent medicine industry. He looked, for example, at the alcoholic contents of some of the products, having sent samples to a chemical laboratory for analysis. Although a few of the items tested had only modest amounts of alcohol, some of them came out with readings in the 40–50 percent range; and a number of them contained grain alcohol, a particularly strong—even dangerous—spirit. Although the recommended dosages might not lead to serious harm, it was clear that these medicines could be overused, especially in "dry" states or counties. In any case, alcohol was hardly defensible as beneficial to one's health. Along the same lines, Adams itemized other potentially damaging substances used in the industry and the false claims made for them by their promoters. His summary finding was that people should believe nary a word from these manufacturers and instead save themselves from grief by avoiding patent medicines altogether.

Published about the same time as Upton Sinclair's landmark exposé of the meatpacking industry, *The Jungle*, "The Great American Fraud" contributed to the development of national reform legislation, the Pure Food and Drug Act of 1906. Under the law, most (but still not all) contents of a purported medicine had to be printed on the label. Manufacturers faced penalties for demonstrated cases of adulteration of contents or the use of false and misleading statements. But whereas meatpacking plants were subject to inspection by government agents, drug makers were able to work around the law in most cases because no strong enforcement mechanism was put in place. Thus, even as reformers celebrated their legal success, manufacturers continued to push the limits. Real change wouldn't come until later in the century. Today's nonprescription, over-the-counter drugs are subject to far more stringent disclosure requirements and are closely monitored for the medical claims stated on their labels vis-à-vis the actual results one can expect based on their ingredients and the science involved in making them. The dietary supplement industry, on the other hand, faces similar but comparatively fewer such restrictions.

Michael Shally-Jensen

See also: Diet Pills and Metabolism Boosters; Folk Medicine; Herbal Remedies; Infomercials and Wellness Promotion; Medicine Shows; Spas and Mineral Waters; Vitamins and Minerals

Further Reading

Armstrong, David, and Elizabeth Metzger Armstrong. 1991. *The Great American Medicine Show.* New York: Prentice Hall.

Tomes, Nancy. 2016. *Remaking the American Patient: How Madison Avenue and Modern Medicine Turned Patients into Consumers.* Chapel Hill: University of North Carolina Press.

Young, James H. 1972. *The Toadstool Millionaires: A Social History of Patent Medicines in America.* Princeton: Princeton University Press.

PHRENOLOGY

Although not created solely for the purposes of healing, phrenology nevertheless played an outsized role in 19th-century medical thought and was hugely popular among the U.S. public. Its animating idea was that the mental and temperamental characteristics of an individual could be discerned by examining the bumps and depressions on his or her skull.

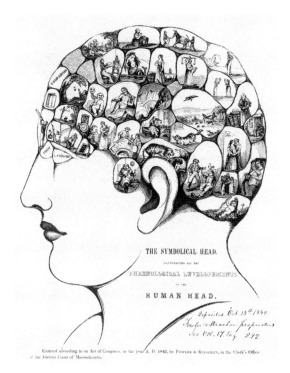

THE SYMBOLICAL HEAD.

PHRENOLOGICAL DEVELOPEMENTS

HUMAN HEAD.

Entered according to an Act of Congress, in the year A. D. 1842, by FOWLER & STRACHAN, in the Clerk's Office of the District Court of Massachusetts.

An 1842 illustration of the various phrenological regions of the cranium and their corresponding subjects (as regards the human personality). (Library of Congress)

The Furor over Phrenology

The concept originated with the work of the German physician Franz Joseph Gall (1758–1828), who thought of the brain not as a single organ but as a complex of many specialized organs operating inside the cranium. Each organ was said to be linked to a particular mental or emotional function, or "faculty." In its modern, greatly revised form, such a statement is more or less true (although today we speak of cortical "areas," not "organs," in discussing neuronal "localization"). Gall also correctly identified the gray matter of the brain as the active and crucial part and the white matter as the supporting tissue, and he put to rest the ancient idea that the emotions and personality were rooted in the internal organs—as part of the soul—rather than in the brain. For all of this Gall is to be recognized as a pioneer. Where he went too far was in claiming that certain abstract human qualities, like vanity, greed, dignity, or industry, were tied to specific locations (or "faculties") in the brain. He believed that an enlargement of a particular segment of the head, as evidenced by a protrusion of the skull at that site, showed that an excess of brain tissue existed there and therefore an excess of the property or quality associated with it. Similarly, a slight indentation of the skull's surface indicated that the underlying brain was lacking in substance and must also be lacking in the associated emotional or intellectual quality. In developing his theory, Gall came up with 27 innate human "faculties" inside the brain as reflected by the shape of the skull.

Gall's writings and live demonstrations made him something of a scientific celebrity in Europe. Yet it was another German physician, Johann Spurzheim (1776–1832), who helped to systemize Gall's new "science" and popularize it in Europe and the United States. Spurzheim was a one of Gall's students and the person, in fact, who coined the name "phrenology" (from the Greek, meaning "science of the mind"). He, like Gall, believed that the outlines of the skull reflected the development of the brain organs and their associated functions, but he differed with Gall over the classification of the various qualities and over the goal of phrenology itself.

Sample List of Phrenological "Organs" or "Faculties"

Although different practitioners employed different lists at different times and places, or used different terms to identify the various human faculties, the practice of phrenology was more or less consistent throughout its history. This particular list, from a revised American edition of an early work by Johann Spurzheim, features a set of thirty-five faculties.

1. Destructiveness
2. Amativeness (i.e., connubial love and affection)
3. Philoprogenitiveness (parental and familial love)
4. Adhesiveness (social attachment)
5. Inhabitiveness (domesticity or home feeling)
6. Combativeness
7. Secretiveness
8. Acquisitiveness
9. Constructiveness
10. Cautiousness
11. Approbativeness (desire for praise)
12. Self-esteem
13. Benevolence
14. Reverence (respect, devotion)
15. Firmness
16. Conscientiousness
17. Hope
18. Marvellousness (sense of the sublime)
19. Ideality
20. Mirthfulness
21. Imitation
22. Individuality
23. Configuration (recognition of forms)
24. Size (size perception)
25. Weight and Resistance (perception of)
26. Coloring (color sensitivity)
27. Locality (geographic sense)
28. Order (neatness, systems, methods)
29. Calculation
30. Eventuality (narrative sense)
31. Time
32. Tune (musicality)
33. Language
34. Comparison
35. Causality

Source: J.G. Spurzheim, *Phrenology, or, The Doctrine of the Mental Phenomena,* rev. 2d American ed. Philadelphia: J.B. Lippincott Co., 1908.

Gall regarded the new science as largely a diagnostic and exploratory tool, rather like a PET scan or an fMRI today, something that could help researchers understand the brain and its functions. Spurzheim, in contrast, took a more pragmatic view and saw phrenology as a way to direct individuals toward self-improvement in the areas in which they fell short, or, in other words, as a means of life guidance. People, he felt, could strengthen their good or bad brain organs under the proper guidance; they could develop their potential along the most desirable pathways of growth and advancement. To that end, Spurzheim modified Gall's classifications of human qualities (or faculties) and added several new categories of his own, to make a total of 33. His categories were generally more positive and open-ended than Gall's, and his brand of phrenology came to be known as "practical phrenology."

Unfortunately, during Spurzheim's 1832 American tour, the popularizer fell ill with typhoid and died. Businesses in Boston, where he had met his end, closed for the day and a crowd numbering in the thousands showed up for his funeral. His brain was preserved in a laboratory at Harvard's medical college.

Fowl Play

Around the same time, phrenology in the United States got a boost from a new group of practitioners organized around the Fowler brothers, Orson Squire and Lorenzo Niles, in New York City. The Fowlers advanced the idea, among other things, of self-instruction in phrenology—every person his or her own phrenologist! They issued numerous publications and advertisements to that end and delivered many lectures and demonstrations. As with Spurzheim, it was all about "mental progress" and pursuing a path of "perfectionism" whereby one could be all that one could be. Once a person's unique character traits were phrenologically identified, they could be augmented or guarded against through personal effort and learning. On the other hand, the Fowlers' system of practical phrenology was designed to be mostly flattering toward the subject. It was akin to a basic psychic reading or review of an astrological chart: it tended to confirm what one already knew or simply missed the mark in places and appeared inapplicable in a harmless way. Through the Fowlers' efforts, nonetheless, America became phrenology crazy for a time in the mid-1800s. It was not uncommon to find plaster skulls displaying the various mental "faculties" in people's homes, along, perhaps, with written summaries regarding the owner's head and personality. The expression "to get one's head examined" is thought to have come from the golden age of phrenology. And many famous people did indeed get their heads examined by the Fowlers, including impresario P. T. Barnum, newspaper publisher Horace Greeley, poet Walt Whitman, writer Mark Twain, women's rights advocate Susan B. Anthony, and Red Cross founder Clara Barton. Other literary figures, including Edgar Allan Poe, Stephen Crane, and Louisa May Alcott, incorporated phrenology into their published stories.

In 1838, the Fowlers launched *The American Phrenological Journal* (*APJ*), which soon became one of the most popular magazines in the United States; it lasted until 1911. Along with other family members, the brothers also participated in and actively promoted new movements developing around vegetarianism, temperance, mesmerism, and hydropathy; they took over the publication of *Water-Cure*, hydropathy's main journal, in 1848. A phrenology school run by the Fowlers and others opened in New York City around the same time. Moreover, a stream of additional applications for phrenological science, ranging from education to vocational guidance to the management of children, was devised by devotees. Various customer outreach schemes were put in place too, such as inviting people to send in photos of their heads to be read by an expert and published in the *AJP*. A great increase was seen in the number of traveling "bump doctors," as phrenologist were derisively called, before the end of the century.

Feels Like Folly

Throughout phrenology's history, the idea of deducing intelligence and character from the size and shape of a person's brain was questioned by many in the medical establishment. As time passed—as medicine advanced while phrenology merely grew in popularity—the differences between the two branches of knowledge became more obvious. Mark Twain, among others, found his skepticism about phrenology increased after he received not one, not two, but three very different readings of his temperament and traits at different times. How could these all possibly be right, he wondered? How could they all so clearly be wrong? Another critic, noted doctor and writer Oliver Wendell Holmes (Sr.), compared the braincase to a steel safe from which no one could glean any information regarding its internal contents. Indeed, the showmanlike tricks employed by the Fowlers and their ilk invited the wrath of many a "regular" physician. By the end of the 19th century, with a more detailed understanding of the nervous system and the brain having been developed, the theories and methods of phrenology came to seem outmoded and absurd. The era of phrenology as a mass phenomenon was soon over, even as it continued to sputter along in the early 20th century as a kind of cultural roadshow, encouraging happy participants, if only for fun, to go ahead and get their brains scanned. By then, the hottest new method of reading the mind was the Freudian one, or the "talking cure." The interpretation of dreams seemed to offer more to clients than the interpretation of cranial bumps and dents.

One of the main legacies of phrenology, in fact, was the development of the equally dubious field of anthropological criminology, or the study of the "criminal type" based on the shape of the criminal skull. Italy's Cesare Lombroso (1835–1909) was the founding figure here, and he gave credit to Franz Gall and phrenology for inspiring his research. The premise was that criminality is inherited and is evident in certain physical signs of degeneracy in an individual or group. In France, Alphonse Bertillon (1853–1914) employed similar methods of measurement in developing his system of criminal identification, including the standard mug shot. But whereas Bertillon's work had important implications for modern criminology (including what we today call biometrics), most of Lombroso's theories fell into disrepute and are now of historical interest only.

Michael Shally-Jensen

See also: Alternative Diagnostics; Craniosacral Therapy; Lobotomy and Other "Psychosurgeries"; Psychoanalysis; Reflexology

Further Reading

Janik, Erika. 2014. *Marketplace of the Marvelous: The Strange Origins of Modern Medicine.* Boston: Beacon Press.

Lyons, Sherrie Lynne. 2009. *Species, Serpents, Spirits, and Skulls: Science at the Margins of the Victorian Era.* Albany: SUNY Press.

Tomlinson, Stephen. 2005. *Head Masters: Phrenology, Secular Education, and Nineteenth-Century Social Thought.* Tuscaloosa: University of Alabama Press.

Wrobel, Arthur, ed. 2015. *Pseudo-Science and Society in 19th-Century America.* Lexington: University Press of Kentucky.

PURGATIVES AND EMETICS

Although purgatives (generally laxatives) and emetics (items given to cause vomiting) are still a part of the medical arsenal today, their current medical use is focused on a limited number of conditions. Prior to early 20th century, however, these items, especially purgatives, were widely used to treat almost every condition imaginable. Much of this was owing to the faulty medical theories of the times; the rest was due to the successful salesmanship of those who marketed and sold such products.

When humans first started trying to understand the causes of disease, they had two basic ideas. One was that spiritual beings were the source of health problems, because they either had failed in their duties to keep things normal or were intentionally causing problems out of spite. The other major theory that developed, and eventually carried the day in the Western world, was that diseases occurred when the natural fluids, or "humors" (also spelled *humours*), of the human body became imbalanced. The goal of the physician, then, was to restore the correct balance to the four principal humors present in each person.

Use in Connection with the Four Humors

Beginning in ancient Greece, when Hippocrates and others rejected spiritual explanations for disease in favor of a physical, natural explanation, the idea was put forward that human health depended on a balance of four internal humors: black bile, yellow bile, phlegm, and blood. (The first reference to this type of diagnosis actually occurred a few decades prior to Hippocrates, but that person, Croton, was not an "antispiritist" in the same way that Hippocrates was.) Several centuries later, Galen, a Roman-era Greek physician, wrote so exhaustively about these humors that the theory was accepted throughout the Western world for another 1,500 years.

Table of Correspondences among Temperaments, Humors, and Other Characteristics

Temperament	Humor	Main Organ	Element	Qualities	Complexion & Physical Type	Personality
Choleric (P)	Yellow bile	Spleen	Fire	Hot, Dry	Red-haired, Wiry, Thin	Violent, Vengeful, Volatile, Ambitious
Melancholic (A)	Black bile	Gall bladder	Earth	Cold, Dry	Thin, Pale	Introspective, Sentimental, Apathetic
Phlegmatic	Phlegm	Lungs	Water	Cold, Moist	Overweight	Sluggish, Lazy, Cowardly
Sanguine (I)	Blood	Liver	Air	Hot, Moist	Ruddy, Chubby	Amorous, Happy, Generous, Carefree, Optimistic

With each humor were associated certain physical qualities, organs, emotions, and activities as well as various other components such as one of the four elements (earth, fire, water, and air), a season, and sometimes one or more animals (see Table). While an overabundance of certain humors was preferable for certain professions (such as yellow bile for soldiers), in general one's health depended on a balance of the four. Thus, when an individual became ill, something was out of balance. One solution was to purge the person's system of the humor that was thought to be in excess. This could be accomplished through bloodletting, which targeted certain areas; or it could be done through the introduction of a strong laxative, which rid the system of humors via the bowels. Similarly, emetics could cause the patient to discharge humors (from the stomach) by vomiting. What was thought to be the key for the individual practicing medicine in this period was understanding which humor was out of balance, and using the correct remedy. The fact that most of the patients who received the treatment got better was accepted as proof that purgatives and emetics worked. What was not well understood at the time was that patients usually improved *in spite of* the treatment, not *because of* it. Humoral therapy was based on weak medical science, though that was the only science available to (Western) healers in this era.

The purgatives and emetics used tended to be natural cathartics, although some had to be refined in certain ways. Now recommended only for external use, Epsom salts, for example, was used by many doctors as a purgative. (The poet Byron, who held highly unorthodox views on diet and health, used Epsom salts, claiming it affected him like champagne.) Another purgative, which has recently made a comeback as a health product (albeit without any proven benefits), was gamboge, a tropical plant (*garcinia cambogia*) brought to Europe and North America from Southeast Asia, where it served as a treatment for worms. However, local plant-based purgatives, like the one from the sap of the European ash tree, were more commonly used. Minerals, such as calomel, mined in Germany, and then refined as it was separated from other compounds, was another cathartic that saw widespread use, even though the mercury it contained was quite toxic. Castor oil, too, refined from the castor bean, was used as a purgative; and it too contained a strong poison, ricin, in its solid residue. Another widely used emetic, at least until the 17th century, was powdered mummy wrappings from Egypt; the chemicals used in the original wrappings functioned as an emetic, though one wonders whether patients weren't also naturally revulsed by the idea of swallowing mummy matter.

Use Relating to Early Germ Theory

Between the 18th and 19th centuries, belief in the four humors began to be replaced by new ideas. The human body was being studied in greater detail, for the purposes of both art and medicine, and one result was a better understanding of human anatomy and physiology. Disease, it came to be seen, was not always due to an imbalance of humors; rather, other factors, including external influences, could play a role. Some medical professionals held that the seeds of disease floated in the air (rather like *germs*), whereas others surmised that an undetectable gas, or "miasma," lay behind the contraction of disease. Some believed that disease developed more or less spontaneously, depending on the characteristics of the individual, while for others it came from the consumption of spoiled food or by "filth" in the home or neighborhood. Some of these suspicions would, of course, later be shown to be correct—for certain types of disease, at least.

These new theories did not immediately cause purgatives to be discarded, but it did put a dent in their use. It was now understood that when a person became ill, the disease organism, whatever it might be, must have been internalized by the patient; it was not there in the body from the beginning. Thus, one way that a patient might be rid of a disease was to flush the system by means of a purgative or, perhaps, even a combination of purgative and emetic. Records indicate that even as physicians began to understand that "purging and puking" their patients did not always help them to get better, often leaving them in a weakened state, patients nevertheless sometimes asked for the traditional therapy. They did so mainly because, with purging and vomiting, they could *see* the positive effects of treatment: something was being done about their condition. Sales of patent medicines, or commercial purgatives and emetics bought by consumers, continued to thrive. Eventually, however, with the rise of germ theory in the late-19th century, people began to understand the nature of disease and illness better and to appreciate the dubiousness of purging and vomiting as a cure for all conditions.

Use by Modern Medicine

By the start of the 20th century, biologists and physicians understood about germs (at least bacteria), and vaccinations were made available for some infectious diseases. Although antibiotics were not developed until the first third of the 20th century, some treatments for specific diseases, such as quinine for malaria, were found to work, and antiseptics became the norm in hospitals and, to a lesser extent, around the home. In the modern era, medical science sought to confront disease directly as the cause of human illness, not to treat the patient in the same way *regardless* of the specific illness. This was a great paradigm shift in medical history. The use of purgatives and emetics as "cure-alls" became largely a thing of the past. Today, selected purgatives, that is, laxatives, are still used to treat constipation, their logical use. Emetics, meanwhile, are used primarily in emergency situations involving the ingestion of poisons.

Donald A. Watt and
Michael Shally-Jensen

See also: Bloodletting and Leeching; Folk Medicine; Herbal Remedies; Medicine Shows; Patent Medicines; Sanitation Campaigns and Public Health

Further Reading

American Chemical Society. 2000. "Patents & Potions." In *The Pharmaceutical Century: Ten Decades of Drug Discovery.* Washington, DC: American Chemical Society. uah.es/farmamol/The%20Pharmaceutical%20Century/Ch1.html

Breslaw, Elaine G. 2012. *Lotions, Potions, Pills, and Magic: Health Care in Early America.* New York: New York University Press.

Discovering Lewis & Clark, Inc. n.d. "Lewis's Medical Chest." *Discovering Lewis & Clark.* Washburn, ND: Lewis & Clark Fort Mandan Foundation. lewis-clark.org/channel/352

Strange, Matthew. 2010. *Bleeding, Blistering, and Purging: Health & Medicine in the 1800s.* Daily Life in America in 1800s. Broomall, PA: Mason Crest Publishers.

Whorton, James C. 2000. *Inner Hygiene: Constipation and the Pursuit of Health in Modern Society.* Oxford: Oxford University Press.

SANATORIUMS

The dreaded disease tuberculosis, also known as "The Great White Plague" because it was perceived to mostly affect white Europeans and Euro-Americans, reached epidemic proportions in the 19th century. With the growth of urban industrialization, cases of tuberculosis grew exponentially, particularly among the laboring classes. People were compelled to work long hours in poorly ventilated factories, thus providing a medium for the spread of this deadly infectious disease. Workers arriving from rural areas, where there was no presence of tuberculosis and therefore no immunity to it, quickly succumbed to the illness. Caused by the bacteria *Mycobacterium tuberculosis*, tuberculosis (TB) had at the time no known cure—except, that is, for the sanatorium, an institution designed to offer isolation, rest, and fresh air to sufferers.

Historical Background

Accounts of tuberculosis of the lung go back at least to Hippocrates (ca. 460–ca. 377 BCE). The Greek word *phthisis* ("to shrivel or waste away") is reflected in the English word *consumption,* meaning "a progressive wasting of body tissue." The latter term was, until the modern era, the common name for tuberculosis.

It is now recognized that a number of distinct and seemingly unrelated ailments described in early accounts are in fact tuberculosis in one or another of its different forms. For example, tuberculosis of the skin (lupus vulgaris) is one such, as are consumption of the lungs (phthisis), tuberculosis of the neck glands (scrofula), and tuberculosis of the spine (Pott's disease).

A few key figures are responsible for developing our understanding of TB before the advent of modern medicine. The first is the French physician René Laënnec (1781–1826), who made careful observations of TB in hundreds of cases and described the course of the illness over time. In his 1819 treatise *De l'auscultation mediate* (On mediated listening, or Remote sensing), Laënnec presented his invention of the stethoscope and described its use in the examination of the chest. Until the discovery of X-rays some 75 years later, the stethoscope, together with the thumping of the chest by a trained practitioner, was the only means to determine the extent of exposure to TB.

Another significant contributor was Jean Antoine Villemin (1827–1892), a French army surgeon who proved that TB was a communicable disease and not something passed on genetically within a family or otherwise contracted. Villemin's extensive studies, published as *Études sur la tuberculose* (1868), came at a time when the new germ theory of disease was coming into the fore. Although he did not identify the precise microorganism involved, Villemin conclusively demonstrated the epidemiology of tuberculosis.

The discovery of the organism at the root of TB, *M. tuberculosis,* is attributed to the German physician and microbiologist Robert Koch (1843–1910). Koch's findings, for which he later won the Nobel Prize, were published in 1882. Koch also identified the causative agents behind cholera and anthrax and for this reason is regarded as the founder of the modern science of bacteriology. Yet even with knowledge in hand concerning the tubercle bacillus, physicians had no way to treat TB until the mid-20th century. For all of those years before and after Koch's discovery, the only treatment option was the sanatorium.

The Rise and Fall of the Sanatorium

In the late 19th century the sanatorium was developed as a strategy to combat TB. Although an early variety of sanatorium opened in Poland in 1863, the sanatorium movement as such was launched 10 years later, when the U.S. physician Edward Livingstone Trudeau, himself a TB sufferer, spent a season in the Adirondacks—on the advice of his own doctor—to take in the fresh air. Soon after, Trudeau decided to devote himself to establishing a 16-acre site at Saranac Lake, New York, for the treatment of people suffering from TB. Trudeau's

Adirondack Cottage Sanatorium was designed to heal patients through a combination of fresh air and a healthful daily regimen, which included three square meals, horseback riding, walking, and a good deal of rest. The latter, which ultimately proved to be the most beneficial, consisted of lying on reclining chairs that were set out on the broad porches encircling each of the sanatorium's "cure cottages." By 1900, Trudeau had secured enough money to erect more than 20 cottages at the site, along with an infirmary, a library, a chapel, and a laboratory for TB research. Unfortunately, Trudeau's "cures" did not stop the progression of the disease within his own body, and, despite having offered himself as a model of recovery, he died from tuberculosis in 1916.

Before his death, however, other public health advocates came to admirer Trudeau's efforts. Officials from the New York Department of Public Health visited the Saranac Lake site and began building comparable facilities to house New Yorkers afflicted with the disease. The Otisville Sanatorium in the Catskills was established in 1906. State and local governments built similar institutions in Rutland, Massachusetts; Boonville, Arkansas; Green County, Texas; and Cass County, Michigan. The number of private sanatoriums grew in parallel with the state-run facilities, producing a great expansion of the "sanatorium idea" across the United States. At the start of the 20th century, there were some 35 sanatoriums located across the country, with a total of about 4,500 beds; by 1925, the number of facilities had increased to nearly 550, the bed count to almost 675,000.

Not all of this growth can be attributed to pure motives on the part of Progressive-era social reformers and, especially, city officials. As historian Sheila Rothman has observed, one key driver among policy makers concerned with public health was to prevent the rise of new cases of TB in order to demonstrate that the contagion was under control. One way to do that was to *remove* cases from the city's jurisdiction. Moreover, the method of implementing treatment at the sanatoriums involved experts exerting strong control and regulation over those who suffered from the disease. The curative routines administered at the sanatoriums dictated every aspect of daily life. There were rules regarding coughing on the premises, sneezing, spitting, and even talking—basically any act involving vapor/spray from the lungs, throat, or mouth. Patients were instructed never to get out of breath (as through exercise), never to engage in activity when temperatures were hot, never to be in contact with others if the sputum was streaked, and always to work steadfastly toward the realization of one's own cure. Over the years, the treatment regimen in sanatoriums moved quickly from light exercise mixed with rest to complete and utter rest, at times even strict bed rest. Many patients, who typically spent several weeks or even months at these facilities, found the level of control inside them stifling and repressive. Nevertheless, the sanatoriums achieved the goals of physicians and reformers alike. TB victims were confined to out-of-the-way institutions, thereby helping to improve the city's health outlook, and victims could feel that they were making progress in controlling the progression of their illness. It was a kind of "win-win" situation, even if the final *prognosis* (often, death) was not changed.

Indeed, Rothman also points out that *death* was the overriding theme of all such institutions, dealing as they were with what was in many cases a terminal illness. "However much the sanatorium resembled other institutions, it had one unique feature—the omnipresence of the shadow of death. Apart from it, nothing can be understood about sanatorium life, whether it was staff enforcing rules or patients seeking sexual pleasure. Staff tried to brush it off with aphorisms about being strong and determined. But in countless ways, some personal, others collective, the sanatorium experience was at its core an encounter with mortality" (Rothman 1995, 238).

Sanatoriums did not, then, provide a comprehensive solution to the tuberculosis problem. Not only was little or no long-term cure available through them (except in relatively few cases), but not everyone was admitted. Some sufferers were deemed too sick to benefit from the curative regime. Others—mostly from minority populations—were considered not "appropriate" candidates for it and turned down. (This, even though death rates for TB among African Americans were two to three times higher than they were for whites.) Many, obviously, could not pay on their own for extended stays at private institutions. At the opposite end of the spectrum were those who preferred *not* to be removed to a sanatorium. Many TB sufferers gave state officials false information to avoid being relocated to a sanatorium because they did not want to be separated from their families, particularly those responsible for supporting children or relatives. Others simply disliked the discipline involved or preferred to carry on, and perhaps die, in the security of the home. Thus, even as the sanatorium movement grew, many of the afflicted continued to pursue their own remedies for their illness. One prominent such solution, for those who could manage it, was to move west, particularly to New Mexico.

In 1943, a researcher at Rutgers University, Selman Waksman, discovered a fungus that was capable of retarding the growth of certain types of bacteria, including *M. tuberculosis*. Within the next decade, three drugs had been developed that, administered together, could effectively cure tuberculosis. Also, preventive therapy with the drug isoniazid came to be used to prevent the progression of the illness from initial infection (class II TB) to full-blown disease (class III). So successful were the new medical treatments that by the mid-1960s TB sanatoriums were virtually gone from the scene.

Michael Shally-Jensen

See also: Homeopathy; Hydrotherapy; Spas and Mineral Waters; Sweat Lodges and Saunas

Further Reading

Bates, Barbara. 1992. *Bargaining for Life: A Social History of Tuberculosis.* Philadelphia: University of Pennsylvania Press.
Bynum, Helen. 2015. *Spitting Blood: The History of Tuberculosis.* New York: Oxford University Press.
Rothman, Sheila M. 1995. *Living in the Shadow of Death: Tuberculosis and the Social Experience of Illness in American History.* Baltimore: Johns Hopkins University Press.

SANITATION CAMPAIGNS AND PUBLIC HEALTH

In 1842, in Britain, a lawyer, journalist, and public health researcher named Edwin Chadwick published a landmark study, *Report on the Sanitary Conditions of the Labouring Population.* In it, Chadwick showed that nearly half of all working-class children died before reaching the age of five. Moreover, in major industrial centers, the average age of death was 36 years for the relatively well-off landed gentry, 22 years for working tradesmen, and a mere 16 years for ordinary laborers. The author stressed the need for regular removal of waste, the directing of sewage into gutters and drainage systems, and the elimination of cesspools, among other improvements. Chadwick's report so alarmed public officials that a new national board of health was created and a doctor, John Simon, was appointed as Britain's first public health officer. As a result of increased awareness, people came to recognize the value of sanitation—that is, the maintenance of more or less clean and healthy living environments, the protection of water supplies, the safe disposal of sewage, the removal of rubbish, and the availability of adequate housing with proper ventilation and other safety features.

A few years later, in 1850, a similar report appeared in Boston. Written primarily by the historian and statistician Lemuel Shattuck, the *Report of the Sanitary Commission of Massachusetts* revealed that life expectancies in the United States at the time were even shorter than those in England, and that there was a strong correlation between declining life expectancy and increasing industrialization in the cities. Among the various recommendations in the report was that Massachusetts establish a state board of health and that local governments do likewise. Shattuck urged more detailed investigations in urban communities and the publishing of vital statistics (i.e., birth and death information broken down by age, gender, race, locality, occupation, and economic status). He also proposed widespread health education, well-child care, and the monitoring of food safety and drug manufacture. Although it was not until 1869 that Massachusetts instituted a state health board and other measures, Shattuck's report came to be recognized as an important watershed in the development of community health systems.

Historical Precursors

The Greek medical practitioner and teacher Hippocrates (460–370 BCE) exemplified the early ideal of the Western physician. He emphasized the four humors or bodily fluids—blood, black bile, yellow bile, and phlegm—and the need to balance them. Over the decades and centuries after Hippocrates's death his followers continued to publish important works on medical subjects. Among the most notable of them were *Airs, Waters, and Places,* a treatise on the significance of ecological factors in disease; *Epidemics,* an account of instances of selected illnesses, including fevers; *Regimen,* a consideration of dietary and lifestyle factors in health; and *Nature of Man,* about the human physical constitution generally.

In the early Christian era, health conditions declined within the Roman Empire. Increased contact with commercial interests in the East brought a variety of new

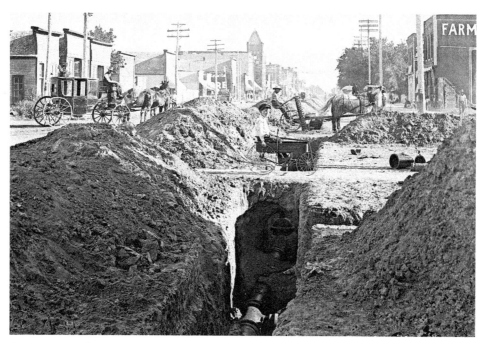

Construction of a sewage system in Nebraska, ca. 1889. By the late 1800s, population pressure had led most industrialized cities around the world to create sanitation departments to deal with the rapidly increasing need for waste disposal. (Library of Congress)

diseases, including bubonic plague. Ongoing wars and ever-expanding cities in the Mediterranean and beyond led to the spread of epidemics. As a result, the Romans undertook to institute a number of programs concerning public health, including checks of freshwater supplies, sewage management, and personal hygiene. The famous public baths were an outcome of the latter concern. (In retrospect, however, the baths may also have helped to spread disease.)

In Byzantium, Christian views of health as a godly gift and disease as a punishment operated alongside older Greco-Roman medical traditions. Byzantine medical practices were often conducted inside a new Christian institution—the infirmary, designed to attend to the sick. These infirmaries grew out of earlier houses for travelers and sick people, including special accommodations for lepers. Later, Byzantium's leaders established a network of hospitals, each containing separate wards and small cadres of physicians.

During the late Middle Ages in Europe, population increases and continued urbanization, together with expanded trade and the movement of religious pilgrims, boosted the rate of spread of infectious diseases. The great pandemic of bubonic plague that hit Europe between 1348 and 1350 and known as the Black Death killed around 25 million souls and created economic and political chaos. Some hospitals built on the Byzantine model were erected, but the primary institution for care of the sick was the church—or, more specifically, the various monastic orders and lay brotherhoods. These groups, however, did virtually nothing to help *prevent* illness, nor did they administer medicine. Rather, sickness was deemed a divine trial: the sufferer would either be saved or face eternal damnation, depending on god's will.

In the Renaissance era there was a revival of Greek learning and the start of new approaches to medicine. The Italian physician Girolamo Fracastoro surmised that infection was passed between objects and people through a kind of foul emanation, or contagion. Some invisible particles and/or unknown substances were thought to play a role, and they were understood to affect the body internally and even propagate there. Fracastoro's ideas, in other words, represented an early version of germ theory, and they contributed significantly to public-health science by impacting the way sick people were treated: those who were ill—from contagion or from other maladies—were generally isolated to prevent the spread of noxious matter.

Under the influence of Enlightenment ideas, governments in the 18th century increasingly undertook public-health measures. Such measures included regulations aimed at safeguarding health and reducing incidences of illness. The most aggressive programs established a force of "medical police" whose duty it was to monitor and enforce personal and public hygiene, from infancy to old age. The overall effect, however, was minimal. More important, in 1796 the British physician Edward Jenner developed the first vaccination—for smallpox. Within a brief period, the new preventive method proved successful, curtailing significantly the incidence of that disease.

The Emergence of Public Health

By the early 19th century, the Industrial Revolution was at its height. Rapid population growth in both European and U.S. cities began to far exceed the capacity to supply adequate housing, clean water, healthy food, and proper garbage and sewage disposal for urban residents. Overcrowding and unsanitary conditions prevailed, particularly in the expanding slum districts. This created ideal conditions for the regular outbreak of epidemics such as typhus and relapsing fever, both tick-borne illnesses. Other diseases, such as dysentery, came from contaminated water supplies. A series of lethal cholera epidemics ravaged European and North American cities in the latter half of the 19th century.

Additional problems associated with factory work and slum dwelling at this time included industrial pollution, long work hours under terrible conditions, child labor, poverty, and malnutrition. Mortality in some industrial cities reached 30 percent in the 1830s. Tuberculosis, a deadly lung disease spread by coughing or sneezing (or even talking), claimed thousands of victims. Conventional medicine was completely inadequate to deal with such a horrendous wave of illness and death. The lack of understanding of the underlying mechanism of disease transmission—"germs"—compounded the problem. At least, though, people began to think that sickness might be both a biological *and* a social problem.

This is the context in which the landmark 1842 report by Edwin Chadwick was produced. Traditional quarantine and isolation measures had largely failed to help, so reformers like Chadwick were led to consider social and environmental problems as contributing factors. As a result, more directed efforts started to be made, in England and elsewhere, against foul water, overflowing sewage and garbage, compromised food, inadequate fresh air, and general filth. Lemuel Shattuck's 1850 report had much the same effect in the United States, with the added benefit of advocating for the ongoing collection of vital statistics and health data. Shattuck also recommended research on tuberculosis, the examination of mental health, the treatment of alcoholism, more physician training in the area of illness prevention, and routine physical examinations for all populations. Change, however, was slow going in the United States, owing to the traditional suspicion of government involvement in social and commercial affairs.

With the development of germ theory in the latter part of the 19th century, public health concerns were put on a proper scientific footing. In the beginning, however, it was difficult for many physicians to believe that something so seemingly innocuous as microscopic organisms could significantly impact human health, being responsible for major and minor illnesses alike. It was simpler to imagine poisonous fumes, weak constitutions, or "miasmic" disturbances caused by bile and other bodily fluids as causes of illness than to credit tiny entities coursing through the bloodstream or lodging in the cavities and organs of the body. Such, however, by the 1880s, was beyond dispute. By the start of the 20th century, public health started to emerge as an academic discipline; the first school devoted to the subject was opened at Johns Hopkins University in 1916.

In the late 20th century the focus of public health began to shift from preventing the spread of infectious diseases (which became a medical specialization in its own right) to addressing chronic conditions such as stroke, cancer, and heart disease. Ending cigarette smoking, treating drug and alcohol addiction, reducing the number of violent and accidental deaths, combating HIV/AIDS and other sexually transmitted diseases, creating awareness around toxic wastes, advocating for a healthy diet, examining health disparities (between groups), and ensuring health care delivery for infants and mothers all continue to be core public health concerns. And in many developing nations, traditional sanitation campaigns remain important tools of public health.

Michael Shally-Jensen

See also: Diet and Exercise; Sanatoriums; Sex, Sexology, and Sex Therapy; Spas and Mineral Waters

Further Reading

Leavitt, Judith W., and Ronald L. Numbers. 1997. *Sickness and Health in America: Readings in the History of Medicine and Public Health*. 3rd ed. Madison: University of Wisconsin Press.

Rosen, George. 1993. *A History of Public Health*. Baltimore: Johns Hopkins University Press.

Turnock, Bernard J. 2015. *Public Health: What It Is and How It Works*. 6th ed. Sudbury, MA: Jones and Bartlett.

SPAS AND MINERAL WATERS

The discovery of natural mineral water, and its use for medicinal purposes, probably occurred in the prehistoric era. Native Americans, for example, developed a tradition of using springwater for healing. By the earliest times of Greece and Rome, as well as of South and East Asia, mineral water was in use as a therapeutic substance. Mineral water is water from a natural spring that contains dissolved salts and other minerals from the rocks and soils through which it flows. Such water may be effervescent, or "sparkling," owing to captured gases that it contains. It can also be hot, due to its origin deep below the surface, and collected in pools to be used for healthful bathing, or "soaking." In the context of the healing arts, then, mineral water may be either drunk or applied externally—or both—for the benefit of the consumer.

History

The sulfurous thermal springs at Tiberias in Lower Galilee (Israel) have been used by rheumatism sufferers at least since biblical times. The hot springs in Greece and the Aegean Islands likewise functioned as healing sites. The Greek physician Hippocrates, writing around 400 BCE, completed a work called *Airs, Waters, and Places* in which he described the watering places and other natural features of his times. The Roman author Pliny (23–79 CE), too, wrote a natural history in which he described some of the mineral springs of Europe. The Romans made such extensive use of the thermal springs of Italy that they cultivated a culture of restorative bathing that survives, in one form or another, to this day. They spread the idea of public baths, or spas, built around mineral springs to other sites in Europe, notably at Aachen (Aix-la-Chapelle) and Baden-Baden, Germany; Vichy, France; Baden, Switzerland; Bath, England; Spa, Belgium; and Carlsbad (Karlovy Vary), Czech Republic.

In Asia, a bathing culture developed around Buddhist temples in India, from which it spread east to other parts of the continent. A form of religious bathing employing steam baths emerged in Japan in the 800s. Originally made use of only by priests and acolytes, Japanese bathhouses were later frequented by those seeking relief from illness. Public bathing in hot waters has remained an essential part of Japanese culture ever since. Rules regarding separation by sex have varied over the centuries, with mixed-sex bathing generally being the norm, albeit often in combination with the use of dividing screens and separate male and female dressing areas.

After the collapse of the Roman Empire in Europe in the fifth century CE, the number of spas decreased. It was not until the Renaissance that they once again began to be utilized. As cities grew, along with urban crowding and unsanitary conditions, people of means sought access to spas as a healthful retreat and a social interlude set in pleasant surroundings. Many well-known resorts—even small cities—were built around mineral springs. Some of the mineral waters associated

---

Bath in English Literature

In classic English literature, when someone is ill, they often travel to "take the waters" in the city of Bath. Bath itself is in the English county of Somerset. The city was founded by Romans in 60 CE, though Bath Abbey itself wasn't built until the seventh century. The waters of the hot springs were said to cure leprosy as well as many other more minor ailments and illnesses.

Jane Austen, one of the best known British authors of the 19th century, set two of her books (*Northanger Abbey* and *Persuasion*) in the city of Bath. Although her characters seemed to enjoy the city, Austen herself wrote to friends that she was relieved when her family moved on to Clifton. Still the city is home to a Jane Austen Centre, where interested fans can learn more about her life and work within Bath.

Several other authors, however, have written about or referenced Bath in their works. In Chaucer's *Canterbury Tales*, the Wife of Bath is one of the most intriguing characters the hero meets. Georgette Heyer is a modern writer of Regency romances, and many of her entertaining novels have been set in the city.

---

with these springs, including Seltzer water (from the Selters area of Germany) and Perrier (the name of a French doctor and spa owner), achieved international renown and are now sold widely as bottled sparkling-water products.

In the United States, a spring at Saratoga Springs, New York, was shown by Mohawk guides to the British superintendant of Indian affairs, William Johnson, in 1776. Saratoga became a major resort town in the last half of the 19th century, serving a posh clientele from East Coast urban centers for many decades. Another site, Hot Springs, Arkansas, was believed by some to have been the "Fountain of Youth" that the 16th-century Spanish explorer Ponce de León had sought. It became the first federal reserve in the United States, in 1832, and was made a national park in 1921. Unlike most of the private spas that developed around natural springs, the spa at Hot Springs served not only wealthy clients but average citizens seeking health benefits; it became known as The American Spa. White Sulphur Springs, in West Virginia, was first used by Euro-Americans in 1778. By the mid-19th century, it was beginning to draw elites from all over the South and eventually became known as the Queen of the Watering Places. All in all, some 500 springs came to be used commercially in the United States by the late-20th century, either as spa areas or as sources of bottled mineral water. The spots for "taking the waters"—a reference to dipping and soaking in spas—became highly fashionable, featuring elaborate facilities to entertain wealthy patrons in the manner to which they were accustomed. Fine dining, stage entertainments, ballroom dancing, horseback riding, boating, golf, and lawn tennis—not to mention servants aplenty—were but a few of the amenities on offer.

Treatments

As suggested above, the therapeutic treatments undertaken by spagoers, at least in the grand era of the spa in the late 19th and early 20th centuries, were often secondary to the social life. European spa guests, in particular, were not usually subject to strict guidelines regarding their diet, therapy regimen, and other activities. (This is one area where spa therapy differed from its cousin, hydrotherapy.) On the American side, too, there was flexibility; but in the United States by the mid-20th century a trend emerged in which spa guests were provided with comprehensive programs covering each person's diet, baths, physical therapy, exercise, and recreational activities. Along with a hotelier to oversee the facilities, a medical director would be on staff to manage health and wellness operations.

Mineral waters are generally clear, although sometimes they have a whitish, more or less cloudy appearance due to suspended calcium carbonate or sulfur. Some waters are noticeably bluish, usually because of suspended slate or clay. Others have a reddish tint because of iron oxide. Mineral waters containing high amounts of hydrogen sulfide (often present at volcanically active sites) give off an odor of rotten eggs.

Externally, mineral waters are used in a number of health treatments. These treatments include mineral baths, whirlpool baths, steam baths, sitz baths (for the buttocks, thighs, and lower torso only), jet sprays (for douches of various sorts), wet packs and rubs, and CO_2 baths (carbonation baths). The clay or silt from the bottom of a natural mineral pond is often smeared over the head and skin to treat eczema or other skin conditions. Mud packs using the same material can also be applied indoors. Heat from hot water springs, or in the form of a sauna (a heated room with low humidity), is a standard remedy in the case of rheumatism of the joints or certain muscular conditions. Cold-water hydrotherapy might also be prescribed to help stimulate the circulation.

The usual one-to-three-week stay at a spa, which may include massages, yoga, physical exercise, and so on, is designed to address any specific ailments that the consumer hopes to find relief from, as well as to cultivate a sense of well-being. More important, a spa visit often functions as a training session to impart awareness of better health habits generally and how to continue them in the home. A premium is placed on the prevention of common chronic conditions such as heart disease and metabolic disorders through the development of good eating habits and daily exercise, as appropriate for individual consumers. In many ways, spas have helped transform the perception of health in the United States and elsewhere.

As a beverage, mineral water is consumed for a variety of health reasons as well for the sheer enjoyment if its fresh, bubbly qualities. Prescribed mineral waters have traditionally included alkaline waters for gastrointestinal ulcers and magnesium-containing waters for liver conditions. Certain types of mineral waters can function as laxatives, while others are diuretics, serving to increase production of urine. Mineral waters are also occasionally recommended for use in enemas or as vapor or mist for inhalation. A bitter taste in mineral water is generally attributable to the presence of magnesium sulfate—used as a laxative but also to treat heart conditions and asthma. A salty taste is due to the presence of sodium chloride (salt)—the main ingredient of saline. Alkaline waters have a smooth mouthfeel and can be neutral, slightly brackish, or even a bit "soapy" to the taste. Iron-containing waters—traditionally said to be "good for the blood" (i.e., in cases of low iron)—have a sharp, astringent taste.

The history of mineral water as a drink includes the creation, often under less than acceptable conditions, of artificially manufactured products. In the United States, in particular, the production of imitation mineral water, made by the addition of mineral salts to plain water, was a thriving industry in the 19th century. All manner of charlatans roamed the country making claims about their "miracle" water and the vast array of illnesses it could cure, from "vitalizing" one's debilitated nerves to "purifying" one's blood. Only when the Pure Food and Drug Act of 1907 went into effect did most of such businesses cease to exist. The sale and consumption of good-quality mineral water has only gained strength in the early decades of the 21st century, as an increasingly health conscious public seeks out the natural benefits of the earth's resources.

Michael Shally-Jensen

See also: Bottled Water; Hydrotherapy; Neurasthenia, or Nervous Exhaustion; Sanatoriums; Sweat Lodges and Saunas

Further Reading

Adams, Jane M. 2015. *Healing with Water: English Spas and the Water Cure, 1840–1960*. Manchester, UK: Manchester University Press.
Chambers, Thomas A. 2002. *Drinking the Waters: Creating an American Leisure Class at 19th-Century Mineral Springs*. Washington, DC: Smithsonian Institution Press.
Large, David Clay. 2015. *The Grand Spas of Central Europe: A History of Intrigue, Politics, Art, and Healing*. Lanham, MD: Rowman and Littlefield.
Porter, Roy, ed. 1990. *The Medical History of Waters and Spas*. London: Wellcome Institute.

SPIRITUALISM

As traditionally understood, *spiritualism* refers to a set of beliefs and practiced centered on the idea that the spirits of the dead survive as personalities and can communicate with the living through individuals known as mediums. Although spiritualism as practiced in the United States has roots in Christianity and mysticism (Christian mysticism), the connection has never been absolute, and in recent decades the religious aspects have tended to give way to the mystic. Thus, spiritualism has long encompassed a variety of ideas and practices, such as the belief that mediums are able to cure diseases, sometimes with the aid of spirit "guides" or "controls" (i.e., spirits who work on "the other side" on behalf of the medium). Some mediums specialize in such spirit healing. Others work with clients to give counsel on personal affairs and practical decisions, drawing on their apparent broad knowledge of and insight into the world and into each client's special lot in life; here, of course, spiritualism overlaps with the familiar areas of palmistry and Tarot. Clairvoyance regarding the hidden aspects of life is assumed to be among a medium's powers, as is prophetic awareness of future events.

The Living and the Dead

Mediums who deal primarily with what are believed to be messages from disembodied persons made up the great majority of spiritualists when the phenomenon first gained popularity in the mid-19th century United States. A smaller number of mediums produced various sorts of physical "effects" said to be caused by spiritual presences. The most famous example of the latter are the "rappings," or knocks, produced by the Fox sisters, Leah, Kate, and Margaret, of Hydesville, New York, beginning around 1848. These noises—from under tables, in walls, around interior corners, from floors, and the like—were taken to be the work of spirits who wished to communicate with the living. With the development of a meaningful code, these rappings became the standard method of communication between the Fox sisters and their clients, and that practice was inherited by the sisters' spiritualist descendants. In their own case, however, it later came out that the sisters had surreptitiously created the rappings themselves using a variety of means, among them the cracking of a big toe inside a boot. Ever since the rise and demise of the Fox sisters, the claims of spiritualists have been subject to scrutiny by critics and to a certain amount of hesitancy on the part of the public, who only hope to avoid being duped by impostors. Ultimately, one either believes in spiritualism as a legitimate undertaking or one does not, just as one either believes in a particular medium as spiritually "gifted" or one does not.

The spiritualist movement as it arose in the 19th century owed a debt to the teachings of the Swedish scientist, philosopher, and mystic Emanuel Swedenborg (1688–1772). In his *Journal of Dreams* and numerous other works, including his magnum opus, *Heavenly Mysteries,* Swedenborg detailed how he would enter into a trancelike state and commune with the spirits, returning with messages of both religious and practical natures. Another spiritualist predecessor was the French physician Franz Mesmer (1734–1815). Mesmer and his followers found that inducing a hypnotic state in their patients seemed to bring out certain powers that were not available under ordinary conditions. They used this psychic energy, this "animal magnetism," to diagnose and treat diseases. Mesmeric trances also caught on in social circles, demonstrating that there is no great distance between this practice and that of spirit healing by an entranced medium or that of holding a séance to communicate with the dead.

Contributing to the emergence of spiritualism, too, was the growth of science and the new historical-theological criticism, at a time when blind adherence to faith and authoritarian religious doctrines were beginning to break down. People began more and more to seek evidence rather than accept assertions of authority. The spiritualists could satisfy that desire by offering revelations of the hidden world. To the open-minded, such demonstrations had a powerful appeal. As a result, a host of notable figures from the 19th century dabbled in spiritual encounters, including Arthur Conan Doyle, Horace Greeley, Camille Flammarion, Edvard Munch, Elizabeth Barret Browning, Arthur Balfour, Lewis Carroll, and Mary Todd Lincoln. The last-named serves to remind us that the Civil War left close to three-quarters of a million dead, and in the war's aftermath, tens of thousands of bereaved survivors sought contact with their fallen loved ones through the use of spiritual mediums. The demand for women's rights also played a role, as women sought areas in which they could express themselves outside the confines of domestic life. (Women probably made up the majority of spiritualism's followers.)

So intense was the interest in spiritualism during the second half of the 19th century that some mediums became quite famous throughout the land. One such was Henry Slade (1835–1905), a kind of automatic-writing medium, or someone who is compelled by a spirit to write down the departed's communications to the living. Slade was eventually exposed as a fraud, although some aspects of his practice remain obscure. Another popular practitioner was William Mumler (1832–1884), who invented spirit photography. Mumler took portrait photographs that featured the ghostly image of lost loved ones alongside his living subjects. He was such a sensation that many affluent and influential figures visited his studio, including, in 1872, Mary Todd Lincoln, who received a now famous photograph of herself, sitting, with an apparition of her husband Abraham Lincoln standing behind her and comforting her with his hands on her shoulders. Mumler, too, was later identified as a technological manipulator. His wife, Hannah, though, continued in his footsteps, manufacturing a "clairvoyant remedy" called Mesmerine and working as a medium.

Sittings and Séances

Although there are a variety of different types of mediumship, certain basic characteristics can be noted. Some mediums go into a state of trance. The depth of the medium's psychological and physiological involvement with the trance state, however, can and does vary. Some mediums—the minority—more or less journey, shamanlike, into "the other world" to commune with the dead, while other mediums—the majority—keep a firmer grip on present realities and interactions with the client, or "sitter." Generally, the medium closes his or her eyes, makes some mildly convulsive movements, and thenceforth behaves as if possessed by the spirit "control" (aide) or other disembodied personality that has been called up by the sitter. Messages are then delivered as if issuing from the possessing spirit agent; the medium is understood to be serving as an "empty vessel," or instrument of interconnection between the living and the dead. In some cases, the entranced medium will begin the process of automatic writing, or recording the messages of the spirit on paper. (Occasionally, today, automatic keyboarding and onscreen displays are used instead.) In other cases, only the voice is used, as utterances from beyond the grave spill from the mouth of the medium or, alternatively, come from independent, incorporeal persons thought to be present in the room.

Fewer mediums today use the trance state than was the case during the heyday of spiritualism. The more common practice is for the medium to report that she sees or hears spirit forms and that they communicate to her the messages they want relayed. Even in a normal, nontrance state some mediums state that they are able to write automatically; they do it, it is said, without being conscious of the contents. Others claim to perform automatic speaking without the need for trance; the spirits talk through them "on demand," as it were, under the appropriate circumstances.

Visual phenomena as well as auditory ones are typical in many séances. For example, "spirit lights" are reported as occurring in darkened rooms (the "Tinkerbell" syndrome), as are entire luminous figures. Deceased relatives or friends may be identified by their materialized form or by their voice or characteristic turns of phrase. Different mediums may specialize in visual contact with apparitions or in verbal or written messages. The specialty chosen is usually said to be the result of a "gift" the medium has been imbued with rather than any deliberate preference.

Objective studies of the activities of spiritual mediums overlap with similar studies of extrasensory perception, telepathy, clairvoyance, and precognition. The field as a whole falls into the category of parapsychology, or psychical research. For the most part, the scientific community remains dubious. Skeptics, for example, point to what they call "stimulus leakage," whereby information is obtained from the sitter by the medium through the reading of subtle yet revealing facial expressions or changes in breathing. The effectiveness of a good medium, in other words, can be accounted for by abilities that are part of the normal makeup of certain individuals. While occasionally a "sham" practitioner is caught out by legal investigators looking into complaints made by consumers, most often psychics and sitters come together because they share a common worldview, one defined by openness to alternative experiences. Most often, too, mutual satisfaction is the result.

Michael Shally-Jensen

See also: Alternative Diagnostics; Anthroposophic Medicine; Astrology; Faith Healing and Prayer; Mesmerism and Hypnotherapy; Past Life Regression Therapy; Reiki and Therapeutic Touch Shamanism and Neo-Shamanism; Voodoo and Santería

Further Reading
Brandon, Ruth. 1983. *The Spiritualists: The Passion for the Occult in the 19th and 20th Centuries*. New York: Knopf.
Cox, Robert S. 2003. *Body and Soul: A Sympathetic History of American Spiritualism*. Charlottesville: University of Virginia Press.
Manseu, Peter. 2017. *The Apparitionists: A Tale of Phantoms, Fraud, Photography, and the Man Who Captured Lincoln's Ghost*. Boston: Houghton Mifflin Harcourt.
McGary, Molly. 2008. *Ghosts of Futures Past: Spiritualism and the Cultural Politics of 19th-Century America*. Berkeley: University of California Press.

WITCH TRIALS AND EXORCISMS
While it is not widely known, the persons most often accused of being witches—the great majority of them women—were individuals who were thought to have

---

How *The Exorcist* Changed Popular Understanding of Exorcisms

The 1973 movie *The Exorcist* is said to have changed cinema forever. Adapted from the 1971 novel of the same name by William Blatty, the movie shows the possession and eventual exorcism of 12-year-old Regan. Throughout the movie, two priests attempt to save the young girl from her possession by a demon; she is eventually rescued only by an act of heroic self-sacrifice from the younger priest, Father Karras.

The film has been considered one of the most terrifying movies ever created. Both the cast and crew of the movie reported dramatic techniques used by director William Friedkin to create genuine and severe reactions from the actors. Actors were jerked around in harnesses to create screams of pain and horror; when actor Jason Miller (playing Father Karras) was to be hit with the famous pea soup, he was told that it would hit him in the chest. The shot in fact hit him directly in the face, causing a reaction of disgust.

There were also several accidents and problems on set that led some crew members to believe the production was cursed. For example, one crew member's toddler was struck by a motorbike and hospitalized.

Several viewers fainted or vomited during the movie's viewing and needed to leave the theater. Modern reviewers still list the movie as one of the most terrifying of all time. While *The Exorcist* is the most well-known movie about exorcisms, popular interest in the phenomenon hasn't faded; in fact, Pope Francis's frequent references to the devil in his speeches is said to have increased interest in the religious ceremony.

---

powers capable of affecting the health and welfare of others. In fact, often the accused witch was an actual healer, midwife, or potion maker. She might also be a diviner, charmer, soothsayer, enchanter, juggler, or an intermediary. On the idea that the messenger is often blamed for the message, those identified as practitioners of the "cunning arts" frequently were called out during periods of economic hardship or historical change and accused of evildoing. They were named as witches essentially in order to provide the community with a scapegoat, or an emotional outlet. The presence of a witch, or witches, in other words, helped "explain" the community's troubles to itself. If a witch could be held responsible for the difficulties they faced, a sense of relief could be had. The "cause" would be identified, and a way out perceived. All that was needed was to rid the community of the witch—say, by burning her at the stake or banishing her. In this way the community could be "healed." This, in a nutshell, represents the phenomenon of the "witch craze" that beset Europe and America, particularly between the mid-16th and mid-17th centuries.

Witches of the World

The word *witch* is derived from the Old English *wicce*, meaning "a female magician or sorceress." You may recognize wicce, or Wicca, as the name of the modern-day

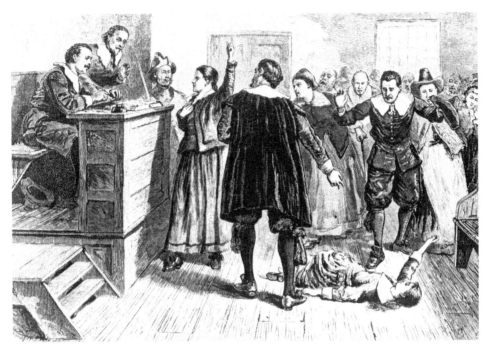

An afflicted girl demonstrates in court how she has been bewitched, during the Salem witch-craft trials. (Library of Congress)

pagan-revival form of the phenomenon. Although the terms *witch* and *witchcraft* can be applied to both sexes and their magical activities, the usual connotation, at least in Western cultures, is a female practitioner.

In many cultures, both Western and non-Western, accidents, sickness, death, and other troubling events have been thought to be caused by witches—those individuals who have magical powers that can be used for nefarious purposes. Sometimes these powers can also be used for good: a variety of cultures distinguish between beneficial, or "white," magic, and evil, or "black," magic. Early Protestant clerics held that white witches were worse than their evil counterparts because they drew in innocent villagers and made them complicit in the irreligious sin of magic. Throughout the world, practitioners of the magical arts have used their skills to assure the safe passage of travelers, protect property from harm, secure a successful harvest, and so on; yet some of these same do-gooders might, for a fee, perform dark magic to produce misfortune or death to an enemy of the client. There are even paid witchfinders, people who basically use magic to identify witches in their midst and report them to the authorities.

In Europe, witchcraft has a long history. Early Greek literature refers to witch-craft. Perhaps the best known is the legend of Circe, who had the power to trans-form men into beasts. Hecate, Greek goddess of sorcery and witchcraft, haunted crossroads and graveyards and wandered by night, when dogs warned of her approach by barking. A one-time midwife, she could pass between the land of the living and the land of the dead and could raise the dead if she wished to. In Egypt, Palestine, and adjacent areas of the Near East, a variety of itinerant tricksters known as *goetae* employed wild shrieks and howls in their incantations; they were feared for their malevolent powers and sold love potions and poisons for money. Legend held that the *goetae* were originally physicians who had become corrupted by their own power.

In Western Europe, witchcraft likely represents a phenomenon of the pre-Christian era that survived into later ages. There is evidence that pagan religious rites were not significantly impacted by the arrival of the Romans and were often practiced in Roman temples in Britain and Gaul. The Romans themselves did at one point (in 184 CE and again around 181 CE) execute some 5,000 people, mostly women, for causing an epidemic in the homeland. Later in Christianized Europe, a number of pre-Christian rites, including baptizing infants quarterly at so-called witches' sabbaths—on February 2 (Candlemas); April 30 (May Day Eve or Walpurgis Night); August 1 (Lammastide); and October 31 (Halloween or All Hallow Eve)—became associated with Christian ritual. Marriages, too, were sanctioned at quarterly sabbath (sabbat) ceremonies, and the religious rites included the distribution of bread and wine, as in the Eucharist. As late as the 17th century, it was said in France that "the greater part of the priests are witches" (Murray 1970, 18). Although initially the church was tolerant of popular religion, by the 14th century it sought to stamp out the pagan cults that flourished beside and even within the church.

The church equated the pagan deities with the notion of evil, epitomized by the devil, and popular rites with witchcraft. A biblical exhortation, "Thou shalt not suffer a witch to live" (Exodus 22:18) was invoked to justify the witch-hunt that flourished for several centuries. In 1431 Joan of Arc was burned at the stake for witchcraft, and in 1484 Pope Innocent VIII issued a bull against witches. It has been estimated that during the next three centuries a half million to 2 million persons were executed as witches. It is difficult to know how many of the victims were dabblers in pagan rites, "white" witches turned "black," midwives or healers thought to possess strange powers, or ordinary people who simply were not well liked in their communities. Certainly many innocent people lost their lives. In Salem, Massachusetts, in 1692, a witch-hunt was begun by a group of teenage girls who may have been inspired by vudú tales told by a West Indian slave woman. Claiming to have fallen ill, the girls started making accusations of witchcraft, and, aided by adults, found it easier to continue doing so than to pull back. A mass hysteria, of sorts, ensued, in which many blameless people were tried as witches and executed or threatened. The collective remedy was worse than the supposed disease.

Before any trial of a witch, or, often, in lieu of a formal trial, it was customary in many cultures to force suspects to undergo an ordeal or test. In England, they might be "swum" to see if they sank or floated—the latter being a sign of guilt. In western India, suspects were hung upside-down over a fire. In parts of Indonesia, the suspect was required to draw up a stone from boiling water without developing blisters. At other times and places suspects were flogged, starved, or deprived of sleep. During the Inquisition, religious persecutors assumed that the witch's loyalty was to the devil and that that relationship had to be broken. A variety of tortures were devised to achieve this, leading to a confession (the "queen of proofs"). The witch's power, in the eyes of the church, derived above all from her sexuality: it was believed that the witch began her career with sexual intercourse with the devil. Therefore, any perceived acts of immorality, blasphemy, subversion, or magicality on the part of a woman were taken to be signs of witchcraft.

Belief in witchcraft persisted in the West long after the classic witch-hunts subsided. The use of charms to cause illness or death has not died out: there were cases of people dying from witches' spells in New York City in the 1980s, in connection with the Santería syncretic religion. That someone could die in this manner seems strange to those who are not susceptible to such beliefs, but it is a well-established fact among believers and the anthropologists who study the subject that such deaths can and do occur. Knowing that one is a victim of witchcraft can be as psychologically damaging as any actual malign magic.

Possession and Exorcism

Exorcism is the driving out of evil spirits, or the warding off of the spirits' presence in the first place. An exorcistic rite might be performed to prevent maleficent spirits from inhabiting a person or place or object. If the spirit is thought to have truly possessed a person, the rite will be designed to drive out the evil being and return the person to a normal state. Professional exorcists existed in ancient Mesopotamia, Egypt, and Greece, as well as in the Judeo-Christian world. Additionally, so-called witch doctors have existed in many African societies, as have shamans among American Indians and their ancient counterparts in Siberia. In indigenous Australia, traditional healers known as *ngangkari* work to banish bad spirits from the body and at the same time remain part of modern health practice.

Belief in demons and exorcism was widespread among the ancient Jews. The Jewish Bible refers to possession of a human by an evil spirit and the means of redressing the situation (1 Samuel 16:14–16). The New Testament, too, contains a number of different accounts (e.g., Matthew 8:28–32; Luke 6:18; Luke 13:32). Jesus claimed power over all demons and conferred that same power on his disciples. The early church used this power extensively, instituting an office of exorcist in the third century CE. The Roman Catholic Church still has a ritual for driving out a demon from a person believed to be possessed, encoded in a document entitled *Of Exorcisms and Certain Supplications*. Not frequently used today, the rite entails the use of prayers, blessings, and invocations to return the victim to good order. In the modern Greek Orthodox Church, a type of exorcism is part of the baptism ceremony. The parent or godparent, besides renouncing Satan and praying for God's protection of the infant, blows three times into the air and spits three times to show contempt for the devil.

In sum, the aim of witch trials and exorcisms was to rid the person or community of foul spirits and begin the process of healing.

Michael Shally-Jensen

See also: Astrology; Folk Medicine; Hysteria; Native American Traditional Medicine; Shamanism and Neo-Shamanism; Voodoo and Santería

Further Reading

Ehrenreich, Barbara, and Dierdre English. 2010. *Witches, Midwives, and Nurses: A History of Women Healers.* 2nd ed. New York: Feminist Press.

Ginzburg, Carlos. 1991. *Ecstasies: Deciphering the Witches' Sabbath.* New York: Pantheon.

Hutton, Ronald. 2017. *The Witch: A History of Fear, from Ancient Times to the Present.* New Haven, CT: Yale University Press.

Murray, Margaret A. 1970. *The God of the Witches.* Oxford: Oxford University Press.

1900–1950s

INTRODUCTION

American medicine had already begun to change substantially by the end of the 19th century. Among the breakthroughs of that era were X-rays, the theory of germs (microorganisms), and the idea of hygiene in general and of sterile surgery in particular. These innovations had the effect of keeping the ball rolling toward continued professionalization of the medical field. They also began to move the practice of healing, at least in urban areas, out of patients' homes and into hospital rooms with trained staff on hand. (This was a gradual process, however.) The new "scientific" medicine that emerged near the turn of the century was built on better understandings of human anatomy and physiology and, to a lesser extent, biochemistry.

At the same time, Americans did not lose their faith in "irregular" healers or in the principle of self-reliance. Some irregulars denied that there was any major difference between themselves and the new class of formally educated physicians, which only tended to make the irregulars look out of touch and ill prepared for the modern world. Still, most alternative therapies were too popular, and their practitioners too well established, to see them overtaken entirely by conventional medicine. Hoping to distinguish themselves, doctors sought stricter licensing laws through state medical associations and legislatures; in most cases, however, they could not succeed in getting them passed without also permitting homeopaths, eclectics, and the like access to licenses of their own.

Battle Lines

A historic study of medical education, prepared by the field researcher Abraham Flexner and published in 1910, set out new standards for teaching institutions. Flexner visited regular, eclectic, homeopathic, and osteopathic schools in the United States and Canada, evaluating them on their ability to turn out regular doctors trained in contemporary methods. Of the 155 schools he visited, 124 were recommended for closure by him. Flexner found most of these institutions to be commercial enterprises or proprietary operations having little or no connection to hospitals or laboratories and marked by liberal admission policies. Flexner noted that irregular schools, in particular, had little to justify themselves and might even pose a danger to society. On the other hand, the criteria Flexner used in his assessment were developed by the American Medical Association (AMA), and he was accompanied in his work by an AMA official. Thus, it is hardly surprising under the circumstances that irregular schools were found to fall short in the preparation of *regular* doctors. Fortunately for the irregulars, Flexner also came down hard on most of the regular schools.

Osteopathy had been developed by a magnetic healer and bonesetter, Andrew Taylor Still (1828–1917). His original conception was based on removing obstructions to the flow of body fluids by manipulating bones, especially vertebrae, that had fallen out of alignment. Still opened the American School of Osteopathy in Kirksville, Missouri, in 1892, though it took decades to build up the field from that beginning. Another magnetic healer and itinerant philosopher, Daniel David Palmer (1845–1913), explored the idea of using spinal adjustments to relieve pinched nerves that, similarly, were thought to disrupt the flow of energy, or what Palmer called "Innate Intelligence." Palmer opened up the first school of the new field of chiropractic in 1897 in Davenport, Iowa. He and his son and inheritor, B. J. Palmer, later backed off of the notion of Innate Intelligence and focused on misaligned bones, joints, and nerves in the spine and elsewhere as the basis of chiropractic. Osteopathy also evolved over time.

Meanwhile, sanitation campaigns that also had begun in the late 19th century continued to be pursued in the early 20th. City public health departments embraced the science of bacteriology and infectious disease and went after the sources of public health crises such as mosquitos (yellow fever), impure water (cholera), and spoiled food and milk (typhoid fever). At the same time, citizens were increasingly advised to follow good personal habits at home and in public: people should not spit on city streets, they should wash their hands before meals, they should refrigerate their food (i.e., use an icebox—since electric refrigerators did not come into wide use until the 1940s), and they should change their underwear twice a week. A number of home disinfectants and mouthwashes began to be marketed around the time of World War I, roughly the same time that several major vaccines also began to be deployed on a large scale. (Even so, influenza would kill millions worldwide in the great epidemic of 1918.)

Also by the early 1920s, medical researchers were making the first significant advances in the areas of nutrition, metabolism, growth, and reproduction. Researchers discovered various vitamins, for example, or compounds that seemed to be essential to human health. They studied the chemical reactions that were needed for the body to process carbohydrates, proteins, and electrolytes. They identified insulin as key in the regulation of glucose. And they found viruses (bacteriophages) that could infect bacteria, suggesting a future line of attack in the control of bacterial infections. Yet, except for the packaging and selling of vitamins, most of these discoveries had little immediate impact on people's lives. It would take years before practical applications were available for most, although insulin began to be marketed by the mid-1920s.

Yet, in these first decades of the 20th century, the bulk of health care continued to take place outside the reach of the new scientific medicine. In the 1930s, for example, about 20 percent of household medical expenses went to the purchase of patent medicines (i.e., over-the-counter tonics) and home medical supplies and equipment; an additional 10 percent or so went to irregular practitioners such as chiropractors along with midwives (Marks 2001). Indeed, despite a mean-spirited campaign by the AMA against them, chiropractors fought hard against the imposition of uniform training and licensing standards on the grounds that it would exclude promising but less-well-off students from becoming doctors. Under Flexner's proposed plan of requiring a four-year college degree as a prerequisite for medical training, careers in professional health care would be off-limits for most working-class Americans and would also tend to be unattainable for minorities, women, and immigrants. The alternative systems were cheaper to train in and to maintain as businesses.

One nonconventional form of care, Christian Science, was able to steer clear of legal restrictions on religious grounds. Among physicians, Christian Science was regarded as one of the more deplorable approaches because it denied all practical care and relied on faith alone. Some critics saw the morality of Christian Scientists as skewed; they allowed people, even children, to suffer and die needlessly, claiming that everything was in God's hands. Members of the faith would occasionally be arrested for practicing medicine without a license, but once their cases went to court, they usually were found to be exercising their constitutional right to practice a religion. In some states that maintained stricter laws against the use of Christian Science for medical treatment, practitioners managed to avoid prosecution by claiming that they did not charge for their services but were there simply as voluntary aides; they would later collect a "gratuity" from the client. Surely no one could object to "healing through prayer" in such a context.

Meanwhile, other religious denominations had their own brands of healing. The Pentecostal movement grew in the first half of the 20th century, in part on the basis of faith-healing crusades. These were particularly popular in rural areas. Other Protestant groups, too, sponsored massive "tent revivals" in which faith healing played a central part. Usually, no questions were raised in these cases about "practicing medicine without a license."

A more esoteric variety of spiritual healing took place under the name of anthroposophic medicine. An import from Austria, via the mystic Rudolf Steiner (1861–1925) and his supporters, anthroposophic medicine mixed cosmic philosophy and medieval alchemic principles with homeopathy and an eclectic assortment of other ingredients. It tended to have limited appeal at first but grew and evolved over time, eventually contributing to such fields as art therapy and rhythmic exercise. A parallel kind of esotericism, based on Eastern philosophy, informed the Russian mystic Helen Blavatsky's (1831–1891) and her spiritual descendants' similarly titled field of theosophy. Theosophy's message of karma and reincarnation, borrowed from Hinduism, enjoyed a worldly popularity in the early 20th century and was revived in a somewhat different, and even more influential form in the 1960s and again in the New Age movement of the 1980s.

Mind versus Body

In the area of mental health, by the start of the 20th century, most states and many large cities had at least one public psychiatric hospital—and the numbers increased in the decades before 1950. As they did so, hospital superintendents found themselves dealing with overcrowded wards filled with the more severe, chronic cases. Both the level of care and the image of the state asylum as a shining example of modern institutional care began to suffer as a result. It was evident that there were serious problems ranging from who was admitted and why to the type and amount of care patients received. Patients were often simply warehoused and forgotten, and the use of constraints and solitary confinement occurred regularly. The hospital administration system was patriarchal and hierarchical to the extreme. Patients were treated less as individuals with lives and rights of their own than as inmates in a penal institution run by a group of elite psychiatric experts. Yet, despite their many failings, public mental hospitals stood with their doors open as places to which people experiencing mental and emotional difficulties could go to get help.

In fact, even at the height of the era of the large psychiatric hospital, these institutions served only a small portion of the many millions of Americans who suffered from the likes of depression, anxiety, manic-depressive illness (bipolar disorder), and milder forms of schizophrenia. The hospitals, besides housing patients living with chronic mental illness, took mostly people in the throes of a psychotic episode. That is, people who experienced single instances of major mental breakdown or distress, or perhaps recurring episodes of serious illness, were admitted and treated. They were discharged when they responded to treatment or improved on their own and were permitted to return to their lives on the outside. People who experienced milder forms of mental illness, on the other hand, did not have a lot of options available to them—unless they were wealthy enough to be admitted to a private institution. The latter, too, experienced growth in the early to mid-20th century.

Even as state hospitals grew, much of the important psychiatric research that took place in the early twentieth century was connected with special research institutes, university laboratories, and private practice groups. Psychiatrists were generally less interested in severe, chronic cases of the kind handled by public asylums, preferring to treat the "walking ill," or those cases that might see an improvement. In the face of such willful blindness on the part of physician-researchers, and the continuing problems with funding inside hospitals, hospital administrators turned, in the 1940s, to new treatments that might help to control their patients if not actually treat them. They used electroconvulsive treatments in far greater numbers than were warranted by the patient population and their conditions, and they experimented with such measures as insulin shock therapy and prefrontal lobotomies (removal of part of the brain).

The prevailing model for psychiatric understanding and treatment, from roughly 1910 through the midpart of the century, was psychoanalysis. Much of the structure of the brain and the nervous system, much of the biological roots of insanity, remained unknown. But, as brought to the United States by its founder Sigmund Freud (1856–1939), psychoanalysis was a system ready to uncover the psychosocial roots of mental illness and deliver the means with which to understand and address it. In this era, psychiatrists began to pay great attention to the neuroses, or those disorders that affect only part of the personality and are accompanied by a variety of mental, emotional, and physiological symptoms. In other words, the crushing anxieties, phobias, and depressive symptoms that hospitals were ill equipped to deal with could now be examined through psychoanalysis. The methods used in this new "talk therapy" included dream interpretation and a focus on fearful or traumatizing events in the patient's childhood, particularly those involving unconscious sex drives.

Psychoanalysis would go on to spawn a host of offshoot schools of thought and practice, and it would reign supreme in U.S. psychiatry for decades. Only after the 1950s did it start to face challenges from other approaches, such as the behavioral psychology (behaviorism) explored by B. F. Skinner (1904–1990) and the budding field of biological psychiatry. Sex research took on a new dimension in the 1950s through the work of Alfred Kinsey (1894–1956) and the research team of Masters and Johnson (William H. Masters, 1915–2001; Virginia E. Johnson, 1925–2013). Not that theirs was the final word on the subject, however; the field would continue to evolve.

Further Reading

Grob, Gerald. 1994. *The Mad among Us: A History of the Care of America's Mentally Ill.* New York: Free Press.

Janik, Erika. 2014. *Marketplace of the Marvelous: The Strange Origins of Modern Medicine.* Boston: Beacon Press.

Marks, Harry M. 2001. "Medicine: From the 1870s to 1945." In *The Oxford Companion to United States History*, edited by Paul S. Boyer, 488–89. New York: Oxford University Press.

Robinson, Paul 1989. *The Modernization of Sex: Havelock Ellis, Alfred Kinsey, and William Masters and Virginia Johnson.* Ithaca, NY: Cornell University Press.

Whorton, James C. 2002. *Nature Cures: The History of Alternative Medicine in America.* New York: Oxford University Press.

ANTHROPOSOPHIC MEDICINE

Anthroposophic medicine is considered an alternative or integrative medical system that, although incorporating parts of conventional medicine, draws on a holistic view of humanity, nature, and spirit in its approach to healing. It was founded in the early 1920s by the Austrian esoteric philosopher Rudolf Steiner (1861–1925) and a trained medical associate, Ita Wegman (1876–1943). Anthroposophic medicine has had its largest impact in Europe but is also present in the United States. It is practiced by specialized physicians, therapists, and nurses who provide treatments such as medicinal remedies and art, movement, and massage therapies along with nursing techniques. Its medicines are derived from plants, minerals, and animals and are generally homeopathic in nature. It builds on a concept of different levels of life forces and on the model of a threefold human constitution or makeup. The key to anthroposophic healing is treating the whole patient, awakening in him or her latent spiritual insights, and guiding both the body and the mind together to another plane of operation. While patients have reported high satisfaction with anthroposophic health care, establishment medical professionals have raised questions about its underlying concepts and methods.

Steiner and Spiritual Science

After studying science, mathematics, and philosophy in Vienna, Steiner was commissioned at the age of 22 to edit the scientific works of Johann Wolfgang Goethe, who influenced him greatly. Steiner began developing anthroposophy in 1901, founding the Anthroposophic Society in 1912 and the first school, or Goetheanum, in 1922. According to the "spiritual science" of anthroposophy, the human mind has the ability to contact spiritual worlds and benefit from that relationship. The present intellectual capacities of humankind, observed Steiner, evolved from an earlier mode of consciousness that participated in the spiritual world directly. While previous philosophers, such as Immanuel Kant, had proposed that there were limitations to human understanding based on the material world and the nature of scientific explanation, Steiner suggested that human beings could expand their cognitive capacities by developing the faculty of spiritual perception.

In Steiner's view, there are four "formative forces" that lie behind both matter and life. These are (1) basic, or elemental, forces, (2) growth forces, (3) animating forces, and (4) spiritual forces. Making up the human constitution, in addition, are three interactive systems: (*a*) the nerve-sense system (perception, sensation), (*b*) the motor-metabolic system (internal processes), and (*c*) the rhythmic system (movement, coordination). In human beings, these distinctive forces and systems overlap and combine in various ways to maintain the body and mind—as one—and produce such qualities as imagination, inspiration, and intuition. These qualities and others can, moreover, be cultivated in order to advance the individual along the spiritual-evolutionary plane, as it were. The idea is to achieve an enhanced consciousness that can perceive and interact with spiritual worlds.

Anthroposophy ultimately proved to be both a philosophy and a new way of approaching certain human endeavors. Besides schools of spiritual science, it established alternative methods of education (the Waldorf schools), rehabilitation centers (for those with disabilities), a system of movement (eurythmy), and a greater awareness of the educational and therapeutic value of such artistic practices as recitation, drama, painting, sculpture, and architecture. Even a type of agriculture, biodynamic agriculture, resulted from anthroposophic research. Nevertheless, it remains a minority view on the world, and critics from establishment science, medicine, and education regard it as a suspect, even occult, field whose tenets are unsupported by evidence. The Anthroposophical Society in America, which naturally would dispute such a characterization, is located in Ann Arbor, Michigan, and stands at the head of some 22 branch groups in 14 different states. There are also associations of Waldorf schools, eurythmy groups, and so on.

Basics of Anthroposophic Medicine

Anthroposophic medicine is informed by alchemistic, esoteric, and homeopathic concepts and concerns itself with the spiritual nature of living as much as with conventional understandings. It takes into account metaphysical relations between planets, substances (metals, etc.), human organs/systems, and spiritual elements in the diagnosis of illness and the development of therapeutic strategies. Diseases are in some cases deemed to be related to actions in previous lives. A range of therapeutic methods and techniques are employed in anthroposophic medicine, including herbal remedies, art therapy, massage, movement therapy, and others.

A guiding principle of anthroposophic healthcare is the recognition of the autonomy and dignity of the patient and thus the need to help people to help themselves. A key therapeutic goal, therefore, is to stimulate self-healing—or, rather, (1) *hygiogenesis*, which means to establish effective autonomic regulation of the organism; and (2) *salutogenesis*, which means to establish effective psycho-emotional and spiritual self-regulation (Kienle et al. 2013). The treatments are intended not merely to restore a previous healthy condition but rather to produce a new level of the organism's, and the individual's, "inner strength" (ibid).

Anthroposophic medicine thus employs a holistic approach to healing. Rather than concentrating on a singular pathological issue, the aim is to strengthen the overall constitution of the patient, taking into account all the various dimensions: physical, mental, emotional, social, and spiritual. Treatments often are necessarily multimodal. They are typically tailored to the individual so as to optimize the effects of the various modalities used and to enhance the chances for (self-) improvement.

Anthroposophic Therapies

Anthroposophic medicine employs, in addition to some conventional treatments, special medications and special therapeutic procedures, including eurythmy therapy, rhythmical massage, anthroposophic art therapy, and counseling. In addition, there are special anthroposophic nursing techniques. The therapies can be used alone or in combination with one another.

Medications

Medications are developed in accordance with the anthroposophical view of the human being and the natural world. They are based largely on homeopathic principles and the established homeopathic pharmacopoeia of Western Europe. The medications are administered orally, rectally, vaginally, topically, or by injection. Conventional pharmaceuticals may also be used in anthroposophic medicine, if appropriate. The best-known anthroposophic remedy is fermented mistletoe extract, which is used to treat cancer. The idea is that mistletoe is a parasitic plant that ultimately kills its host, and so it can be used against cancer to kill that unwanted malignancy.

External Applications and Rhythmical Massage

External applications—such as liniments, compresses, hydrotherapy, and medicinal baths—are used as elements of nursing care and therapy to stimulate, strengthen, or regulate hygiogenic (autonomic) processes. For this purpose, etheric or fatty oils, essences, tinctures, and ointments are used, as well as carbon dioxide in baths. Of particular importance is rhythmical massage, which augments traditional massage with lifting movements, undulating or gliding movements, and other techniques such as working from core areas out to the periphery. In addition to the standard effects of massage (on skin, tissues, and muscles), rhythmical massage is thought to increase general vitality and to aid in the amelioration of specific disease conditions.

Art Therapy

Anthroposophic art therapy, developed by Margarethe Hauschka (1896–1980) and others, is similar to conventional art therapy. It employs one or more of the following: therapeutic sculpture (often using softer, more pliable materials); therapeutic drawing and painting; therapeutic musicmaking; and anthroposophic speech therapy, which is used to address a range of medical, psychiatric, or leaning/developmental conditions or issues. Art therapy can be used in individual or group settings. Based on a patient's medical history and diagnosis, he or she may be assigned a particular medium or be encouraged to participate in a variety of art-therapeutic modalities and sessions.

Eurythmy Therapy

Eurythmy therapy (from the Greek for "harmonious motion") is an exercise therapy intended to be supportive of both physical and mental/emotional health and wellness. It is conducted by eurythmy therapists in small group or individual settings. Participants are instructed to perform particular movements of the hands, limbs, feet, and/or whole body. Eurythmy movements are associated with certain vocal elements (vowels, consonants, etc.), with music intervals, and with the flow of time generally and are captured in different "gestures of the soul." Specific movements can be prescribed for specific patient conditions, or an individual can participate in general eurythmy sessions. A session usually lasts 30 to 45 minutes. In between formal sessions, the patient may be asked to practice the prescribed exercises regularly.

Anthroposophic Psychotherapy and Counseling

Psychotherapy in the anthroposophic vein is designed to augment other forms of psychotherapy or, in some cases, to supplant them. The goal is to improve the patient's condition through "soul work" and the exercise of imagination, inspiration, and intuition. Separating the self from ordinary sensation/perception and engaging the spiritual dimension is a key focus. Similarly, anthroposophic counseling concerns itself with giving guidance on lifestyle, nutritional, social, mental, and spiritual matters in the pursuit of health and wellness.

Anthroposophic Nursing

In anthroposophic nursing, the aim is to become acquainted with the whole patient and perceive him or her as a physical, psychological, and spiritual being. Developing a caring relationship is key as the nurse seeks to assist the patient in healing in both the existential and metaphysical senses.

Michael Shally-Jensen

See also: Alternative Diagnostics; Art and Music Therapy; Astrology; Dance Therapy; Drama Therapy; Homeopathy; Hydrotherapy; Mind–Body Medicine; Past Life Regression Therapy; Spiritualism

Further Reading

Kienle, Gunver S., et al. 2013. "Anthroposophic Medicine: An Integrative Medical System Originating in Europe." *Global Advances in Healthcare and Medicine* 2(6): 20–31. https://www.ncbi.nlm.nih.gov/pmc/articles/PMC3865373/

Singh, Simon, and Edzard Ernst. 2008. *Trick or Treatment: The Undeniable Facts about Alternative Medicine.* New York: W. W. Norton.

Steiner, Rudolf. 1999. *Introduction to Anthroposophic Medicine.* Hudson, NY: Anthroposophic Press.

Wilson, Colin. 1985. *Rudolf Steiner: The Man and His Vision.* Wellingborough, UK: Aquarian Press.

ANXIETY AND ITS TREATMENT

Although not easily defined, anxiety is generally taken to be a state of emotional and physical disturbance caused by a real or imagined threat. In the field of abnormal psychology, the term refers to a disturbance brought on by a threat that is experienced in such a way as to be out of proportion to the true situation, or as something that only the subject experiences. Unlike the relatively mild, brief anxiety felt by many people in connection with stressful events—from test taking to a job interview—anxiety disorders of a clinical nature last six months or more and can worsen if not treated. As the anxiety increases, moreover, the person's behavior becomes more disorganized and ineffective.

Anxiety is one of those conditions that is widely experienced and can become quite severe even in otherwise healthy individuals. Yet different people seem able to withstand differing degrees of anxiety in their lives, some succumbing readily to their fears, imagined or otherwise, while others endure and move on. Thus, there is not always a sharp boundary between "normal" stress and anxiety and "clinical" anxiety requiring a medical remedy. This is one reason why anxiety medications are prescribed so widely in the United States. Some 40 million adult Americans suffer from an anxiety disorder.

One of the common emotional symptoms of severe anxiety is a feeling of constriction. The person may also feel distanced from reality or other people, and he or she may become depressed, agitated, or unable to concentrate. Physiological symptoms include palpitations, pounding in the head, profuse sweating, and tightness of the chest. In addition, anxiety is almost always accompanied by increased muscle tension, which in turn may cause a headache, tiredness, overbreathing (hyperventilation), and various bodily aches and pains. Insomnia and digestive disorders can also develop. If it comes to facing all that, a person would be wise to seek professional advice.

Types of Anxiety Disorders

Anxiety may arise in a specific situation that the person seeks to avoid. Such a state is called a *phobia*. Phobias can develop, for example, around spiders or snakes, around heights or enclosed spaces, or around interacting socially with other people. These kinds of phobias affect about 5 percent of people in the United States and Europe. They can vary somewhat by culture, with different cultures having different fears—as well as a few shared ones. Regarding such specific fears, scientists have found that the mammalian "fight or flight" response, centered in the limbic system of the brain (especially, the amygdala), is generally involved; but there remains some uncertainty as to the exact causes of phobic anxiety in many cases.

People may suffer, too, from a persistent feeling of dread that has no apparent cause. This type of anxiety is called generalized, or free-floating, anxiety. In serious cases, it can greatly hinder daily functioning, as the sufferer worries irrationally about any number of disasters that await him or her in the course of a day. Persons with such *generalized anxiety disorder* (GAD) find it difficult to control their worry. The worrying intensifies over a period of weeks and months, especially during times of stress. Individuals may agonize over the arrangements for a party or the best gift for a celebration. The heightened worry may interfere with the person's ability to concentrate and with sleep patterns. The world can seem a dark, threatening place. GAD as a condition also has a developmental component; more than half of those who seek treatment for it report having had symptoms in childhood and adolescence. Women experience GAD with nearly twice the frequency of men—up to 8 percent of women versus fewer than 5 percent of men.

Panic disorder, another anxiety condition, is characterized by a sudden, overwhelming wave of fear. Symptoms appear abruptly and for no apparent reason. They may include racing or pounding heartbeat, nausea and dizziness, difficulty in breathing, feeling smothered, and numbness or tingling in the limbs. Individuals report feeling intense terror and a need to escape from some impending disaster. These distressing symptoms may last for several minutes, but a longer time still is usually needed for the individual to calm down.

Another anxiety-related disorder is *posttraumatic stress disorder*, or PTSD. Here, a specific stressor, or stressful event from the past, causes an extreme form of anxiety or panic. PTSD often arises from encounters involving violence—combat, domestic violence, automobile accidents—either experienced directly or witnessed firsthand. However, with the publication of the latest "bible" of psychiatry, the *Diagnostic and Statistical Manual of Mental Disorders* (DSM) in 2013, PTSD was removed from the Anxiety category and placed in a different one, Trauma and Stressor-Related Disorders.

A similar shift occurred in the case of *obsessive-compulsive disorder* (OCD), which involves obsessive thoughts and/or compulsive, repetitive behaviors. Previously regarded as a specialized form of (hyper)anxiety, OCD too now has a category of its own.

Depression, as well, is very common among sufferers of anxiety. Yet, strictly speaking, depression is a *mood* disorder and thus is often dealt with as a separate but related—or "comorbid"—condition. The term *anxious depression* is sometimes used to denote the presence of symptoms of both conditions in a single person.

The Age of Anxiety

Before the era of modern medicine, anxiety and its cousins—nervousness, fear, tension, worry—were thought to be signs of a weak disposition, a corrupted spirit, a failure of courage, a lack of willpower. By the late 19th and early 20th centuries, the term *neurasthenia*, or "tired nerves," was being applied to cases of what today we might consider anxiety of one form or another. Various "nerve doctors" rose to prominence by dispensing remedies that ranged from bogus patent medicines to hydrotherapy (water treatment) to electrical treatments. These were all prescientific solutions that nevertheless may have had some positive effects, if only as a result of the placebo principle. It was more beneficial to have someone address one's symptoms, or something with which to address them, than to have no recourse at all.

Sigmund Freud (1856–1939) developed the theory that anxiety arises when the memory of unsettling childhood experiences or emotions is so intolerable that it is repressed, or forced from the person's consciousness. The memory is kept in the unconscious by defense reactions—thoughts and behaviors that are developed to continue repressing the anxiety-provoking content. According to Freud, the unconscious memory, along with the resulting defense reactions, forms a complex. This complex can be unraveled only by undergoing psychoanalysis.

In contrast to Freud, the behaviorists of the mid-20th century held that anxiety is a learned reaction that develops when the emotion evoked by a frightening event is generalized or attached to surrounding circumstances. Sometimes such generalization brings together remotely related circumstances. For example, a child who cuts his foot while playing in a sandlot may thereafter be afraid of any patch of sand, including beaches.

Unfortunately for sufferers of anxiety, neither psychoanalysis nor behaviorism alone proved to be a satisfactory solution in many—perhaps most—cases. Both of these remedies operated on the basis of limited understandings of the human brain and nervous system, even as they served to tap into some of the underlying mental, emotional, and physiological components of the condition.

The modern breakthrough in the treatment of anxiety came from the field of psychopharmacology, or the use of (prescription) drugs to treat mental conditions. In the late 1940s pharmaceutical companies began marketing new varieties of barbiturates, or sedatives, for the control of anxiety and related conditions. Barbiturates had been around for decades, but only in long-acting forms that were used on psychiatric patients in mental hospitals. The newer varieties—Amytal, Seconal—were shorter-acting but still came with serious side effects, such as heavy sedation, addiction, and, frequently, death from overdose. Then, in 1955 a new class of pill was introduced, a benzodiazepine drug called Miltown. Although scientists at the time did not have a perfect understanding of how it worked, they knew that it interacted with neurotransmitters in the brain and had a notably less sedating effect than barbiturates. Miltown quickly became a sensation, the first blockbuster medication for a psychiatric ailment. The drug's success, moreover, altered public perceptions of anxiety and its treatment. It suddenly was okay to see a doctor for drugs to make one feel better mentally and emotionally—to make one *live* better.

After Miltown came a number of other popular pharmaceutical remedies, chief among them the tranquilizer Valium. Dubbed "mother's little helper," Valium became the most widely prescribed pill in the Western world between the late 1960s and early 1980s. By then, taking a tranquilizer to cope with life had become something of a status symbol, a sign that one had entered the adult world and was living the modern dream, even if the dream also contained nightmares that required the use of medication. Moreover, benzodiazepines were not without problems of their own. They often produced unwanted side-effects such as dizziness, sluggishness, headaches, confusion, nausea. The pills built up physical dependency, too, and withdrawal after extended use was difficult and painful.

In response, a new class of drugs was presented in the 1980s. These were SSRIs—selective serotonin reuptake inhibitors, which block certain receptors in the brain in order to keep more of the neurotransmitter serotonin available. The first popular SSRI, Prozac, came out in 1987, followed by Paxil, Zoloft, and others. Meanwhile, improved brands of benzodiazepine (Xanax, Ativan) were marketed as well, becoming bestsellers in their own right. In fact, of the 71.4 million U.S. prescriptions written for anxiety disorders in 2006, most—more than 40 million—were for benzodiazepines (Tone 2009). Both of these classes of drugs, however, carry some of the same side effects as earlier varieties, albeit perhaps more manageable in some cases. Recently, the early enthusiasm over SSRIs has begun to subside over concerns about both common side effects and the (largely unknown) long-term impacts. The fact is that scientists still don't entirely understand how or why these psychotropic medications work, apart from the idea that they increase levels of key neurotransmitters (dopamine, norepinephrine, and serotonin).

Meanwhile, psychotherapies, often used in combination with medications, continue to be utilized. Cognitive-behavioral therapy (CBT) can be useful in treating anxiety disorders in general. This approach helps people change the way they think about their fears and teaches healthier responses to anxiety-provoking situations. CBT can assist those dealing with obsessive-compulsive disorder, as well. Meditation, relaxation therapy (massage), and aromatherapy may be employed to help anxiety sufferers relax and relieve their worries. There are also kava kava and other herbal remedies for the relief of stress and anxiety. The modes of therapy used to deal with posttraumatic stress disorder are somewhat more wide-ranging and include behavioral techniques, sedatives or tranquilizers, group therapy, and individual psychotherapy.

In sum, we appear still to be living in the Age of Anxiety, though now better armed with an array of remedial solutions. The science has advanced notably but is not fully there yet. Whether the huge increase in antianxiety prescriptions represents the medicalization of nervous jitters or the uncovering of undiagnosed millions, one cannot properly say at this point.

Michael Shally-Jensen

See also: Behavioral Theories and Therapies; Depression and Its Treatment; Hydrotherapy; Hysteria; Meditation and Mindfulness; Neurasthenia, or Nervous Exhaustion; Psychoanalysis; Spas and Mineral Waters; Stress and Stress Management

Further Reading

Kurth, Charlie. 2010. *The Anxious Mind: An Investigation of the Varieties and Virtues of Anxiety*. Cambridge, MA: MIT Press.
Nydegger, Rudy. 2016. *Dealing with Anxiety*. Santa Barbara, CA: Praeger.
Peterson, Andrea. 2017. *On Edge: A Memoir of Anxiety*. New York: Crown.
Tone, Andrea. 2009. *The Age of Anxiety: A History of America's Turbulent Affair with Tranquilizers*. New York: Basic Books.

ART AND MUSIC THERAPY

There is good evidence from both the historical record and more recent studies that creativity can benefit one's mental and emotional well-being. Creative expression allows people to articulate their thoughts and feelings, often in ways that are not available to them in the course of daily living. It is widely recognized, as well, that the passive *consumption* of creative works—literature, art, music—can prove beneficial. Seeing, reading, or listening to creative works seems to stir complex emotions inside us and perhaps echo our own experiences at some level—or should do so, anyway, when we appreciate the work before us.

Art and music *therapy*, conducted by accredited professionals, is a 20th-century development that draws on both the active/creative and the passive/receptive aspects of art and creativity to achieve individualized therapeutic goals for those in need of or otherwise seeking health and wellness support.

Expressive Interventions

Art therapy generally tends toward active participation on the part of the individual. According to the American Art Therapy Association (AATA), art therapy is

> an integrative mental health and human services [practice] that enriches the lives of individuals, families, and communities through active art-making, creative process, applied psychological theory, and human experience within a psychotherapeutic relationship. Art therapy, facilitated by a professional art therapist, effectively

supports personal and relational treatment goals as well as community concerns. Art therapy is used to improve cognitive and sensorimotor functions, foster self-esteem and self-awareness, cultivate emotional resilience, promote insight, enhance social skills, reduce and resolve conflicts and distress, and advance societal and ecological change. (AATA 2017)

Those are fairly lofty claims, but they reflect the growth of art therapy in recent decades and its increasing acceptance as a standard treatment modality.

At a more concrete level, art therapy is often used for people experiencing trauma or physical illness, seeking personal development, or struggling to deal with the day-to-day trials of living. Through the act of creating art and thinking about the process and the medium, people are able to develop skills that, so the research shows, improve cognitive ability, increase awareness of self and others, and help them cope with the symptoms or limitations imposed by illness,

---

Awakening to Music

The noted neurologist Oliver Sacks, as he recorded in his best-selling book *Awakenings,* which later was made into a popular movie starring Robin Williams, explored the use of music in treating victims of a rare brain disease. The patients Sacks worked with had suffered for years, even decades, from an uncommon form of Parkinson's disease (Encephalitis lethargica), "sleeping sickness," that prevented them from making any movements or any speech. They were essentially "frozen." Along with medication, Sacks introduced music, which had a salutary effect. Suddenly, his patients were able to dance, sing, and interact socially. Especially with rhythmic, period music from the time of their youth, the patients experienced a remarkable recovery (although it was not, unfortunately, permanent). Sacks surmised that it was all owing to the fact that musical memory is lodged in parts of the brain that are immune from amnesia and other effects of mental and physiological disorders. Himself a pianist and longtime music aficionado, Sacks observed that humans are naturally musical, going back to the early development of our species. Today, music therapy continues to be used to help Alzheimer's patients and others to tap into their memories and experience the rhythm of life.

Music can also be a problem, as described by Sacks in another of his books, *Musicophilia.* Some people experience what is called "broken-record syndrome" or "earworms." In these cases, the music in one's head never stops: short passages from familiar tunes repeat themselves over and over. In the more serious cases, the music interferes with one's ability to operate on a day-to-day basis, drowning out everything else. In minor cases, the situation is simply annoying, with snippets of musical favorites thrumming quietly in the background as one goes about one's business. The phenomenon is little understood, and there is no ready remedy.

Sources

Oliver Sacks. 1987. *Awakenings.* New York: Summit Books.
Oliver Sacks. 2007. *Musicophilia: Tales of Music and the Brain.* New York: Knopf.

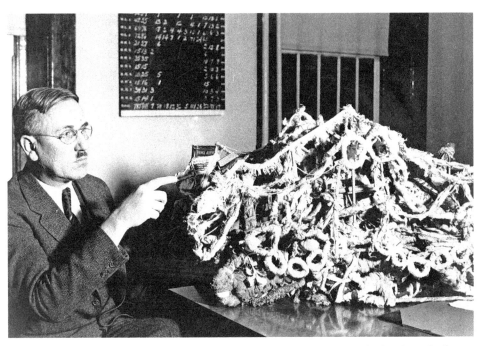

Dr. John Lind of St. Elizabeth's Hospital in Washington, D.C., displays the handiwork of one of his psychiatric patients, a piece entitled "dimensional divertissement," c. 1950. (National Library of Medicine)

disability, or disease. Algaze and colleagues (2013, 44–45), describing research on the use of expressive writing as therapy, note the following:

> Creative expression can . . . help us bring certain difficult experiences to consciousness where they can be more rationally processed. The work of [some researchers] indicates that expressive writing can help people organize and process complex emotional experiences, thereby significantly improving emotional and physical health. Without structure, painful experiences can lead to unconscious distress, rumination, and more. Forming a coherent narrative may give people a sense of control over painful events in their lives, leading to resolution instead of unproductive defending.

The primary purpose of art therapy, then, is to help patients heal their mental, emotional, and, to some extent, physiological wounds or challenges as much as possible. Apart from *written* expression, as described above, art therapy uses visual and symbolic expression to get participants to move beyond the limitations of language and give voice to their experiences in new and meaningful ways.

Art therapy is also sometimes used in conjunction with a mind–body therapy known as guided imagery, or visualization. This involves using imagination or mental images to promote relaxation, encourage healing, and bring about a change in mood or attitude. Sometimes the patient is encouraged to record an image or visualization using an artistic medium, but most often visualization is a mental exercise aimed at reducing fear and anxiety surrounding an illness by focusing on the process of recovering in one's "mind's eye"—for example, by picturing the body free of a problematic condition. Guided imagery, although regarded as a complementary or alternative therapy, is increasingly used in "mainstream" settings to help patients work through their conditions and feel better about their prospects—which is a proven strategy for benefitting health.

Music therapy, according to the American Music Therapy Association (AMTA), is

> the clinical and evidence-based use of music interventions to accomplish individualized goals within a therapeutic relationship by a credentialed professional who has completed an approved music therapy program. Music therapy is an established health profession in which music is used within a therapeutic relationship to address physical, emotional, cognitive, and social needs of individuals. After assessing the strengths and needs of each client, the qualified music therapist provides the indicated treatment including creating, singing, moving to, and/or listening to music. Through musical involvement in the therapeutic context, clients' abilities are strengthened and transferred to other areas of their lives. Music therapy also provides avenues for communication that can be helpful to those who find it difficult to express themselves in words. Research in music therapy supports its effectiveness in many areas such as: overall physical rehabilitation and facilitating movement, increasing people's motivation to become engaged in their treatment, providing emotional support for clients and their families, and providing an outlet for expression of feelings. (AMTA n.d.)

Music can influence both physical and mental health. Music therapy may be used in either an individual or group setting to achieve a state of relaxation or to enhance awareness. In addition to its effects on physiological health, studies have shown that music therapy improves sleep quality and reduces anxiety. Music therapy has been used successfully to help mitigate or modulate the effects of, for example, Alzheimer's disease, autism, depression, and stress. It can also prove beneficial to those with physical illnesses or people recovering from surgery. Like art therapy, music therapy is sometimes combined with other approaches such as guided imagery to achieve the desired goals. Overall, the results of music therapy have been promising, the consequence, as described by Ernst and colleagues (2008, 84), of its unique impact on the brain:

> Sensations that accompany music therapy may activate limbic or other areas of the brain related to the reward and motivation circuitry (limbic-cortical circuits). Secondary physiological changes and bodily reactions may follow, . . . such as changes in autonomic nervous system activity, relaxation effects on vital functions such as breath, respiratory rate, blood pressure, and cardiac output. Analgesic [i.e., pain-relieving] and anxiolytic [i.e., anxiety-reducing] properties of music are mainly due to the lowering of stress levels and stress hormone production similar to the relaxation response.

An associated form of treatment is known as "ambience therapy." Researchers have explored whether playing natural sounds—rain, waterfalls, ocean waves, winds, sounds of the rainforest, and the like—in hospital recovery rooms might help improve recovery rates by relieving anxiety and encouraging relaxation and healing.

Historical Dimensions

Music therapy and, to a lesser extent, art therapy began after World War I and then again after World War II, when community musicians and artists/teachers, both amateur and professional, went to veterans hospitals in various parts of the country to play for and/or artistically encourage veterans suffering from the physical and emotional traumas of war. In the 1940s, three people emerged as leaders in the development of music therapy. The psychiatrist and music therapist Ira Altshuler promoted music therapy in Michigan for three decades. Willem van de Wall pioneered the use of music therapy in state-funded facilities and wrote the first "how to" music therapy text. E. Thayer Gaston, known as the "father of music therapy," was instrumental in organizing the profession and developing educational standards for music therapists. The first major academic training program in music therapy was established at Michigan State University in 1944; other university programs followed. The National Association for Music Therapy (NAMT) was founded in New York City in 1950 and operated until 1997. The American Music Therapy Association (AMTA), which continues in operation today, was formed in 1998 as a merger between NAMT and another organization.

Formal art therapy in the United States was pioneered in the 1940s by the psychologist and educator Margaret Naumburg and the German American painter and psychoanalysis follower Edith Kramer, both of New York City. Naumburg, like Kramer, was psychoanalytically oriented and argued that art expression functioned as a form of symbolic speech, thereby aiding the patient who was experiencing difficulties. Kramer, similarly, considered the creative process as key to overcoming psychological defenses; the idea was to relieve anger, anxiety, and pain through expressive means. Other early proponents of art therapy in the United States were Elinor Ullman, of George Washington University; Robert Ault, of Emporia State University in Kansas; and Judith Rubin of Pittsburgh. The American Art Therapy Association was founded in 1969.

Michael Shally-Jensen

See also: Anthroposophic Medicine; Dance Therapy; Drama Therapy; Gestalt Therapy; Mind–Body Medicine; Psychoanalysis

Further Reading

Algaze, Daphne, Dennis K. Kinney, and Ruth Richards. 2013. "Creativity and Mental Health." In *Mental Health Care Issues in America: An Encyclopedia,* edited by Michael Shally-Jensen, 138–48. Santa Barbara, CA: ABC-CLIO.

American Art Therapy Association (AATA). "About Art Therapy." https://arttherapy.org /about-art-therapy/

American Music Therapy Association (AMTA). "What Is Music Therapy?" https://www .musictherapy.org/about/musictherapy/

Ernst, Edzard, Max H. Pittler, Barbara Wider, and Kate Boddy. 2008. *Oxford Handbook of Complementary Medicine.* Oxford: Oxford University Press.

BEHAVIORAL THEORIES AND THERAPIES

Behavioral theory is a classic psychotherapeutic approach that focuses on analyzing and altering human behaviors based on a pattern of actions and related consequences. This theory operates under the basic premise that human behavior is learned. Thus, through the use of proven techniques, undesirable behavior can be replaced by teaching new, more desirable behaviors. Several behavioral therapies are commonly accepted as effective treatments for a wide range of mental health needs, including disruptive child and adolescent behavior, spousal abuse, irrational fears and phobias, and mood disorders such as anxiety and depression.

Key Concepts

All behavioral therapies have certain elements or characteristics in common. First, all such therapies rely on models of behavior change that are based on empirically supported learning principles. Learning theory asserts that changes in thinking can alter internal processes, and overt behaviors will consequently be altered (Vargas 2009). This process occurs through respondent or operant conditioning. *Respondent conditioning* describes the process whereby behaviors are completed in response to a stimulus. *Operant conditioning* refers to the process by which a behavior is completed in anticipation of an often desirable consequence.

Second, behavioral therapists reject the idea that mental health issues and daily difficulties are the result of a disease. In fact, they place no emphasis on why or how problems develop; they care only about factors that currently influence a behavior and its continuation. Behavioral therapists do not believe it is fruitful to work on developing a client's insight. They believe that with behavior change alone, people will begin to feel better and that as they do, greater self-awareness may be developed. Thus insight is never a goal of behavioral therapy because even without insight, people are generally able to make required changes to their behavior.

All behaviorists have a commitment to the scientific method and value its use in helping clients change their behaviors. They also believe in the use of the scientific method as a means of assessing the efficacy of treatments and specific interventions. In other words, particular behaviors are targeted for change, and specific interventions are used to overcome these behaviors with a constant eye toward evaluating their effectiveness.

Additionally, behavioral therapists believe that the counseling relationship is necessary to create enduring client change. In other words, without a strong client-counselor relationship, a foundation for change is not present, and clients may not optimally benefit from treatment interventions. However, behavioral therapists do not believe that enduring client change is achieved solely through the therapeutic relationship; rather, this relationship is only a vehicle for change to occur. Through this relationship, behavioral therapists believe that clients come to trust the mental health counselor, and thus they are open to their interventions. Because behavioral therapy requires clients to be active and complete assigned homework, a solid client-counselor relationship is important.

Related to this idea, behavioral therapies are "active": they require clients to be active participants in the counseling process. Clients need to be participatory and learn new skills and ways to create behavioral changes. Clients need to track and monitor their behaviors and apply skills and new behaviors learned in session to situations outside of the session.

Conditioning and Behaviorism

Classical conditioning (i.e., respondent conditioning) was first demonstrated by Russian physiologist Ivan Pavlov (1849–1936) in the early 20th century. Pavlov's initial research on the digestive system of dogs switched to focus on salivation after he observed that the dogs began to salivate every time a laboratory assistant opened the door to feed them. As a result, Pavlov conducted a series of experiments that showed how respondent behavior such as salivation occurs in response to a specific stimulus such as food. To begin the experiments, Pavlov presented a neutral stimulus (e.g., a bell) to the dogs and found that this had no effect on their salivation. Next, he paired the sound of the bell (i.e., neutral stimulus) along with the unconditioned stimulus (UCS) of food, which elicited the unconditioned response (UCR) of salivation. After pairing the bell and food for several trials, the dogs began salivating in response to the bell. As a result the bell became a conditioned stimulus (CS), and the conditioned response (CR) of salivation was established.

John Watson (1878–1958), the early 20th century American psychologist who helped to spread Pavlov's ideas, is given the most credit for founding modern behaviorism. He was dissatisfied with the psychology of the time, complaining that psychology was slipshod compared to other sciences such as physics, chemistry, and biology. Watson was disenchanted with two aspects of psychology: the subject matter and the methods of study or research. In 1913, Watson published a paper titled "Psychology as the Behaviourist Views It," which is nicknamed the "Behaviorist Manifesto." The paper outlined his vision of the field, stating that only behavior should be the object of study in psychology (the study of emotions, thoughts, etc., would be the realm of another field such as philosophy), and study procedures should be objective. He added a third goal for the field: research in psychology should always be applied; that is, when a psychologist pursues a research question, he or she should have a particular application in mind for the research rather than studying simply for curiosity's sake.

Operant conditioning, traditionally associated with B. F. Skinner (1904–1990), is the conceptual underpinning of modern applied behavior analysis (ABA); it refers to the process and effects of *consequences* (i.e., reinforcement or punishment) on behavior. A consequence in this sense is a result that follows a given behavior and alters the frequency of that behavior in the future. If the frequency of a behavior has increased in connection with a consequence, then positive or negative reinforcement has taken place. Positive reinforcement occurs when a stimulus (or "reward") is added to the environment immediately following a behavior, while negative reinforcement occurs when a stimulus (particularly an undesirable stimulus) is removed from the environment immediately following a behavior. By contrast, if the future frequency of a behavior has decreased, positive or negative punishment has taken place. Generally, operant conditioning is most often referred to as the strengthening of behavior and should focus on the use and effects of reinforcement. Skinner, through his experiments and provocative writings, did much to establish and popularize the field of behaviorism from the 1950s through the 1970s.

Therapeutic Techniques

Applied Behavior Analysis

Applied behavior analysis (ABA) is a science in which the principles of behavior are applied to improve socially significant behavior to a meaningful degree. The framework of ABA encompasses many interventions, including reinforcement, prompting, stimulus control, shaping, and fading (Dunlap et al. 2008). ABA methods are used to teach new skills, to reinforce and maintain already learned skills, and to restrict or minimize conditions under which interfering behaviors occur. In addition, data are continuously collected and analyzed to evaluate intervention effectiveness and to formulate treatment decisions.

Relaxation Training

The essence of relaxation training is that an individual cannot be anxious and relaxed at the same time. Therefore relaxation training is the gradual tensing and relaxing of major muscle groups (i.e., legs, stomach, chest, shoulders, arms, neck, and face) combined with deep breathing in an attempt to become increasingly more relaxed. These techniques are often taught to individuals experiencing more than expected amounts of stress, fear, and/or anxiety. Relaxation training can be done as a stand-alone intervention or in conjunction with the process of systematic desensitization.

Systematic Desensitization

Systematic desensitization is a behavioral treatment grounded in classical conditioning that is used for fears, anxieties, and phobias. To begin the process, a client must identify a hierarchy of situations from least to most fearful in conjunction with being taught relaxation and coping strategies. Next, the client is prompted to imagine anxiety-producing situations beginning with the least fearful. The goal of the systematic desensitization process is for the client to use relaxation and coping strategies to gradually extinguish anxiety-producing fears. Client treatment traditionally begins with visualization procedures and gradually progresses to in vivo ("live") situations.

In Vivo Exposure

In vivo exposure, also called flooding, refers to the re-creation of a situation that occurs in an individual's actual environment and that creates a great deal of anxiety, fear, and/or stress. The individual desires to overcome the debilitating nature of these situations, and through the aid of a mental health clinician can do so through the re-creation of that situation in a controlled environment. There are two types of in vivo exposure: (1) gradual exposure and (2) direct exposure (i.e., flooding). In the gradual approach, individuals learn and practice relaxation techniques as they are gradually exposed to stressful or anxiety-provoking things or situations. This process systematically builds up to the anxiety-provoking situations or things over the course of many sessions. In direct exposure (i.e., flooding), the individual is presented all at once with the stressful or anxiety-provoking stimulus. The rationale for this approach is that an individual's anxiety level will reach an apex and then dissipate. This realization will provide the individual with an experience for overcoming his or her fear, stress, or anxiety.

Social Skills Training

The central aim of social skills training is to facilitate and improve an individual's ability to communicate and interact with other human beings. Behaviorists contend that since social skills are learned behaviors, individuals can improve and correct those patterns of behaving (i.e., socialization) through operant conditioning, modeling, and role plays. The intention behind utilizing social skills training is that if individuals correct their maladaptive behaviors in social situations, they can reduce their level of stress and anxiety and begin to resolve their social interaction problems. Such training is used, for example, in cases of social anxiety disorder (social phobia).

Strengths and Limitations of Behavioral Therapies

Behavioral theory is a classic psychotherapeutic approach with empirically supported value in the mental health community. Behavioral therapies are effectively used to analyze and alter undesirable human behaviors. All behavioral therapies are based on learning theory and share a similar foundation. Behavioral theory can be applied in a variety of settings and is effective with a broad range of mental health difficulties ranging from mood disorders to antisocial behaviors. However, behavioral therapy is most effective in the presence of a trusting therapeutic relationship and it does not address past events or insights that may be important to the client's success. Overall, behavioral theory is accepted as a valuable addition to the mental health field. In the 1980s and 1990s, some of its core principles and techniques were "merged" with those of cognitive (or "mentalistic") therapies to form the extremely productive and promising field of cognitive-behavioral therapy (CBT).

Nicole A. Adamson, Matthew J. Paylo, Leah Gongola,
Victoria E. Kress, and Gretchen Reevy

See also: Anger and Anger Management; Biofeedback; Stress and Stress Management

Further Reading

Cooper, J., T. Heron, and W. Heward. 2007. *Applied Behavior Analysis*. 2nd ed. Upper Saddle River, NJ: Prentice-Hall.

Dunlap, G., E. G. Carr, R. H. Horner, J. R. Zarcone, and I. Schwartz. 2008. "Positive Behavior Support and Applied Behavior Analysis: A Familial Alliance." *Behavior Modification* 32(5): 682–98.

Mills, J. A. 1998. *Control: A History of Behavioral Psychology*. New York: New York University Press.

Skinner, B. F. 1976. *About Behaviorism*. New York: Vintage.

Vargas, J. 2009. *Behavior Analysis for Effective Teaching*. New York: Routledge.

CHIROPRACTIC

Chiropractic is a form of therapy in which manipulation of the spine and related parts of the musculoskeletal system is the main method of treatment. The somewhat odd-sounding name, *chiropractic* (kī-rə-prak'tik), is derived from the Greek words *cheir*, meaning "hand," and *praktikos*, meaning "practical"; together they suggest "done by hand." Chiropractic practitioners maintain that the nervous system, particularly that part of it running through the spinal column, is key to the body's healthy functioning. Thus, if the central nervous system is impaired in any way, as by pressure on a nerve, it will operate poorly and cause damage to tissues, organs, and other physiological systems—including, according to some, the immune system. Chiropractors use vertebral manipulation to ensure proper "alignment" of bones, nerves, and related components.

Critics, mainly from the medical mainstream, have long maintained that chiropractic is a pseudoscience based on faulty principles and questionable practices. In recent decades, however, there has been a "rapprochement," of sorts, whereby medical doctors have come to see that chiropractic can serve a legitimate health purpose in some cases while chiropractors, in turn, have come to rein in the more extravagant claims about what their form of therapy can accomplish.

The "Discoverer" and His Discovery

One point of controversy in the history and practice of chiropractic is the character of its founder, Daniel David (D. D.) Palmer (1845–1913). Born in a rural area outside of Toronto, and having only a modest education, Palmer took a variety of odd jobs before settling into life as a "magnetic healer"—one who seeks to control electromagnetic forces said to be causing a patient's illness—in Davenport, Iowa. Palmer prided himself on his drugless methods and the increasing popularity of his practice, as people came to him with all manner of complaint and seemed, moreover, to improve over the course of a series of magnetic treatments. In due course, Palmer shifted the focus of his healing efforts from magnetism to bodily manipulation. The inaugural moment is supposed to have occurred when a janitor in Palmer's office building, someone known to have been hard of hearing following an accident years before, was discovered by Palmer to have a vertebra out of position. Palmer thereupon brought it back into alignment, and allegedly the man could hear normally thenceforth. Afterward, Palmer continued investigating the subject of spinal misalignment and disease in other of his patients, ultimately claiming a strong linkage between the two. In 1896, therefore, Palmer announced the founding of a new healing science called *chiropractic,* "the grandest and greatest science the world has ever known" (quoted in Whorton 2002, 166).

The theory of chiropractic was developed largely after the fact of its founding. Palmer, in other words, developed his understanding of the processes involved in manipulative healing into the early years of the 20th century, after having practiced on patients for over a decade. His 1910 textbook, *The Chiropractor's Adjuster: The Science, Art, and Philosophy of Chiropractic,* laid out his main thesis. The book ranged widely over spiritual and metaphysical matters as well as medical practicalities. Central to the new science was the idea of nervous "tone," or the degree to which a person's nervous tissues and organs reflected normal "vigor, tension, activity, strength" (169). Being off in tone—being ill, essentially—meant having nerves that were either too "slack" or too "tense." To exhibit the correct tone or vitality, in contrast, was to be the embodiment of life itself, for life, according to Palmer, was basically a matter of vital spirit. Palmer went on to discuss vibratory mechanics, or how a nerve might vibrate above or below the golden mean. Moreover, he regarded the totality of vital energy flows within the body as a kind of "intelligent life-force," something that was part of a greater whole but the basis of existence nevertheless. This innate force was thought to function like the "soul," then; it held the body and mind together within a grand design. It also required tender loving care by its owner.

According to Palmerian theory, the most common way that health is compromised is through skeletal *subluxation,* or the partial dislocation of a bone in a joint. The most serious luxations—that is, those that impact other segments of the body—are found in the spine, with its 33 stacked vertebrae, numerous shock-absorbing vertebral discs, and a vast complex of major nerves, including, of course, the spinal cord. An opening known as the intervertebral foramen at the intersection of each vertebra, together with other, similar openings, allow elements of the nervous system to pass through the surrounding bone and connect with the body's physiological systems. Palmer theorized that these foramina were the most likely sites of impinged nerves when minor spinal dislocations (subluxations) were present. A nerve need not necessarily be *pinched* to be affected, however, as any improper pressure or imposition on it might cause it to become enlarged or contracted, too taut or too loose, overly sensitive or numb. Furthermore, any such impingement could affect the organs or tissues to which the nerve was connected, resulting in the development of disease or ill health. In his book, Palmer stated that he was able to correlate specific ailments with specific vertebrae (and with the nerves emanating from them). Thus, heart disease was linked to the fourth dorsal vertebra; impotence, to the first lumbar; insanity, to the third cervical; smallpox, to the fifth cervical, and so forth (One feature of Palmer's system was that the germ theory of disease was regarded as insignificant compared to the "life-force" theory and the complications of the spine.)

Chiropractic, as defined by Palmer, is "the science of adjusting by hand any and all luxations of the 300 articular joints of the human body, more especially of the 52 articulations of the spinal column, for the purpose of freeing any and all impinged nerves, which cause deranged functions" (quoted in Lerner 1952, 110). Treatment, which entails manually "resetting" the backbone or any affected bodily joints, is aimed at eliminating nervous interference and allowing the body to address, by itself, the ailment or physiological "derangement" in question.

The public in Palmer's day seemed to welcome chiropractic and wanted to see more of it. Palmer founded the first college of chiropractic, the Palmer School and Cure, in Davenport in 1897; by the time of his death, in 1913, dozens of other schools had opened throughout the United States. Three weeks of training was all that was needed to obtain a certificate. Additionally, there were more than 100 chiropractic infirmaries or clinics in the country at the turn of the century. Palmer's son, Joshua Bartlett (B. J.) Palmer, was especially talented not only in chiropractic technique but in the art of promotion. He helped raised the profile of the new method and drew in patients and practitioners in the United States and abroad. He also clashed with his father over methods and goals; in the end, the son ended up killing the father in an auto accident.

Conflict and Evolution

As chiropractic continued to grow, it drew the ire of "regular" medical professionals as well as those practicing in the relatively new field of osteopathy, which similarly was bone-centered yet had a rather different philosophy (namely, disease as a loss of structural integrity). The American Medical Association (AMA) early on undertook to challenge chiropractic as unscientific in its approach and substandard in its training and practices. In fact, the AMA maintained, chiropractic was *hazardous* to a patient's health because of the risks it posed to the nerves and blood vessels in the vicinity of any bones or joints undergoing adjustment. (Some adjustments can be quite severe.) Medical doctors took grim delight in reporting cases of alleged death or permanent harm caused by chiropractors, including stories of patients who never woke up after falling asleep following their treatment. Most of these stories were unreliable, but they had an effect. Osteopathic practitioners, likewise, lamented the brief training and false precepts that underlay chiropractic as against their own superior science. Professionals in both camps derided the grand claims made by the more shameless commercial boosters of chiropractic, sometimes filing complaints against chiropractors for practicing medicine without a license. This was a professional war—about which many consumers knew or cared little. They just went to whichever practitioner they were comfortable with.

Chiropractors, meanwhile, fought back by arguing that charges against them were motivated by fear of competition and based on a misunderstanding of the aims of reputable chiropractors. In 1987, the chiropractic community won a major legal victory when a federal judge ruled that the AMA and two allied groups had improperly campaigned against chiropractic for decades, seeking to contain or eliminate it. In doing so, the court said, the physicians' groups had violated anti-trust laws designed to preserve market competition.

Thus, since that decision the two fields have come to coexist more or less peace-fully, with chiropractors referring patients to medical doctors when a condition lies outside their own realm of expertise, and doctors referring patients to chiro-practors when certain musculoskeletal issues arise—particularly lower back pain. Most chiropractors today have dropped the notion of innate "life-force" and no longer see bone and joint complications as the sole source of disease. Instead, they favor more traditional views of human anatomy and physiology. Still, there is a fair amount of variability among practitioners, some of which (called "mixers") take a more holistic approach and others of which (called "straights") rely on a stricter approach centered on spinal and pelvic manipulations. According to the American Chiropractic Association, there are more than 75,000 licensed chiropractors in the United States, serving over 27 million Americans annually. Training is much more extensive (three–four years) and medically rigorous than before. The field has come a long way since the experimental "bone cracking" of its early years— even as challenges to its principles and methods remain.

Michael Shally-Jensen

See also: Alternative Diagnostics; Craniosacral Therapy; Feldenkrais Method; Magnet Therapy; Mesmerism and Hypnotherapy; Osteopathy; Shiatsu

Further Reading

Folk, Holly. 2017. *The Religion of Chiropractic: Populist Healing from the American Heartland.* Chapel Hill: University of North Carolina Press.

Janik, Erika. 2014. *Marketplace of the Marvelous: The Strange Origins of Modern Medicine.* Boston: Beacon Press.

Lerner, Cyrus. 1952. *The Lerner Report: A History of the Early Years of Chiropractic.* New York: Foundation for Health Research. http://philosophyofchiropractic.com/wp-content/uploads/2011/08/Lerner.pdf

Whorton, James C. 2002. *Nature Cures: The History of Alternative Medicine in America.* New York: Oxford University Press.

CLIENT-CENTERED THERAPY

Client-centered psychotherapy is still going strong—even though it was developed more than 70 years ago and is not all the rage that it once was. Nowadays, it often goes by the name of person-centered therapy, to reflect its humanistic orientation.

Like a number of other popular psychotherapeutic treatments, client-centered therapy is largely the creation of a single person, the American psychologist Carl

Psychotherapy and *Good Will Hunting*

The 1997 movie *Good Will Hunting* was the first major film featuring Matt Damon and Ben Affleck, who also cowrote the script. Featuring Robin Williams as a psychotherapist, the film centers on the character of Will Hunting (Matt Damon) and his interactions both with Chuckie (Ben Affleck) and eventually his therapist, Sean Maguire (Williams).

In the film, Will is a mathematical genius who works as a janitor and hangs out with his Boston "Southie" friends every night. When a math professor recognizes his genius, he tries to get Will help for his antisocial tendencies. Will eventually connects with Sean, and through a shared history and a few heart-wrenching declarations, Will confronts his demons and moves on to what the film tells us will be a happier life.

While the movie is often pointed to as an example of the benefits of talk therapy—Sean and Will discuss many different situations, with Sean giving Will perspective on why he might be making certain choices—there's more to it than that. The reason Will ends up spending his therapy hours with a community college professor instead of a highly paid professional therapist is that Will makes a mockery of every other therapist in Boston. He analyzes therapists faster than they can analyze him, fakes hypnosis, and more.

Good Will Hunting demonstrates the importance of the relationship between the therapist and the client. While it does offer a somewhat simplistic approach to treatment—most clients need more than a declaration of "it's not your fault" and a tearful hug to recover from serious emotional trauma—the film does demonstrate many of the positive benefits of psychotherapy treatment.

Rogers (1902–1987), who both drew on earlier schools of thought and laid out new ideas of his own. Rogers originally termed his approach *nondirective therapy* or the "new" psychotherapy. From its inception, client-centered therapy stressed the role of the patient—later called the "client"—rather than that of the therapist. The term "client" (or "person") emphasizes the value placed on individual autonomy and self-determination and underscores the difference between client-centered therapy and other forms of psychotherapy that grew out of medicine, psychiatry, and behavioral science.

Client-centered therapy focuses significantly on the therapeutic relationship, seeing it as the medium for effecting personality change, and on the client's immediate experience in the therapeutic situation. In a sense, the therapeutic relationship is considered the same as any good human relationship in which a person feels accepted, respected, and valued. The client is seen not as a "sick" individual but as someone whose previous experiences in life have left him or her harmed, defensive, lacking in free and open communication, perhaps separated from his or her peers, and held down in terms of realizing his or her full potential as a functioning human being.

Founding Figure

Carl Rogers was a child of the Midwest (Illinois) and graduated from the University of Wisconsin. He thought he might go on to study theology, attending Union Theological Seminary, but switched to psychology, obtaining his master's and doctorate from Teachers College (Columbia University) in New York. (He later became an atheist.) In the 1930s he was associated with the Society to Prevent Cruelty to Children, in Rochester, NY, and with the University of Rochester. His first published work dealt with the clinical treatment of "problem children." However, Rogers came to doubt the validity of standard diagnostic categories and treatment methods. He felt that the relationship between the patient and the therapist should not be cold and impersonal but, on the contrary, warm and accepting. The therapist, or counselor, should not be controlling and directive but instead appreciative of the patient's (client's) thoughts and feelings. He believed that a counselor who could reflect back the client's feelings, who could communicate an understanding of those feelings and display an unconditional regard for that person, could help bring about positive personality change.

In the early 1940s Rogers became the first therapist to record and transcribe therapy sessions verbatim, a practice that later was adopted as the professional standard. He published his ideas and clinical results in several books, including *Counseling and Psychotherapy* (1942), *Client-Centered Therapy* (1951), and *Psychotherapy and Personality Change* (1954). He became widely known outside of the field of psychology with his *On Becoming a Person* (1961). After teaching at Ohio State University (1940–1945), the University of Chicago (1945–1957), and the University of Wisconsin at Madison (1957–1963), he moved to the Center for Studies of the Person, in La Jolla, California. He died in La Jolla in 1987.

Precepts and Progression

In one of his early works, *Counseling and Psychotherapy* (1942), Rogers identified four main tenets of his new therapy. First, in the normal course of things, the client is viewed as choosing to grow and develop. Psychotherapy involves freeing the client for this natural unfolding rather than giving him or her authoritative direction. Second, client-centered therapy focuses on the more emotional, feeling aspects of a client's experience than on intellectual components. Experience is considered more crucial than intellection, or analytical reflection. Third, the client's present experience is emphasized rather than memories and events from the past. This is the "here and now" element which is shared with other humanistic approaches. Last, the therapeutic relationship is viewed as a potential situation for growth, a situation in which the person comes to learn about and understand him- or herself, thus allowing him to make sound choices and relate successfully to others in a mature fashion.

In his foundational *Client-Centered Therapy* (1951) and in an article published in 1957, Rogers further developed his theory of psychotherapy. He again emphasized that the therapist is not an authority figure; rather, the client is primarily responsible for the course of therapy. He argued that characteristics of the therapist are very important in determining the outcome for the client; in fact, these characteristics may be more important than specific therapy techniques. He identified three important characteristics of the therapist. First, the therapist must experience an "unconditional positive regard" for the client; that is, the therapist is fully accepting of the client, feels warmth, and is nonjudgmental toward him or her. Second, the therapist must have an empathic understanding of the client. This involves, to a point, seeing things the way the client sees them and feeling what it must be like to be the client. Last, the therapist must be genuine, or honest with the client. The honesty does not have to be bluntness or brutality, but a certain level of truthfulness and forthrightness is necessary for the client to trust the therapist.

Client-centered therapy, then, is not made up of a set of techniques designed to produce specific changes but rather is a holistic approach toward experience and interpersonal activity. Respect for the client's autonomy suggests that the therapist should not interfere directly in the client's life. Rather, changes that the client realizes are to a great extent changes in his self-concept and personal world (inner and outer) that the client has identified and undertaken, with the assistance of the therapist. In client-centered therapy, there is no interest in psychiatric diagnosis, in dwelling on the past, or even in close analysis of the client's current life situation. What matters is the client's *experience,* especially in the "here and now," including the experience in the therapeutic encounter. In such a context, the therapist's role is generally a supportive one.

Although client-centered therapy is primarily about creating a certain type of climate in the psychotherapy room—sometimes called "core conditions"—and not primarily about technique, Rogers did mention a couple of techniques for his new therapy. One such method is mirroring. In mirroring, the therapist rephrases what the client has said. This has at least two purposes. First, it shows the client that the therapist understands and is empathic. Second, it is a means of clarification for the therapist to ensure that she indeed understands the client. If the therapist's rephrasing seems to be inaccurate, the client may say so. Another method is to encourage experiencing; that is, the therapist encourages the client to feel his or her feelings in the present, deeply. The therapist will gently guide a client toward focusing on the present rather than the past and toward focusing on emotions rather than intellectual aspects of experience.

Current Status

Client-centered therapy is practiced with individuals as well as with groups and is usually short-term, comparatively speaking. It underwent a decline in popularity with the rise of behavioral approaches in the late 1950s and early 1960s, but then experienced a resurgence in the 1980s with the rise of the New Age/Alternative Medicine movement. Today, client-centered therapy continues to be a popular as well as effective form of therapy, falling generally within the "humanistic" school of thought and practice. Its fruitful person-focused approach has affected the development of other areas including education (student-centered learning), organizational psychology (human relations), and the public square (respect for individual differences, etc.).

Criticisms of person-centered therapy are varied and depend, to some extent, on one's preferred approach or school of thought. One criticism is that with all the focus on the therapeutic situation and setting up proper "core conditions," little can be said about what the therapist, or counselor, brings to the treatment as far as his or her own experiences and philosophies. Is the therapist truly just a springboard or "mirror," echoing the client's experiences? Or in developing a relationship, and ideally a meaningful one, is not he or she, by definition, more than that—someone who also has motivations and expectations vis-à-vis the client? Similarly, what if the client's experiences and goals are not sufficient, in and of themselves, to establish a path to positive growth? Does the therapist then merely "reflect back" those same factors? Or does he or she become more "directive," in contravention of the basic precepts of the client-centered approach, in order to steer the client toward something else, something outside the established pattern? These questions are one reason why the original Rogerian client-centered therapy has evolved toward being a more integrative approach, one that draws on other philosophies and methods as well.

Michael Shally-Jensen and
Gretchen Reevy

See also: Codependency Counseling; Drama Therapy; Encounter Groups; Existential Psychotherapy; Gestalt Therapy; Moral Treatment; Recovery Movement

Further Reading

Cornelius-White, Jeffrey H. D. 2015. *Person-Centered Approaches for Counselors.* Thousand Oaks, CA: Sage Publications.

Rogers, Carl. [1961] 1995. *On Becoming a Person: A Therapist's View of Psychotherapy.* Boston: Houghton Mifflin.

Thorne, Brian. 2003. *Carl Rogers.* 2nd ed. Thousand Oaks, CA: Sage Publications.

Tudor, Keith, and Mike Worrall. 2006. *Person-Centered Therapy: A Clinical Philosophy.* New York: Routledge.

DEPRESSION AND ITS TREATMENT

Depression is a mood disorder characterized by an overwhelming sense of sadness along with inactivity, difficulty in thinking straight, uneven appetite, sleep disturbances, and feelings of dejection and hopelessness. It affects millions of people in the United States—indeed, around the world—and lies behind significant numbers of suicides each year.

Normal human responses to some situations in life include temporary depression. For example, most of us have felt depressed for some length of time over the loss of a family member or friend, the failure of a relationship, a setback in one's career, or some traumatic event. Experiencing transient depression in these situations is to be expected. However, in some cases the emotional and physiological effects of depression persist over an extended period of time and come to display a set of symptoms that psychiatrists then refer to as *major depression*, or depression requiring intervention by a mental health professional. In those cases, the experience of simply "feeling blue" turns to one in which the world appears quite black.

Major depression occurs in 7–11 percent of the U.S. population, or up to one in nine Americans of all ages (NIMH 2017; Yan 2017). Women are more often affected than men, by a nearly two-to-one ratio; this is due to cultural and social factors rather than biological ones, although women are subject to a particular type of depression, postpartum depression, that is exclusive to their sex. The offspring and relatives of individuals with major depression are at some higher risk of becoming depressed, because of genetic linkages, and family members are affected in a secondary way as well, in that they typically must help manage the condition in the patient and learn to cope with it for themselves. Nearly 3 percent of the adult U.S. population suffers from a related condition, bipolar disorder, characterized by cycles of high (mania) and low (depression) moods. A smaller percentage (under 2 percent) suffers from a chronic condition known as a depressive personality disorder.

Depression has long been a theme in literature, the arts, and Western culture generally. Once called melancholia, it has been the subject of everything from philosophical treatises to popular music lyrics (blues, hip-hop, etc.). Elegiac books have even been written about some antidepressant medications, such as Prozac. (Criticisms of those drugs have been offered, too.) Most everyone has come into contact with depression in one form or another. One might say that depression is the new normal—or perhaps the new black.

Symptoms of Depression

Clinical depression is defined by its symptoms. Among the major symptoms are:

- A low mood nearly all of the time
- Loss of interest or enjoyment in almost everything
- Changes in appetite or weight
- Trouble sleeping or oversleeping
- Lack of initiative, with slowed-down or agitated movements
- General tiredness or lack of energy
- Feelings of worthlessness or inappropriate guilt
- Difficulty concentrating or making decisions
- Recurring thoughts of death or suicide.

Because transient emotional responses are common, these symptoms will have needed to be present for two to three weeks before a diagnosis of major depression can be made.

Not all of these characteristics occur in each depressed individual. Moreover, some or all of them may be present and yet the individual may not consider him- or herself depressed. According to the *Diagnostic and Statistical Manual of Mental Disorders*, a person is considered to have experienced a major depressive episode if he or she exhibits a loss of interest or pleasure in all or almost all usual activities and shows at least four of the above symptoms nearly every day for at least two weeks. Professional treatment would be considered essential for such individuals.

Risk Factors and Causes

Clearly, depression is one of the most common mental disorders in the United States. Current research suggests that the condition is caused by a combination of genetic, biological, environmental, and psychological factors.

Depression can occur at any age, but often it begins in adulthood. Although depression is recognized as occurring in children and adolescents, in those cases it usually presents with more apparent irritability than low mood. Thus, both depression and bipolar disorder, as well as various anxiety disorders, often appear in adults who experienced high levels of anxiety as children. Yet, there is no simple, one-to-one correlation here.

Depression, especially in midlife or older adults, can co-occur with other mental illnesses, such as anxiety ("anxious depression"), as well as physical conditions or illnesses, such as serious wounds or dismemberment, diabetes, cancer, heart disease, and Parkinson's disease. These conditions often can worsen and become more difficult to treat when depression is present.

The principal risk factors, then, are: (1) personal or family history of depression; (2) major life changes, trauma, or stress; and (3) certain physical illnesses and/or side effects from medications.

As for causes, the science is indeterminate. In psychological terms, depression has been considered a reaction to some loss of or separation from a valued person or object. This is called reactive depression (or, erroneously, "neurotic" depression). It is contrasted with the more severe type of depression having no apparent cause, called endogenous depression. Another type, accompanied by delusions or hallucinations, is known as psychotic depression. In many cases, however, these distinctions are not clear-cut; the person suffering severe depression for no apparent reason may *feel* that they have experienced a loss of some kind and may or may not become deluded in the course of the illness.

Treatment

Depression is commonly treated with medications and counseling or psychotherapy—or a combination of the two. In more persistent cases, electroconvulsive therapy (ECT) may be tried. Most depressions are naturally time limited, but selected treatment with modern therapies can shorten the duration of the illness by many months. Treatment and hospitalization may also prevent suicide attempts.

The three major classes of antidepressant drugs available are: (1) tricyclic drugs, (2) a group called *selective serotonin reuptake inhibitors* (SSRIs), and (3) the mono-amine oxidase (MAO) inhibitors. All are effective in three-quarters of all cases of depression, and yet each comes with its own set of side effects, withdrawal problems, and overdose risks.

Tricyclics (e.g., imipramine) have been used since the early 1960s. As with the other antidepressants, their exact mechanism of action is unknown; it is believed to involve their effect on the disposition of norepinephrine or serotonin in the brain. They are not stimulants—in fact they often cause sleepiness—and effects may not be apparent until two to three weeks after the start of treatment. Sleep disorders may then diminish, and a lightening of mood becomes apparent; continued treatment is needed for six to nine months before use of the drug ceases, however.

Fluoxetine (Prozac), introduced in 1988, quickly became one of the most widely used of all antidepressants; and antidepressants, as a group, had already become one of the most widely prescribed medications. An SSRI class of drug, Prozac blocks the reuptake of serotonin into brain cells and thus increases the amount of serotonin available in the brain. A number of similar antidepressants, such as sertraline (Zoloft) and paroxetine (Paxil), do the same. Prozac and, to a lesser extent, the other SSRIs, were initially lauded as harbingers of a new age of "cosmetic psychopharmacology," or the use of drugs to make us feel "better than well" (Slater 2018, 164). It was not to be, however, for within a decade or so, negative accounts, many by users, started to come out. Apart from withdrawal issues and side effects, both of which could be considerable, a major complaint was drug resistance, or the need to continually increase the dosage to attain the same results. Moreover no one, least of all the drug companies, understood what the long-term effects might be. (Few studies have been done.) Some critics labeled the whole Prozac/SSRI phenomenon as "the manufacture of depression," because the marketing campaigns for these drugs were so massive and because doctors so readily prescribed them for their patients (Greenberg 2010).

The other major group of drugs, the MAO inhibitors such as phenelzine, prevent the formation of monoamine oxidase, an enzyme that breaks down biogenic amines in the brain and intestinal tract. Their effectiveness is attributed to normalizing the amount of amine in the brain. Because the enzyme ordinarily breaks down food amines that would otherwise cause an increase in blood pressure, however, the body is no longer protected from this effect when the drugs are used. Patients given the drugs must control their diets accordingly. MAO inhibitors can also interact with other drugs (including the other antidepressants) and cause serious side effects; patients receiving them should, therefore, ask to be provided with instructions about necessary precautions.

Certain methods of psychotherapy, such as cognitive-behavioral therapy, can help in the treatment of some cases of depression. No evidence exists, however, that traditional, insight-oriented psychoanalytic therapy is effective in acute cases, such as those accompanied by suicidal thoughts or attempts. Psychiatric hospitalization is often necessary in such cases, which are usually treated by drug or electroconvulsive therapy.

In depressions severe enough to need psychiatric treatment, electroconvulsive therapy (ECT) has been found effective. It has been so misused and overused in the past, however, that a public aversion to it exists. Nowadays, it is most often used in cases of severe (endogenous and delusionary) depression. Although ECT is at least as effective as any of the drugs, it comes with significant short-term side effects (e.g., confusion and memory loss) and continues to carry a stigma outside of the hospital setting.

Other, more recently introduced types of therapies used to treat medicine-resistant depression include the brain stimulation techniques of (1) repetitive transcranial magnetic stimulation (rTMS) and (2) vagus nerve stimulation (VNS), both of which use medical technologies to introduce or enhance electromagnetic activity at specific sites in the brain. These techniques and others continue to be under study even while offering some early practical results and prospects for the future.

Michael Shally-Jensen

See also: Anxiety and Its Treatment; Biofeedback; Electroconvulsive Therapy; Mental Hospitals

Further Reading

Greenberg, Gary. 2010. *Manufacturing Depression: The Secret History of a Modern Disease.* New York: Simon and Schuster.
NIMH (National Institute of Mental Health). 2017. "Major Depression." https://www.nimh.nih.gov/health/statistics/major-depression.shtml
Nydegger, Rudy. 2016. *Understanding Depression.* Santa Barbara, CA: Praeger.
Slater, Lauren. 2018. *Blue Dreams: The Science and the Story of the Drugs That Changed Our Minds.* New York: Little, Brown.
Yan, Jun. 2017. "Percentage of Americans Taking Antidepressants Climbs." *Psychiatric News (American Psychiatric Association).* https://psychnews.psychiatryonline.org/doi/full/10.1176/appi.pn.2017.pp9b2

DIANETICS

The main source for the early development of Scientology, Dianetics represents a set of concepts and practices concerning the relationship between the mind and body as set forth by Scientology's founder, L. Ron Hubbard (1911–1986). Hubbard, a science fiction writer, published the book *Dianetics: The Modern Science of Mental Health* in 1950. In it, the author described a self-help system that went beyond the usual understandings of the causes of ill health and the remedies to be applied. Instead, Dianetics, as a system, incorporated many novel ideas and methods that Hubbard believed could both cure individuals and, if practiced on a global scale, reconstitute humanity itself.

Teachings and Expansion

One of the key concepts of Dianetics is the *engram*, an unconscious memory, or imprint, of past trauma (emotional or physical). The engram stands as a barrier

---

Scientology and *South Park*

The irreverent adult cartoon *South Park* debuted in 1997. With new episodes continuing to be aired 20 years later, the show, by Matt Stone and Trey Parker, has taken potshots at just about every social situation that exists—including Scientology.

In Season 9, episode 12 ("Trapped in the Closet"), the character of Stan joins the Church of Scientology. He is found to be the reincarnation of L. Ron Hubbard, the founder of Scientology, and is revered by well-known Scientologists such as Tom Cruise and John Travolta. The episode contains a condensed version of the story of Xenu, drawn from the organization's own texts, and has a running caption of "This is what Scientologists really believe." Later, the president of the church admits to Stan that Scientology is just a big moneymaking scheme.

The episode generated a fair amount of controversy. Isaac Hayes, the actor who portrayed the prominent character of Chef, asked to be released from his contract, finding the episode offensive. Due to the church's litigious reputation, the credits for the show were only made-up names like John Smith and Jane Smith.

The episode's title, "Trapped in the Closet," is actually a reference to rumors around Tom Cruise's sexuality. Many fans wondered if Cruise would sue the show creators, but no such lawsuit appears to have occurred. There were also rumors that Cruise refused to participate in a press junket for the film *Mission Impossible III* if the episode was reaired on a scheduled date; the show was pulled, but Cruise and his representatives denied that they had made any such threat. The episode has occasionally been reaired, but notably, Cartoon Network has not stopped the episode from proliferating online.

---

between the individual and his or her intellectual and spiritual growth, interfering with one's sense of freedom, happiness, and success. Stored in the mind like a kind of silent recording, the engram becomes a source of faulty thinking and irrational behavior. Other key concepts that play a major role in Dianetics are the *reactive mind*, a mostly unconscious mechanism in which engrams are stored and that functions reactively, or in a stimulus-response fashion; the *analytical mind*, which is the opposite of the reactive mind and can reflect on conscious thought processes and memories; *auditing*, a process whereby engrams are brought to the surface, typically by means of an *E-meter*, which is a device comparable to a lie detector (it measures physiological responses to statements during the auditing process); and, finally, *Clear*, the state of being free from the reactive mind and any irrational behaviors stemming from engrams. Although in some ways it may remind readers of psychoanalysis, Dianetics is different in that the reactions of the subject are not interpreted but simply monitored—treated as signals indicating the subject's status vis-à-vis the path to becoming "Clear." Followers of Dianetics/Scientology, in fact, have been among the most determined critics of psychology in general and psychotherapy in particular. They hold that their system is far more objective and beneficial, and that psychology and psychotherapy are distortive.

By the mid-1950s, Dianetics had begun to evolve from what was originally a self-help method into a broader *religious* system—or what its followers call an "applied religious philosophy." Thus was Scientology proper—a philosophy of mind and a spiritual quest—born. Reportedly, as people undergoing auditing began accounting for their engrams in terms of seeming past lives that they had led, Hubbard felt it necessary to expand the metaphysical dimensions of Dianetics to reflect this alternative conception of human nature and the universe. In the end, he advanced a cosmology that was not unlike that of ancient Gnosticism. The universe, said Hubbard, was made up of eight concentric circles called the Eight Dynamics. Human beings were said originally to have been divine beings known as *thetans*. The thetans had fallen into a state in which they were enmeshed in matter-energy-space-time, or MEST. Being tied up in material existence, they had lost sight of their true capacities. It is the goal of Scientology to restore to thetans the knowledge of their true selves and their full capabilities, at which point they become known as *Operating Thetans* (OTs). Hubbard described a hierarchy of mental and spiritual stages ranging from "pre-clear" and "Clear" to OT I, OT II, and beyond. An individual advances through the different levels by taking progressive Scientology courses, for which, usually, substantial fees are charged. Critics therefore claim that Scientology is a perverse kind of religion, or even a kind of cult. Scholars sometimes group Scientology with UFO groups because both essentially claim the existence of a deep "truth" that has yet to be discovered by the mainstream community. Moreover, Scientology's belief system features alien beings and space travel.

Among the most controversial beliefs in Scientology is the concept of *body thetans*, known from the various accounts Hubbard left of them. A body thetan is a disembodied thetan—like a spirit or soul—who exists in or in proximity to a human body; clusters of these thetans infest and/or irritate human individuals, seeking to regain their "free will." In doing so, they leave physical and mental scars on their subjects. According to Hubbard, body thetans were created some 75 million years ago when a galactic dictator named Xenu, seeking to relieve a massive overpopulation problem, brought alien beings to Earth in space vehicles (which happened to be perfect copies of DC-8 airliners) and inserted them into live volcanoes. The souls of these beings were then subject to additional abuse. Afterward, they came to attach themselves to ancestral human beings and, ultimately, to us, causing much personal harm along the way.

The "space adventure" aspect of Hubbard's cosmology is viewed by Scientology's own leaders as potentially so controversial that it is treated as a major "trade secret," to be known only by higher-level insiders. In the course of undergoing auditing, Scientologists often reveal that they have led past lives on distant planets and have engaged in space travel and/or intergalactic warfare, and such. Yet, they are not supposed to tell others—even other Scientologists—about their stories. The goal of the practicing Scientologist is to reach the upper OT stages in order to allow one to understand the "whole track" of his or her existence. In Hubbard's view, numerous interplanetary civilizations have existed throughout time. Upon death, therefore, one embarks on another life adventure set in some other universe. Hubbard himself, before he died following a stroke in 1986, observed that he had existed for many *trillions* of years and had twice visited Heaven, among other places.

The Church of Scientology has claimed that it is one of the fastest growing religious movements today, yet estimates have placed the number of Scientologists in the United States at between 25,000 and 50,000, and declining. Worldwide, there are perhaps twice that number. The church's headquarters, called Gold Base, is in San Jacinto, California. There are housed many of the top *Sea Org* members, or those who form the inner command of the church. Sea Org, which operates in a quasi-military fashion (with maritime uniforms, ranks, etc.), got its name from a time in the late 1960s when Hubbard managed church affairs from a fleet of four small ships in order to avoid tax investigators and other federal regulators. Upon Hubbard's death, and following an internal struggle within the church, a relatively young member of Sea Org, David Miscavige, took over as Scientology's head.

Criticism and Reaction

From the beginning, Scientology has had an unusual standing as a religion. Soon after publishing the book *Dianetics,* Hubbard lost the rights to it. (They went to a distributor, instead.) He subsequently argued that Dianetics, his system of self-improvement, was a religion and moreover that he held the rights to Dianetics terminology, its principles, the E-meter, and the mechanics of auditing. These things are collectively referred to as *spiritual healing technology*, or *tech*. Hubbard succeeded in his claim and, today, the Church of Scientology owns and publishes the book (under a separate imprint). The current leader of the church, Miscavige, is known officially as the Chairman of the Religious Technology Center, a corporation that controls the copyrights and trademarks of Dianetics and Scientology. The chief source of income for the church is not charitable donations, as with most churches, but sales of its courses and auditing services. Many Scientologists admit that they spend enormous amounts of their personal earnings on "tech," but that is the only way to advance. For this reason, Scientology has run into problems with a number of governments worldwide that claim it functions more like a business than a faith.

The church, in fact, has been involved in countless court cases, some instigated by critics or former Scientologists and others instigated by the church itself. The church maintains a substantial financial "war chest" for just such suits. Critics have argued that Scientology owes more to Hubbard's particular interpretations of science and psychology than it does to a developing theology. They point to, among other things, the centrality of "tech" in Scientology's doctrines and methods. Scientology has responded to these claims by declaring the movement a religion on the basis of its unique vocabulary, its reliance on a core text, and its use of a creed and various rituals of observance. In its official catechism, Scientology is described as a "the only major new religion to emerge in this undeniably turbulent twentieth

DIET AND EXERCISE   113

century," one whose "approach to the mysteries and problems of life is based on fundamental axioms that isolate and describe the very factors of life." Scientology is said to "encompass the entire scope of life"; and "the answers it provides apply to all existence and have broad-ranging applicability" (Catechism, n.d.).

Unlike most new religions, Scientology is not particularly critical of the older, established religious orders. Instead, it has reserved most of its criticism for the mental health profession, particularly its utilization of antidepressants, antipsychotic medication, and electroconvulsive ("shock") therapy. Scientology sees itself not as lessening people's awareness or making them more tractable, as psychiatry is accused of, but as awakening people and bringing them greater freedom and truth. The church has long targeted the Internal Revenue Service and similar agencies, both in the United States and abroad, in an effort to establish its religious bona fides (and thus qualify for tax-exempt status). These positions have tended only to add to the controversies that seem to have been part of Scientology's history from the beginning. The French government, for example, has declared Scientology a cult, one that cannot enjoy the favored status of a religion. (Indeed, several Scientology officials in France have been convicted of crimes such as fraud and embezzlement.) In the United States, Scientology was given tax-exempt status in 1993. Its critics, however, have questioned that decision. There also have been a variety of reports from church "defectors" who have claimed physical punishment and/or emotional abuse inside the church organization. Here, too, the church has fought back. Individuals who do end up leaving Scientology are shunned by church members, even by those of one's own family.

Michael Shally-Jensen

See also: Alternative Diagnostics; Anthroposophic Medicine; Biofeedback; Electroconvulsive Therapy; Faith Healing and Prayer; Psychoanalysis; Recovered Memory Therapy, "Split Personality," and Satanism

Further Reading

Bednarowski, Mary Farrell. 1989. *New Religions and the Theological Imagination in America.* Bloomington: Indiana University Press.

Church of Scientology. "A Scientology Catechism." www.whatisscientology.org/html/Part12/index.html

Ortega, Tony. 2012. "Why Do Scientologists Accept the Xenu Story?" *Village Voice,* July 12, 2012. www.villagevoice.com/2012/07/21/why-do-scientologists-accept-the-xenu-story/

Urban, Hugh B. 2011. *The Church of Scientology: The History of a New Religion.* Princeton: Princeton University Press.

Wright, Lawrence. 2013. *Going Clear: Scientology, Hollywood, and the Prison of Belief.* New York: Knopf.

DIET AND EXERCISE

Diet and exercise, two main tracks of a healthy lifestyle, became concerns for many people only in the modern era. While in past centuries most people just struggled to survive and worked too hard to think about extracurricular physical activity, a growing segment of the population in the modern period had the luxury of making some choices regarding the way they lived. Even though it was far from perfect, scientific knowledge was beginning to help people have a better understanding of how food and work environments affected their lives. By the early 19th century, advances in transportation allowed a greater range of dietary choice for the typical consumer, especially in urban areas. In addition the gymnasium, a place for indoor sports or exercise originating in ancient Greece, enjoyed a resurgence in Germany during the early-19th century, and emigrants from Germany soon brought the idea to North America. Together, these developments laid the foundation for the creation of a "health and fitness" movement that, in one form or another, has continued into the present.

Diet Plans

The European health and fitness movement began in the gymnasium. In the United States, on the other hand, it began with some religious leaders proclaiming that certain dietary strictures—including temperance—should be followed as part of a lifestyle that promoted morality and helped one to move toward spiritual perfection. (The United States has always been uniquely religious in that way.)

Reverend Sylvester Graham (1794–1851), the first self-proclaimed "national health expert" as well as a temperance advocate and an evangelistic preacher, believed that the American diet was a major contributor to social decline. During the 1820s, he had become a vegetarian, and he urged his followers to do the same—not only in order to have healthier bodies but, more importantly, to have a purer, less "carnal" lifestyle. As part of the bland diet that Graham believed would produce a more harmonious way to life, he advocated using whole grain flour in the making of bread and crackers. His invention came to be known as graham crackers. Although he carried many of his teachings with him to the grave, in their time they achieved some popularity, and he did succeed in making the vegetarian movement widely known.

Other people linked to other religious denominations pushed vegetarianism as part of their own tenets. Individuals like John Harvey Kellogg (1852–1943), a fervent Seventh Day Adventist, followed Graham's ideas about certain foods promoting sexual urges, which in turn cause disease and harm one's physical and spiritual fitness. Operating the Battle Creek Sanitarium, Kellogg, along with his brother, created Kellogg's Corn Flakes as their contribution to the U.S. diet. While temperance, or moderation in the use of alcohol, remained a part of many churches' doctrines, as the 19th century waned, so too did the widespread inclination to connect diet with religion or spiritual health.

In England, concerns regarding diet had to do with weight control, rather than with the spiritual matters that seem to have inspired the Americans. As it happened, the first diet that spread across the United Kingdom and parts of Europe was the opposite of the type pushed in the United States. William Banting (1796–1878) was overweight, and after failing to lose weight by exercise, he tried attending to his diet. Working with a doctor, Banting ended up eating plenty of meat and virtually no starches. Thus, in 1862 he was on a successful low-carb, high-fat diet of the kind that would be known as the Atkins Diet in the 1970s and onward. The Banting Diet was the leading medically recognized diet plan, in both the United States and Europe, for nearly 90 years.

For weight-conscious Americans, however, other ideas were also tried. Horace Fletcher (1849–1919) advocated chewing food until it was as liquid as possible and then swallowing the liquid and spitting out any remaining solids. Calorie counting became possible in the 1920s, when a book listing the number of calories in different foods was published. This became the basis for what were considered "scientific" weight-loss diets in later decades, since taking in fewer calories than one burns can cause weight loss. Nevertheless, the difficulty of counting calories has always made "fad" diets popular, whether or not they work. In recent decades, many promoters have found success by marketing unique, and often short-lived, dietary programs, from the Scarsdale and Atkins diets to the South Beach and Beverly Hills diets, not to mention so-called lifestyle services such as Weight Watchers, Jenny Craig, and Nutrisystem. Research done during these decades has confirmed the health value of not being obese and of maintaining a balanced diet; no easy solutions have been found, however, for helping people to eat only healthy foods and to overcome the desire to eat more than necessary, given our modern lifestyle and given the massive influence of the food and restaurant industries and their tempting products and advertisements.

Fitness

Exercise, or the fitness regimen, represents another side of modern health and wellness, and movements have developed around this activity as well. It started with organized activities for groups in Europe and then moved to the United States and elsewhere. In addition to local gymnasiums, regional activities, such as the Scottish Highland Games, were started during the first half of the 19th century, in part, to promote strength and general fitness. Similarly, at the end of the 19th century the modern Olympic Games were begun, which inspired athletic development by teams and individuals.

In the United States, there were proponents of exercise (including gymnasiums) during the first half of the 19th century, but they produced limited results. J. C. Warren, a Harvard professor of medicine, encouraged exercise, including calisthenics; and the educator Catharine Beecher pushed an aerobic-style exercise regime for women. In the post–Civil War period, exercise and gymnastics became much more common in the United States. Groups like the Young Men's Christian Associated (previously a group organized to study the Bible) added gyms and swimming pools in the 1880s and remains a strong presence today. Dioclesian Lewis was a prime mover in the revived gymnastics movement, as physical education was added to the curricula of many schools. Also adding to the small yet significant fitness boom of the late 19th- century was the beginning of athletic competitions in the new sports of baseball and football, quickly followed by basketball and volleyball. Into the early 20th century, gymnasium exercises and sports were mainly the realm of the upper class.

Virtually all the leaders in the fitness movement adopted what they considered healthy diets, generally skipping highly processed foods and pushing whole grain and raw foods, which they saw as a key to maximizing the benefits of exercise. One of the individuals who began mass-marketing fitness was Bernarr Macfadden. Having health problems when he started working in an office, Macfadden began an exercise and diet regimen that restored his own health and strength. He founded *Physical Culture* magazine in 1899, as a step toward encouraging and enabling the urban masses to exercise and do activities that contributed to a healthy life.

An individual who came to epitomize exercise and fitness for much of the first half of the 20th century was Charles Atlas (Angelo Siciliano), who won Macfadden contests in 1921 and 1922. The exercise program that Atlas developed and marketed, called Dynamic Tension, was used by countless individuals, and his ads originated the term "97-pound weakling" as a foil for the muscular person. His name and commercial style are still sometimes employed in programs promoting fitness regimens involving body-building-type activities and the body builder's physique.

Although he had worked (and owned) exercise clubs prior to the television era, Jack LaLanne became the first superstar of TV fitness programs. His influence on many later icons of fitness was significant. Just as technology progressed in other areas of life, beginning in the post–World War II era technology reshaped exercise and fitness regimes. Television and, more recently, the Internet have allowed theories, techniques, and products that are sponsored by exercise gurus to spread rapidly, whether helpful or not. In the 1980s there was the Jane Fonda Workout, and in later decades there have been any number of similarly branded workout routines, often paired with dietary advice.

Donald A. Watt

See also: Dance Therapy; Detox Diets; Diet Pills and Metabolism Boosters; Fat and Obesity Surgery—and Other Weight-Loss Methods; Infomercials and Wellness Promotion; Juice and Juicing; Macrobiotics; Paleo Diet; Vegetarianism; Vitamins and Minerals; Walking and Jogging; Yoga

Further Reading

Black, Jonathan. 2013. *Making the American Body: The Remarkable Saga of the Men and Women Whose Feats, Feuds, and Passions Shaped Fitness History.* Lincoln: University of Nebraska Press.

Dalleck, Lance D., and Len Kravitz. 2002 "The History of Fitness." In *The University of New Mexico: Exercise Science.* Albuquerque: University of New Mexico. www.unm.edu /~lkravitz/Article%20folder/history.html

Grover, Kathryn, ed. 2012. *Fitness in American Culture: Images of Health, Sport, and the Body, 1830–1940.* Amherst: University of Massachusetts Press.

Segrave, Kerry. 2008. *Obesity in American, 1850–1939.* Jefferson City, NC: McFarland.

Shiprintzen, Adam D. 2013. *The Vegetarian Crusade: The Rise of an American Reform Movement, 1817–1921.* Chapel Hill: University of North Carolina Press.

Wdowik, Melissa. 2017. "The Long, Strange History of Dieting Fads." *Colorado State University: Source.* Fort Collins: Colorado State University. source.colostate.edu/the-long-strange-history-of-dieting-fads/

DREAM INTERPRETATION

Dreams are sequences of images, sounds, and feelings that are experienced by subjects during sleep. They often have a rough narrative form, although that is not an essential criterion. More to the point, dreams are not just witnessed but *experienced*: things happen (or seem to), people appear, actions take place, and emotions are felt. All of this occurs, however, in a fantasy world. Many people forget dreams as soon as they awaken; others retain memories of them and may seek to interpret them.

In earlier eras dreams were conceived of as supernatural communications, prophecies, or wanderings by the soul in the world of the spirits. Peoples and cultures around the globe have each had their own unique approach to interpreting dreams and their meanings. Connecting past actions with the present and/or the future is one common focus, however, as is appreciating, via dreams, the impact of one's actions on "the ancestors." In the West, dreams have long been speculated about by philosophers but were only taken up as a subject of systematic psychological research in the late 19th century. Western theories of dream interpretation often are tied up with questions of (mental) health and pathology, but they also deal with questions concerning social relations, career directions, and other matters that occupy the mind during both the day and the night.

Freud and Jung

Sigmund Freud (1856–1939), the founder of psychoanalysis, was the first major thinker to offer a comprehensive theory of dreams. In his *Die Traumdeutung* (1900; translated as *The Interpretation of Dreams* in 1913), Freud presented his views on the sources, formation, and functions of dreams and his method of interpreting them. The book was revised and enlarged several times during Freud's lifetime and consistently ranks as one of the great books of the Western canon.

Freud believed that dreams served two main purposes: (1) to fulfill repressed, unconscious wishes, especially those that are sexual or aggressive in nature; and (2) to preserve the sleeping state for the subject, since if the disturbing nature of his dreams became known to him, he most certainly would awaken. Thus, according to Freud, dreams often come in disguises. Through a variety of means—such as condensation (the fusion of two or more dream thoughts into one), displacement (the deflection of disturbing thoughts or images onto a neutral object), and symbolization (the use of, e.g., a metaphorical image for the real one)—a dream is distorted in such a way as to become more or less acceptable to the dreamer, even though it can still be powerful. As Freud saw it, then, the *manifest*, or surface, content of the dream is less threatening to the dreamer than the *latent,* or underlying, content. The process of disguising a dream (called dreamwork) is never perfect, however, and such slipups can provide clues regarding the dream's meaning when it comes to interpreting it.

Freud maintained that the contents of dreams are made up of memories but that the impetus behind a dream is inevitably an unconscious wish that links back to the dreamer's childhood. To uncover the childhood wish, one must work through the various distortions present as well as any so-called secondary elaborations, or details and connections added by the subject in the act of remembering or retelling the dream. (We often tend to make our dreams more coherent in reviewing them.) Once the component parts of the dream have been identified by the psychoanalyst, the subject is invited to free-associate on each and every element—that is, to say whatever occurs to him regarding them. In this way the dream as remembered is translated into its latent, or "real," content and used to understand the drives and motivations of the dreamer. As Freud proclaimed, dreams provide a "royal road into the unconscious" because during sleep we reveal our darkest selves to ourselves, albeit only through a flanking maneuver. In any case, dream interpretation is one of the essential apps in the psychoanalyst's cache to understand and treat patients.

Like Freud, Carl Jung (1875–1961) believed that dreams were largely symbolic, and Jung too analyzed the dreams of his patients to get at otherwise unexpressed thoughts and emotions. Jung's view of the function of dreams differed somewhat from Freud's notion of wish fulfillment, for Jung held that dreams served to compensate for aspects of the dreamer's personality that are neglected in her conscious life. That is, whereas Freud understood dreams to be linked to infantile wishes, Jung ascribed them to innate thought patterns, or archetypes, common to all humanity. Such archetypes express themselves in dreams not as cryptic distortions but as symbols, which have a universal quality to them. For Jung, then, dreams seek to reveal neglected elements of the personality, not to conceal disturbing thoughts from the dreamer. Yet, like the twisted dreams of Freud's dreamwork, the archetype-based dreams of Jung's theory of the unconscious employ imperfect or incomplete symbols in any given dream. Therefore, the analyst must explore, with the subject, all possible meanings of an archetypal symbol in order to arrive at the true meaning of a dream. Jungian analysts go beyond childhood memories and make use of mythology, comparative religion, and cultural history in interpreting dreams. His particular concern was with individuation, or how people achieve separate identities while maintaining psychic wholeness. Because each person goes through this process in the course of development, Jung believed that myths and visions held striking parallels with individual experience.

Other Theories

Dream interpretors can also make use of other, surveylike methods of collecting dreams and analyzing large numbers of them to arrive at conclusions regarding individual dreams and their meanings. The main method here is collecting reported dreams from one person over time or from a group of people, and applying content analysis. This consists of categorizing the various elements that appear in dreams and comparing them with another set or another human group. One can look, for example, at characters, objects, events, storylike themes, and so on, as well as which elements are associated with such variables as gender, friend or stranger, aggression, passivity, sexuality, luck, misfortune, et cetera. These variables tend to be stable across time in individuals or groups. Content analysis can then be used to determine similarities and differences among individuals or groups on the basis of age, gender, ethnicity, and, mental and/or general health.

For example, it is generally the case that male dreamers dream as often if not more about other males than about females—a somewhat surprising fact for many (Hall 2012). Women, in contrast, dream equally often of both sexes, more or less—also perhaps surprising. Male dreamers typically have more frequent dreams of aggressive actions toward other males, and of friendly or sexual actions toward females. Female dreamers, on the other hand, have roughly equal proportions of aggression-themed and friendly themed dreams, featuring both males and females. In some, but not all, cases, a male dreamer who experiences a high frequency of dreams featuring hostility toward women could be facing a mental health issue.

One researcher has suggested that dreaming is not necessarily a matter of deep, symbolic expression, or anything like that; rather, it might just be a delirium-like state that serves, merely, to allow the brain to go offline (Hobson 2003). On this view, in sleeping we all intermittently experience a mild form of insanity, for the betterment of our health. In other words, dreaming is a kind of natural biofeedback and perhaps even a crude therapy. Nightmares, too, have been researched for what they might say about the mental state of the dreamer. Some evidence suggests that people for whom nightmares are common may experience anxiety in their waking lives, whereas other research indicates that it is not so much the frequency of nightmares that matters but the degree to which the person is affected by any given nightmare or series of them (see Barrett and McNamara 2012). Trauma, as well, appears to be related to nightmares, yet people who have not experienced trauma may still be subject to bad dreams and nightmares.

Michael Shally-Jensen

See also: Alternative Diagnostics; Dianetics; Gestalt Therapy; Jung and Jungian Analysis; Meditation and Mindfulness; Mesmerism and Hypnotherapy; Primal Therapy and Feeling Therapy; Psychoanalysis; Recovered Memory Therapy, "Split Personality," and Satanism

Further Reading

Barrett, Dierdre, and Patrick McNamara, eds. 2012. *Encyclopedia of Sleep and Dreams.* Santa Barbara, CA: Greenwood.
Hall, Calvin S. 2012. *The Meaning of Dreams: Their Symbolism and Their Sexual Implications.* N.p.: Iconoclastic Books.

Hobson, J. A. 2003. *Dreaming: An Introduction to the Science of Sleep.* New York: Oxford University Press.

Kamenetz, Rodger. 2008. *The History of Last Night's Dream: Discovering the Hidden Path to the Soul.* New York: HarperCollins.

ELECTROCONVULSIVE THERAPY

Electroconvulsive therapy (ECT) is the application of electrical current to the brain to induce a so-called tonic-clonic (or grand mal) seizure and ameliorate the symptoms of mental illness. After ECT was invented in 1938 by the Italian psychiatrist Ugo Cerletti, it became the most successful of the somatic medical remedies invented during the interwar years to combat the chronic and untreatable mental diseases of the era, which included schizophrenia, major depressions, acute manias, and paresis (a neurological disorder). At the time of the invention of ECT, and other somatic remedies, many patients were doomed to a live out their lives in the often inhumane conditions of state mental institutions, which were overcrowded and underfunded. The population of the chronic mentally ill had risen in

ECT and Lobotomy in *One Flew over the Cuckoo's Nest*

In *One Flew over the Cuckoo's Nest*, Randall McMurphy pleads insanity for a crime he has committed; in a mental hospital, he believes he will avoid hard labor and serve his sentence in relaxation. Instead, he finds himself in a ward controlled by the vicious Nurse Ratched. The nurse operates with little medical oversight and uses medication, intimidation, and treatments like electroconvulsive therapy (ECT) and lobotomies to control her patients. Originally a novel written by Ken Kesey, *One Flew over the Cuckoo's Nest* was adapted into an Academy Award winning movie in 1975.

As McMurphy enters a battle of wills with Nurse Ratched, he is first sent for ECT treatments, and later a lobotomy. While the first has no real effect on him, the second leaves him in a permanently altered and diminished state.

One Flew over the Cuckoo's Nest presents ECT as it was performed at the time—with very high doses of electricity that induced severe seizures, and without sedation. Memory loss was common after the procedure; broken bones were possible due to the strength of the seizures. ECT is occasionally used in modern medicine, but under anesthesia, and with much lower doses of electricity.

Lobotomy is the practice of surgically removing the connections between the prefrontal cortex of the brain—the area that controls most of our higher reasoning—and the rest of the brain. In most or many cases, this resulted in severe brain damage; patients were docile and easy to manage, but at the expense of their personalities and apparent intellect.

When McMurphy's friend Chief sees what has been done to the vibrant and lively McMurphy, Chief smothers his friend with a pillow rather than see him remain in this state. The film ends with Chief escaping the hospital, as McMurphy had been encouraging him to do.

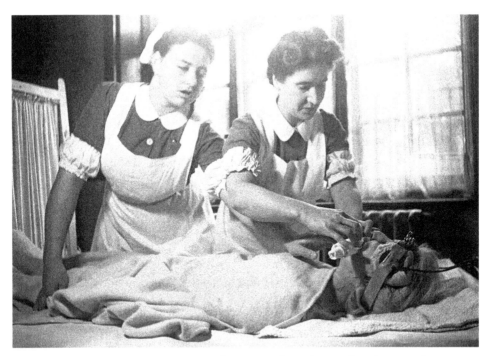

Nurses attend a patient who is receiving electroconvulsive therapy (ECT) to cure depression at a mental hospital in 1946. (Kurt Hutton/Picture Post/Hulton Archive/Getty Images)

the first years of the 20th century, prompting both European and U.S. physicians to seek a remedy for the public health crisis in new somatic interventions or heroic measures to rescue patients from a life of insanity.

Emergence of ECT

The first significant somatic treatment was developed in 1917 when Julius Wagner-Jauregg (1857–1920) discovered that following a high fever, some of his mental patients became calmer and more coherent. To induce fevers he began injecting patients with a benign strain of malaria that generated a therapeutic fever as high as 105°. Fever therapy became a standard treatment for patients suffering from paresis, the end stage of neurosyphilis, before the advent of antibiotics. For his insight Wagner-Juaregg was awarded the Nobel Prize in Medicine in 1927, and his treatment, called fever therapy, was utilized in at state institutions in the United States into the 1950s (Braslow 1997).

Manfred Sakel (1900–1957) discovered, through an accidental overdose, that placing patients with schizophrenia into an insulin coma could alleviate the psychotic symptoms of mental disease. Sakel experimented with insulin shock, as the treatment came to be called, until he discerned that the best practice was to induce a daily insulin coma, lasting for at least an hour, over a period of ten days or longer. Following a course of treatments by insulin shock, Sakel claimed that patients evinced increased lucidity, a markedly friendlier attitude, and enhanced communicative skills. Sakel boasted that his intervention had an 88 percent success rate in treating schizophrenia. In the absence of other therapies, insulin shock was adopted in both Europe and the United States, but was abandoned in the early 1950s with the advent of ECT (Valenstein 1986).

Ladislas von Meduna (1896–1964) was a neuropsychiatric researcher who studied the brain. After conducting autopsies on the brains of both epileptics and schizophrenics, he concluded that schizophrenics had a deficiency of glia tissue in their hippocampus, whereas epileptics had an overabundance. If schizophrenics could be given an artificial grand mal seizure, perhaps they would develop more tissue in this region and diminish the symptoms of schizophrenia. Thus he developed a new convulsive treatment for schizophrenia. After first trying and rejecting camphor in oil, he found pentylenetetrazol (Metrazol or Cardazol) more effective. Clinical trials with the convulsive treatment indicated that schizophrenics did show signs of remission after their convulsive treatments. From its first use in 1936 until the middle decade of the 20th century, this treatment was used frequently on schizophrenics and showed good results for patients who had only recently fallen ill (Braslow 1997).

The Italian psychiatrist Ugo Cerletti (1877–1963) was well aware of the new heroic measures but was most interested in the effects of Metrazol to induce convulsions. Cerletti wanted an even more efficient and controlled method to induce seizures than Metrazol. He and his assistant, Lucio Bini, began experimenting on dogs to determine if a nonlethal dose of electricity could be applied directly to the brain. After a series of successful experiments on dogs, Cerletti tried electroshock, his name for the procedure, on his first patient, a schizophrenic who had been brought to Cerletti's clinic by the local police. To send the patient into seizure, Cerletti tried several combinations of electrical application until he found the proper voltage and duration of electricity to generate a convulsive seizure. The patient was given electroconvulsive treatments from April to May 1938, and after only one month of electroconvulsive therapy, he showed sufficient remediation of his symptoms that he was released from the hospital (Shorter and Healy 2007).

ECT in the United States

The procedure for electroconvulsive therapy has evolved considerably from Cerletti's time. Initially it consisted of sending 70–100 volts of electricity through the brain via two electrodes placed on the temples. The tonic-clonic seizures the electrical current induced sent the body into a thrashing convulsion and patients flailed about on the table, often breaking bones, biting their tongues, and involuntarily urinating, defecating, or ejaculating. Treatments were given daily for upward of two weeks or more, and occasionally more than one treatment was given per day. Although of short duration the procedure was difficult for the untrained to watch, but the results far outweighed any concerns of that time. Treatment provided temporary respite from psychoses and neuroses and allowed institutionalized patients to return home. Thus ECT became a highly prized treatment that replaced nearly every other somatic approach available in the interwar years, including hydrotherapy, fever therapy, insulin shock, Metrazol shock, and lobotomies. Despite fears that the technique caused brain damage and memory impairment, it was adopted for a wide variety of psychoses and neuroses, and for patients as young as 2 or as old as 100 (Kneeland and Warren 2008).

Invented on the eve of the Second World War, ECT was brought to the United States by psychiatrists fleeing the Nazis, including David Impastato, Victor Gonda, Renato Almansi, and Lothar Kalinowsky. Once it was established in the United States, ECT was used to treat a spectrum of illnesses from anxiety and depression to schizophrenia. The treatment was easy to use, was more effective than any competing treatment, and was quickly established as the leading treatment for nearly every mental disease, including such "diseases" as homosexuality, cross-dressing, and nymphomania—behaviors that, at that time, were deemed to be psychological disorders. It was employed by psychiatrists, psychoanalysts, and general practitioners, and it could be found as a therapeutic tool in large state mental institutions, in private hospitals, and at the local doctor's office. Some doctors even made house calls with their portable ECT machines (Kneeland and Warren 2008).

ECT was the gold standard of somatic treatments in the United States until the invention in the 1950s of new drug therapies such as chlorpromazine (CPZ), or Thorazine, for treating psychosis (Healy 2004). Following the development of pharmacological treatments for the management of schizophrenia and major and minor depressive episodes, ECT declined greatly in use. The marketing campaign mounted by drug manufacturers was directed to physicians, psychiatrists, and state legislatures. Chlorpromazine, only eight months after its introduction, was already being used on 2 million patients suffering a range of psychotic ailments. ECT's hegemony in state mental wards began a steady decline (Kneeland and Warren 2008).

Decline of ECT

Electroconvulsive therapy was further challenged when new medications to treat depressive illnesses, the tricyclic and monamine oxidase inhibitors, were introduced (Healy 1999) for depression and anxiety. As a result of the new medications, psychoanalysts, psychotherapists, and psychologists suggested alternate treatments that employed prescription drugs together with occupational therapy, talk therapy, or behavior therapy. This undercut the use of ECT in private hospitals and private practice (Kneeland and Warren 2008).

Following on the heels of new medications in the 1950s, there was an outbreak of antipsychiatry writings in the 1960s. Intellectuals and academics such as Erving Goffman, David Rothman, and Michel Foucault challenged the entire field of psychiatry, which triggered a political and social backlash aimed at state mental institutions and their treatment of the mentally ill. Journalists began to publicly expose institutions for malpractices, including the use of somatic treatments such as ECT as a form of punishment and the physical and sexual abuse of patients by staff. Patients and their families began to challenge the institutions in court and to demand the right to refuse treatment as part of the basic civil rights guaranteed to all citizens. In response, new legislation was passed to provide for patients' rights, and federal policy moved away from building new institutions for the mentally ill to closing them down. The process, sometimes called deinstitutionalization, led to a steep decline in hospitalized patients and increased reliance on drug therapy (Grob 2011).

In the 1960s and 1970s, several former mental patients who had been treated with ECT claimed that they had permanent brain damage resulting from their experience. They attacked the practice of electroconvulsive therapy as barbaric and called for a complete ban on its use. Among the leading figures in this movement was Leonard Roy Frank, who published a thorough and impressive text entitled *The History of Shock Therapy* that attacked ECT and demonstrated its abuses. In 1973 Frank and Wade Hudson founded the Network against Psychiatric Assault (NAPA), which organized to protest all forms of psychiatric abuse. At about the same time, Ted Chabinski, who received shock as a child, started the *Madness Network News*, a publication devoted to patient advocacy. In the late 1970s Marilyn Rice, a former employee with the Department of Commerce, experienced significant memory loss following treatment with ECT and founded the Committee for Truth in Psychiatry (CTIP) in the early 1980s, which sought, among other things, to have the FDA ban electroconvulsive shock machines. After Rice died in 1992, CTIP continued under the direction of another ECT survivor, Linda Andre (Andre 2009).

ECT was indicted in novels such as Ken Kesey's *One Flew over the Cuckoo's Nest* (1962), documentaries such as Richard Cohen's *Hurry Tomorrow* (1975), and the film version of *One Flew over the Cuckoo's Nest* (1975). As a result of growing antipathy to psychiatry and ECT, an increasing number of patients were inspired to speak out about their treatment, which they said left them more damaged than when they were first admitted to the hospital (Shorter and Healy 2007). By the mid-1970s ECT was no longer viewed as a "cure," and psychiatric practice and training shifted away from somatic therapies to pharmacology and psychotherapy (Fink 2002).

Recent Changes and Critiques

ECT was considered disreputable in the media and popular culture through the 1970s and 1980s, but it was never wholly abandoned by practitioners. Led by Max Fink, Richard Abrams, Harold Sackheim, and Richard Weiner, the methods for employing ECT were revised and the treatment was restored and became a reputable treatment for mental illness at the end of the 20th century. New machines and techniques were introduced in the 1970s to deliver the electrical current in a series of brief pulses, to send the electricity through one side of the brain (unilateral), to monitor seizure duration, and to provide patients with muscle relaxers and sedatives prior to the procedure. Given muscle relaxants, patients now remain practically motionless on the table. Medication inhibits their secretions, and only their twitching toes are visible to the naked eye. At one time, practitioners observed the convulsion to assess the effectiveness of the treatment, but now the seizure is unseen and is detected by a series of machines that monitor the patients and assess the effectiveness of the seizure (Fink 2002; Kneeland and Warren 2008).

In addition to the modifications to the practice of electroconvulsive therapy, the return of ECT was aided by the discovery that even as the United States became the "Prozac nation," the pharmacological treatment of mental illness was no magic bullet. Drug therapies have their own set of side effects, can create dependency, and do not work for all patients. Antidepressant drugs work well in only 60 to 70 percent of cases in ameliorating depression. Proponents of ECT claim an 80 to 90 percent response rate. Antidepressants such as Elavil caused blurred vision, dry mouth, intestinal discomfort, sexual dysfunction, weight gain, and sleep disturbance. Prozac may cause sexual dysfunction, and even when taking the prescribed regimen, patients have reported having bouts of severe depression in an effect called "Prozac poop-out." Prozac may be addictive with the symptoms of withdrawal mimicking that of depression. Hence, the need for treatment inspired a renewed use of ECT. ECT is now commonly used on patients who did not respond to drug therapy, have suicidal ideation, or have conditions that contraindicate the use of medication. Currently, the most likely candidates for ECT include elderly patients and pregnant women. Thus ECT has returned and continues to be employed in a variety of mental disorders (Fink 2002).

One of the significant critiques of ECT has been the side effect of memory loss. There are four kinds of memory loss associated with ECT, running the gamut from very mild to significant memory impairment. All patients are subject to a postictal (i.e., postconvulsion) disorientation that lasts for a few hours. Patients are also likely to suffer anterograde amnesia and will not remember any new information received during or after their treatment. More troubling for patients is a short-term retrograde amnesia that may create memory gaps of a few days or weeks leading up to their treatment. The most serious memory damage occurs when patients suffer retrograde memory loss of months or years. The problem of memory impairment continues to generate controversy, and despite the milder procedures for employing ECT, critics of the practice remain unconvinced that "modified ECT" is any less barbaric or dangerous (Andre 2009; Payne and Prudic 2009).

The mechanism for how exactly ECT remediates mental illness remains, even today, unknown. There have been hundreds of ideas suggested as to why ECT works. Ugo Cerletti, who created the practice, continued to believe Meduna's postulate regarding the difference between the brains of epileptics and those of schizophrenics. Believing that he could isolate the source of that difference, Cerletti himself abandoned ECT. Some have suggested that the memory defects created by ECT might be the mechanism of action. Lucio Bini, Cerletti's associate, advocated what he termed "annihilation therapy," or multiple, repeated, daily dosages of shock on psychotic patients to obliterate faulty neural pathways. Other ideas on the efficacy of ECT drew on psychology. Noting that even though patients do not recall their procedure, almost all patients in the 1940s and 1950s expressed dread at the thought of receiving it; one psychologist said that the fear of ECT would lead patients to escape to health rather than face more treatment. One physician suggested that it satisfied a patient's need for punishment, that the seizure released the patient's pent-up aggression and hostility through the violent muscular convulsions (Gordon 1948).

Physiological theories about electroshock have been nearly as speculative. One early theory was that the shock produced some slight brain damage that erased the most recent neurological structures of the high brain area and thereby erased chemical pathways, thus eliminating the cognitive and somatic circumstances that precipitated mental illness. Recent research has centered on the hippocampus, where there has been evidence that ECT encourages the growth of new neurons in this region of the brain. Studies have already shown that mental disorders attack and inhibit neuron growth in this region. Thus ECT might provide a respite and regeneration of neural mechanisms. Researchers have also hypothesized that the efficacy is due to the release of neuropeptides and hormones such as prolactin, thyrotrophin, and vasopressin, which are released following ECT. Studies have also discovered that the brain responds to electroshock by functionally suppressing the convulsive effects, and it has been speculated that the resulting suppression of neural activity may be the key element of the therapeutic effect of electroconvulsive therapy (Payne and Prudic 2009).

Conclusion

Despite current debates over its specific mechanism of action, controversies over its potentially harmful side effects, and the lingering stigma of shock treatment in popular culture, electroconvulsive therapy is increasingly being employed in the practice of psychiatry, not as a measure of last resort but as an alternative to other therapies. Potential clinical uses for ECT are regularly identified in the medical literature and by proponents of the treatment such as Max Fink, thus ensuring its continued and likely expansive use into the 21st century.

Timothy Kneeland

See also: Anxiety and Its Treatment; Behavioral Theories and Therapies; Deep Brain Stimulation; Lobotomy and Other "Psychosurgeries"; Mental Hospitals; Neurodiversity; Psychedelic Drugs; Shamanism and Neo-Shamanism; Witch Trials and Exorcisms

Further Reading

Abrams, Richard. 1997. *Electroconvulsive Therapy*. 3rd ed. New York: Oxford University Press.

Andre, Linda. 2009. *Doctors of Deception: What They Don't Want You to Know about Shock Treatment*. Piscataway, NJ: Rutgers University Press.

Braslow, Joel. 1997. *Mental Ills and Bodily Cures: Psychiatric Treatment in the First Half of the 20th Century*. Berkeley: University of California Press.

Cohen, Richard, director 1975. *Hurry Tomorrow*. Richard Cohen Films. DVD.

Fink, Max. 2002. *Electroshock: Healing Mental Illness*. New York: Oxford University Press.

Forman, Milos, director. 1975. *One Flew over the Cuckoo's Nest*. United Artists.

Foucault, Michel. 1964. *Madness and Civilization: A History of an Idea in the Age of Reason*. New York: Pantheon.

Frank, Leonard Roy. 1978. *The History of Shock Therapy*. San Francisco: Leonard Roy Frank.

Goffman, Erving. 1961. *Asylums: Essays on the Social Situation of Mental Patients and Other Inmates*. New York: Anchor Books.

Gordon, Hirch. 1948. "Fifty Shock Therapy Theories." *Military Surgeon* 103:397–401.

Grob, Gerald. 2011. *The Mad among Us: A History of the Care of America's Mentally Ill*. New York: Basic Books.

Healy, David. 1999. *The Anti-Depressant Era*. Cambridge, MA: Harvard University Press.

Healy, David. 2004. *The Creation of Psychopharmacology*. Cambridge, MA: Harvard University Press.

Kesey, Ken. 1962. *One Flew over the Cuckoo's Nest*. New York: Viking Press.

Kneeland, Timothy. 1996. "The Use of Electricity to Treat Mental Illness in the United States, 1870–Present." PhD dissertation, University of Oklahoma.

Kneeland, Timothy, and Carol Warren. 2008. *Pushbutton Psychiatry: A Cultural History of Electroshock in America*. Walnut Creek, CA: Left Coast Press.

Payne, Nancy, and Joan Prudic. 2009. "Electroconvulsive Therapy: Part I: A Perspective on the Evolution of Current Practice of ECT." *Journal of Psychiatric Practice* 15:346–48.

Rothman, David. 1971. *The Discovery of the Asylum*. Boston: Little. Brown.

Sackheim, Harold. 1985. "The Case for ECT." *Psychology Today* 19:36–40.

Shorter, Edward. 1997. *A History of Psychiatry: From the Age of the Asylum to the Age of the Prozac*. New York: Wiley.

Shorter, Edward, and David Healy. 2007. *Shock Therapy: A History of Electroconvulsive Treatment in Mental Illness*. Piscataway, NJ: Rutgers University Press.

Valenstein, Elliot S. 1986. *Great and Desperate Cures: The Rise and Decline of Psychosurgery and Other Radical Treatments for Mental Illness*. New York: Basic Books.

Weiner, Richard. 2001. *The Practice of Electroconvulsive Therapy: Recommendations for Treatment, Training and Privileging*. 2nd ed. Washington, DC: American Psychiatric Publishing.

FAITH HEALING AND PRAYER

Treating illness or relieving suffering is sometimes accomplished by relying on the mind or spirit—or, in other words, divine intervention. Indeed, the term *spiritual healing* is often used as a synonym for *faith healing* or *divine healing*. A wide range of beliefs and practices is covered by these terms. At one extreme is the belief among some—e.g., Christian Scientists—that illness does not exist except as a spiritual crisis that has affected the body. These believers typically refuse the offer of medical assistance because to accept it would be a sign of a lack of faith. On the other end of the spectrum are those who turn to divine or spiritual help in combination with medical treatment, or only after such treatment has failed them. For them,

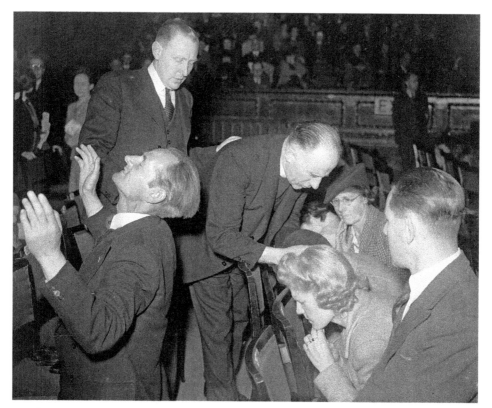

At a faith-healing session in the 1940s, people genuflect in awe and receive sacred blessings as part of the healing rite. (Walter Bellamy/Express/Getty Images)

faith is not the treatment of first resort but should be recognized as an important ingredient in one's overall health and state of mind.

Early Expressions

In traditional cultures, past and present, physical ills and emotional disturbances are usually ascribed to supernatural causes. In such cultures, the full-time healer or other practitioner (such as an experienced woman of the clan) seeks to encourage the departure of evil spirits by means of potions, charms, song, or incantations. Throughout much of the world, the local shaman/priest continues to be sought out as the source of all things medical and spiritual. In India, the classical Ayurveda texts describe the transmission of medical knowledge from gods to sages and then to human physicians. In East Asia, Buddhist, Taoist, and Shinto physicians came to be venerated by the populaces they served. In the world of ancient Egypt, Greece, and Rome, healers and special sites of healing held religious significance; the Greek site of Delphi, for instance, was known as a place for receiving oracles and was considered the navel of the world. In the Old Testament of the Bible, priests and prophets are associated with spiritual healing and the exorcising of demons. In the New Testament, Jesus and the Apostles are described as having healing powers—at least for those who placed their trust in the new Christian faith.

As Christianity developed, both the Eastern Orthodox and the Roman Catholic churches recognized special acts of healing as miracles, the details of which were to be preserved, passed down to later generations, and honored by religious pilgrims. These churches moreover provided prayers and blessings in cases of illness, and through their various religious orders (especially the Catholic orders) they offered medical care to laypersons who fell sick.

After the Reformation, and particularly with the advent of Evangelicalism in the 18th century, believers came to construe the Scriptures more literally than before; they emphasized God's healing power as part of one's personal salvation (dependent on a confession of sins, etc.). This later led to healing "cults" of various kinds. However, *during* the Reformation members of the emerging Protestant sects looked on such practices as the Anointing of the Sick as representing popular superstitions that ran against the Christian faith. Lutheran and Reformed congregations did provide for administering to the sick through nursing and prayer—but without regarding it as a sacramental act.

In subsequent centuries, an appreciation of science and medicine grew as absolute religious faith and devotion subsided. People came to regard disease as a naturally occurring phenomenon, not as a visitation by demons or a result of God's wrath. According to this more modern worldview, disease could be cured through the application of medical science. Nevertheless, sufferers understood that an abiding spiritual faith—a belief in the power of religion—was not necessarily a bad thing as far as one's health went. Thus, a belief in medicinal healing accompanied by faith remained strong in the 20th century and continues to be so today. Faith healing as such, on the other hand, is pursued by an increasingly small number of religious believers together with those who "convert" to a spiritual worldview in the face of death.

Later Variations

One person who looms large in the development of faith healing in the late 19th and early 20th centuries is Mary Baker Eddy (1821–1910), founder of Christian Science. Eddy, in turn, was influenced by one Phineas P. Quimby (1802–1866), a mesmerist, magnetizer, and philosopher who borrowed from the thought of Emanuel Swedenborg (1688–1772), G. W. F. Hegel (1770–1831), and Ralph Waldo Emerson (1803–1882). Quimby was active as a healer in New England in the mid-19th century. Eddy was a student and patient of his, although she later disavowed Quimby's influence on the development of Christian Science.

Eddy and her followers in Christian Science hold that disease, pain, and suffering essentially do not exist; they are merely effects, or illusions, caused by faulty mental processes: a mind that has become overly focused on the visible, material world instead of the spiritual realm. Such mundane evils, according to Eddy, can be eliminated by engaging in "right thinking," that is, by working to root out of negative, delusional thoughts and concentrating on the true and the real—in this case, God and the goodness he brings. Although Eddy faced harsh criticism for her approach to human suffering, and for the quizzical nature of her writings (particularly, *Science and Health,* 1875), Christian Science managed to win a small early following and eventually blossomed into a 250,000-plus member religious community. (Today, that number is much smaller.) Christian Science Reading Rooms, where healing through thought and prayer is supported, are located in thousands of towns and cities across the United States and beyond. They represent, as it were, the "clinics" of the Christian Science mission. Other denominations arising from the same idealistic metaphysics that gave birth to Christian Science emerged, in Eddy's time and after, under the umbrella term of New Thought organizations.

Faith healing began to grow in popularity in the early 20th century, reaching a peak during the 1980s. In the decades between 1910 and 1950, for example, a Pentecostal movement involving the handling of live venomous snakes spread in the Appalachian region. The impetus for this movement lay in the Gospel of Mark: "And these signs shall follow them that believe: In my name shall they cast out devils; they shall speak with new tongues. They shall take up serpents; and if they drink any deadly thing, it shall not hurt them; they shall lay hands on the sick, and they shall recover" (Mark 16:17–18). Thus, those who could hold and release vipers without coming to harm gained a unique power that helped to keep them in good health and allowed them to cure others. On the other hand, those who were bitten and died were regarded either as undeserving of the spiritual gifts or simply as persons whose time was up according to God's plan.

The varieties of faith healing that emerged later in the 20th century differed somewhat from the older versions in that disease was not dismissed as somehow unreal, and healing was thought to be a gift from God rather than any self-directed form of thinking. Healing was often accomplished by the "laying on of hands," by prayer, and by anointing penitents with oil. Certain Protestant "tent revivals," marked by ecstatic expressions of faith and acts of healing, became very popular before the television era and remained popular afterward. With television, however, such "healing crusades" could reach a much wider audience. These programs, and televangelism in general, contributed to the expansion of faith healing in the 1980s.

Skepticism

The phenomenon of faith healing has been examined by both outside critics and ecclesiastical commissions of various sorts. In looking at what are said by believers to be spontaneous cures of physical and emotional ailments, observers have generally taken a sympathetic yet skeptical view. The concern among many is that those who become involved in faith healing can encounter disillusionment later on or may fail to seek medical assistance when it is needed. Another concern is that faith healing may propagate illusions about the reality of death, when in general a healthy reckoning with death is advised. Finally, critics worry that spurious or mendacious healers are common, and it is best to protect the sick and the worried from them and their prodigious "gifts."

Michael Shally-Jensen

See also: Anthroposophic Medicine; Astrology; Dianetics; Meditation and Mindfulness; Moral Treatment; Native American Traditional Medicine; Past Life Regression Therapy; Self-Help; Shamanism and Neo-Shamanism; Spiritualism; Voodoo and Santería; Witch Trials and Exorcisms

Further Reading

Curtis, Heather D. 2007. *Faith in the Great Physician: Suffering and Divine Healing in American Culture, 1860–1900.* Baltimore: Johns Hopkins University Press.

Grazier, Jack. 1989. *The Power Beyond: In Search of Miraculous Healing.* New York: Macmillan.

Offit, Paul A. 2015. *Bad Faith: When Religious Belief Undermines Modern Medicine.* New York: Basic Books.

Opp, James William. 2005. *The Lord for the Body: Religion, Medicine, and Protestant Faith Healing in Canada, 1880–1930.* Montreal: McGill-Queen's University Press.

Robinson, James. 2014. *Divine Healing: The Years of Expansion, 1906–1930.* Eugene, OR: Pickwick Publications.

GESTALT THERAPY

Gestalt therapy grew out of a school of psychology that originated in Germany in the 1920s, entered the United States in the 1930s, and came together as a type of therapy in the 1940s and 1950s. The word *gestalt* (gə-shtält') is German for "form," "shape," or "pattern," and both Gestalt psychology and Gestalt therapy are concerned with the wholeness of perception and experience and with the patterning of thought and behavior. The notion of "the whole," as in a total configuration, is central to the Gestalt approach. A common example of this is the experience of listening to music: one does not merely add together the individual notes to appreciate a piece of music; rather, the music is experienced as a whole, as a complete sound (harmony, melody, etc.), at any given moment. Gestaltists, therefore, argue that human perception and behavior cannot be usefully broken down into artificial bits like rudimentary sensations and responses; rather, they must be examined as wholes. When these components are brought together, in experience, something new emerges from the combination, something that does not exist in the individual parts. Experience is not the sum of discrete elements but rather a dynamic system that is greater—more unitary, more meaningful—than the sum of the parts. Whereas behavioristic approaches, in contrast, treat human beings essentially as passive responders to external stimuli, Gestalt psychologists and psychotherapists view humans as active agents trying to understand and cope with their environment.

Origins of *Dr. Strangelove?*

The 1964 movie *Dr. Strangelove* by legendary director Stanley Kubrick is an iconic film in U.S. history. The protagonist, Dr. Strangelove, is an ex-Nazi who winds up working at the center of the U.S. government's nuclear security apparatus. He suffers from a strange ailment (possibly alien hand syndrome) that causes him to be unable to completely control one arm; it is as if it has a life of its own, and occasionally it tries to give the Nazi salute. Strangelove struggles to suppress it, but it doesn't always work. He fights against his own body.

In a 1951 publication by the founder of Gestalt therapy, Fritz Perls, we find an interesting parallel to Strangelove and his odd arm. Perls, describing how a troubled individual can sometimes struggle against his own bodily urges, writes this:

> When you control an urge to pound someone with your fist by contracting the antagonistic muscles . . . thus immobilizing your arm and shoulder, the [action] does not consist of pounding yourself; it is instead a statically maintained counteraction. It is a doing of one thing and also its opposite at the same time. . . . So long as the conflict endures, the use of the arm for other purposes is impaired, energies are squandered, and the state of affairs is the same as the military situation of a destabilized battleline. Here the battleine is within the personality. (Ehrenwald 1976, 509)

Supposedly, the actor who played Strangelove in the movie, Peter Sellers, improvised his character's "battle" against his arm on the set during shooting; one can wonder, however, whether he or director Kubrick may at some point have come across this popular text of Perls's, or whether this is just a case of an interesting parallel.

Source

Jan Ehrenwald, ed. 1976. *The History of Psychotherapy.* New York: Jason Aronson.

Emergence and Development

The early Gestalt researchers Max Wertheimer (1880–1943), Kurt Koffka (1886–1941), and Wolfgang Köhler (1887–1967) had a major influence on the study of perception, thinking, and learning. Wertheimer developed a number of principles regarding the organization of perception—for example, the principles of proximity and similarity. These principles state that stimuli that are close together or similar to each other tend to be construed as a group. Koffka, for his part, examined what he called the *closure tendency*, or the way in which the mind "fills in the blanks" when presented, for example, with a cartoon or a picture made up of a minimum of lines. The observer brings the whole, the gestalt, into being. The way in which great apes learn through a kind of "Eureka experience," or the sudden formation of an appropriate gestalt, was explored by Köhler.

Koffka relocated to the United States in 1927, where he taught at Smith College in Northampton, Massachusetts. With the growth of fascism under the Nazis in Germany, Wertheimer and Köhler, too, fled Europe and found political and academic freedom in the United States—Wertheimer at the New School in New York

City and Köhler at Swarthmore College outside of Philadelphia, Pennsylvania. All three continued to research the perception and reintegration of relationships within an organized whole, the primary contribution of Gestalt psychology to psychological theory.

The development of Gestalt *therapy* is primarily associated with the German psychiatrist Fritz Perls (1893–1970). As a youth in Berlin, Perls participated in the avant-garde art scene (Expressionism, Dadaism, etc.) and later fought in the trenches during World War I. He completed studies in medicine after the war and trained as a psychoanalyst under the maverick Freudian Wilhelm Reich. After serving as an army psychiatrist in South Africa in the early 1940s, Perls and his wife and sometime collaborator, Laura Perls, left for the United States. His first book (with contributions by Laura), *Ego, Hunger, and Aggression,* originally published in 1942, was reissued in the United States in 1947. In New York City, where the Perlses settled, Perls worked with the influential existentialist author and practitioner Paul Goodman in drafting his second book, *Gestalt Therapy* (1951). The Perlses established the Gestalt Institute in their Manhattan apartment and served clients and students there in the 1950s, before Perls left the marriage and moved to California, where he became interested in Zen and began teaching at the alternative/humanist organization the Esalen Institute in Big Sur. While at Esalen, Perls aided Ida Rolf in the development of the mind–body technique known as Rolfing, or Rolfing Structural Integration. Perls himself, however, remained close to Gestalt practice and in 1969 founded a Gestalt training community on Vancouver Island, Canada. He died in 1970.

Therapeutic Aspects

Gestalt therapy differs from traditional psychoanalysis in that it emphasizes the present—the "here and now"—rather than the past. It looks at the social and environmental contexts of a person's life, the adjustments he or she makes under those circumstances, and the role of personal responsibility. Gestalt theory posits that the natural course of biological and psychological development of the human individual entails a full awareness of physical sensations and psychological needs. Such awareness is said to lead the person to organize his or her behavior in such a way as to be able to fulfill basic needs and allow for the expression of emotions. When a need is satisfactorily met or an emotion satisfactorily expressed, the matter is resolved, thereby permitting other needs and sensations to occupy one's awareness. A new adjustment to the environment is made. But if this process is interfered with, it may threaten the healthy survival of the person. Gestalt therapy rests on the idea that people strive for wholeness and completeness in their lives; a self-actualizing tendency is at work in each of us that seeks to bring that goal about.

Repression is considered the most common form of interference, upsetting the normal process of adjusting to the environment. In some cases repression can lead to a "split," or disturbance, in the personality, as unsatisfied needs linger while behavior fails to address their demands. The neurotic person has in effect separated him- or herself from his or her emotional needs and is therefore unlikely to relate productively to the environment (including to other individuals). Because the human individual, and the human psyche, is regarded as being self-regulating, awareness of needs is basically curative: the person will respond properly once fully aware of the need. The therapeutic effort, therefore, typically stresses sensorimotor awareness and the physical expression—or acting out—of repressed desires. Gestalt therapy emphasizes discovery of the self through experience rather than talk, of action and the assumption of responsibility rather than analysis and linking to the past.

An unusual example of this approach is provided by Perls's work at the Esalen Institute in the 1970s. At Esalen, Perls held "dream workshops" in which participants acted out the parts of people and objects in dreams they had had. Having dreamed of sharing a hot dog with an aunt at a restaurant, for example, a participant might be asked to "be" not only him- or herself and/or the aunt, but also the hot dog and perhaps even the restaurant or some part of it (a counter, a table, etc.). Recall that Gestalt therapy stresses treatment of the person as a whole. The idea behind this example is that every element in a dream is actually part of the self. By taking on the various roles, by identifying with the different elements, the person may gain insight and come to understand his or her condition. Another Gestalt exercise is that of the "empty chair," whereby clients interact with different aspects of their personality as if they were occupying the vacant seats. The effort is geared toward understanding the whole person and integrating any internal splits or dichotomies.

Gestalt therapy, then, aims at expanding clients' self-awareness, bringing them into close contact with their bodily sensations and repression processes, and improving their relationships with the outside world. A variety of sensorimotor and psychological exercises are designed to achieve this aim. The therapist takes an active role in the encounter, seeking to identify perceptional and emotional blockages that blind clients to their "true" feelings, their true selves. The therapist forces clients to attend to psychological and physical stimuli in the environment that had previously been blocked out. Intellectual comprehension of the underlying causes of neurotic behaviors, as with some other psychotherapies, is considered relatively unimportant, for what occurred "then and there" in the past cannot be changed, whereas what happens today in the "here and now" can be.

In group sessions there often is a "hot seat" next to the therapist where group members take turns working closely with him or her. Acting out is encouraged, and a variety of other techniques are employed to promote the ventilation of feelings. Clients are encouraged to express unresolved feelings, assert views that previously may have frightened or offended them, play different roles, and examine personal tendencies to detach, project, split, and deny feelings and attitudes. In this way, it is thought, the client will experience him- or herself as a patterned whole—a gestalt. Such experiential learning can continue outside the therapeutic situation, as people come to recognize thoughts, feelings, and reactions that negatively affect their personal functioning and interfere with living.

Fate

Perls challenged clients to see how they were covering up feelings or avoiding responsibility using a somewhat confrontational, abrasive, and theatric style. A newer version—Gestalt Practice, also known as Relational Gestalt Therapy—allows for more support, kindness, and compassion than Perls's original Gestalt therapy did. A more radical, hard-edged version is represented by Erhard Seminars Training, or est, in which one aggressively "takes responsibility" for one's life. (Yet est has a different origin and philosophy, as well.) While Gestalt therapy has been adapted for use in a group format, it was originally developed for use in individual therapy. It continues to be used for individuals with mood disorders (e.g., major depressive disorder, bipolar disorder), adjustment disorders, somatization disorders (e.g., physical symptoms with no known physical cause), and occupational or interpersonal problems. It is not normally used to treat individuals with severe emotional disturbance (e.g., schizophrenia).

Gestalt therapy offers a relatively flexible approach that helps people integrate all aspects of their lives. It considers the whole individual, in the present moment, within the context of his or her environment and relationships. Critics say that Gestalt therapy lacks a strong theoretical base. Some say that Gestalt therapy is too focused on exercises (technique) and the present experience to allow for solid insight and change. Others have said that Gestalt therapy is self-centered, focusing solely on feelings and personal discovery. A limitation of Gestalt therapy is that it does not utilize formal diagnostic tools or assessment techniques. This makes it difficult to monitor progress and change and could result in an individual receiving an inappropriate type of therapy. Obviously, it is important for Gestalt therapists to be properly trained and supervised, lest they cause harm to clients. While Gestalt therapy still exists as an alternative form of treatment, other approaches—cognitive-behavioral, psychodynamic, and behavioral—are now more popular.

Michael Shally-Jensen

See also: Client-Centered Therapy; Codependency Counseling; Drama Therapy; Encounter Groups; Est and Other "Human Potential" Therapies; Existential Psychotherapy; Mind–Body Medicine; Primal Therapy and Feeling Therapy; Psychoanalysis; Rolfing

Further Reading

Corey, Gerald. 2013. *Theory and Practice of Counseling and Psychotherapy*. 9th ed. Belmont, CA: Brooks/Cole.

Gladding, Samuel T. 2008. *Counseling: A Comprehensive Profession*. 6th ed. Upper Saddle River, NJ: Pearson Educational.

Reevy, Gretchen. 2013. "Humanistic Theories and Therapies." In *Mental Health Care Issues in America: An Encyclopedia*, edited by Michael Shally-Jensen, 336–43. Santa Barbara, CA: ABC-CLIO.

Wheeler, Gordon, and Lena Axelsson. 2015. *Gestalt Therapy*. Washington, DC: American Psychological Association.

JUNG AND JUNGIAN ANALYSIS

Carl Gustav Jung (1875–1961) was a Swiss psychiatrist and one-time associate of Sigmund Freud (1856–1939) who came to be known for his own unique investigations of the human unconscious and mythology. He examined the significance of dreams and religion in relation to problems of the mind, and he developed the idea of the collective unconscious—that is, the belief that people's feelings and reactions are often based on deep memories of human experience in the past. Jung went on to formulate new psychotherapeutic techniques designed to familiarize the person with his or her unique "myth" or place in the collective unconscious, as expressed in dream and imagination. Although his work has been criticized for being rather like a religious system for its lack of objectivity and testability, it nevertheless has proved durable as a specialized form of psychotherapy and, for some, an entire worldview.

The Life of Jung

The son of a poor Protestant clergyman, Jung was a sensitive and imaginative child, who in later life recalled his fascination with stories of Hindu deities and other religious themes that his mother read from an illustrated children's book.

Star Wars and Jungian Archetypes

Western scholars and creators love to look for the story structures that underlie myths and tales as far back as we can remember. From literature analysis to Dan Harmon of *Community* asking "What is a story?" we seek commonalities in the overall structure of stories.

While Jungian psychology has generally fallen out of favor, the Jungian archetypes continue to provide an interesting framework to look at story construction. The original *Star Wars* trilogy, in particular—*Star Wars*, *The Empire Strikes Back*, and *Return of the Jedi*—has often been held up as a perfect example of the journey of a Jungian hero and the overall structure of myth, as conceived by Carl Jung.

For example, a focus of Jung's work is the Shadow; the Shadow is considered to be the dark nature inside of everyone. Jung suggested that when we try to hide from or eradicate our Shadow, we cause ourselves pain and psychological distress. When we embrace and come to peace with our darker selves, however, we are able to be more complete, psychologically content people. The Shadow is easily compared to the light and dark sides of the Force, or to the Jedi and the Sith.

A more specific example of the Shadow happens in *The Empire Strikes Back*. When Luke Skywalker confronts Darth Vader in the cave in Dagoba, he cuts off Vader's head—only to see that Vader is himself. This is a reflection of how Luke needs to see the darkness within himself before he can finally fully embrace the light.

While myth structure is not universal in all cultures, as Jung (and later Joseph Campbell) proposed, the Jungian archetypes do provide an interesting starting place for examining myths—and stories—that have a primarily European origin.

His father taught him Latin at a young age, and he was generally a good student and avid reader. During his youth he was interested in philosophy, history, and archaeology, but a medical scholarship to the University of Basel enabled him to study psychiatry. In 1902 he completed his doctoral dissertation on spiritualism and the occult, based on his study of a young cousin who was a medium. Such subjects continued to have a place in Jung's thought throughout his career.

From 1900 to 1909, Jung was an assistant physician at the Burghölzli Psychiatric Hospital in Zurich, headed by the noted psychiatrist Eugen Bleuler, who developed the concept of schizophrenia. During 1902–1903, Jung studied briefly in Paris with the psychologist Pierre Janet—noted for his research on dissociation and trauma. In 1903 Jung married Emma Rauschenbach,

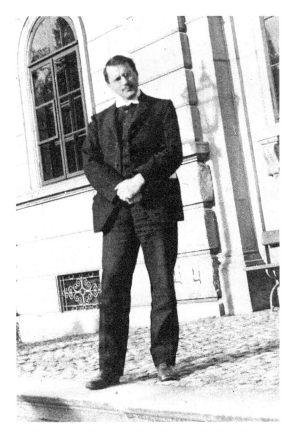

Carl Jung in 1910, shortly before his break with Freud and his development of analytical psychology. (Library of Congress)

and the couple eventually produced five children. During this period Jung's studies of schizophrenia and his development of a word association test for identifying unconscious mental blocks established his reputation as a rising professional in the field.

In 1906 Jung began corresponding regularly with Freud, and the following year he visited the great founder of psychoanalysis in Vienna. Their respect and admiration for one another was mutual at first, and for a time Freud considered Jung as his likely heir. From 1911 to 1914, Jung served as first president of the International Psychoanalytic Association. Relations with Freud became increasingly strained, however, as Jung's intellectual independence and theoretical divergence from orthodox psychoanalysis became evident. In particular, Jung was dubious of Freud's exclusive focus on the sexual origins of psychiatric symptoms and felt that Freud's interpretation of dreams and symbolism was too limited. In 1912, Jung presented his own ideas in *Psychology of the Unconscious*, whose title was changed in later editions to *Symbols of Transformation*. In this work, Jung interpreted a variety of mythological themes and uncovered parallels between ancient myths and psychotic fantasies.

After his break with psychoanalysis, Jung developed his own system which he called *analytic psychology*. For the next half century he explored and wrote about human personality, especially its symbolic, mythological, and spiritual dimensions. Although his work life appeared normal on the surface, Jung was in fact engaged in a quest of self-discovery, seeking to get at the psychic elements and forces that made him up and that he would later elaborate in his writings. In 1921 a major work, *Psychological Types,* presented Jung's theory regarding the division of humanity into extroverted and introverted personality types, along with a few others. Other books included *Psychology and Religion* (1938) and *Memories, Dreams, Reflections* (1962). Health problems forced Jung to retire from practice and teaching in 1947, although he continued to publish. He died in Zürich in 1961.

Jung's Thought

Jung held that individual consciousness develops out of a prior unconscious psyche that continues to function together with yet apart from conscious awareness. In addition to the ego, or the "I" of the conscious mind, Jung believed there is a personal unconscious made up of the individual's repressed memories, thoughts, and feelings as well as a collective unconscious shared by all humankind. The latter finds expression in the emotionally charged symbols, images, and themes that emerge spontaneously in fantasies, dreams, delusions, and myths, which vividly express and reflect basic human urges and experiences. Jung argued that evolutionary history has established deep psychic predispositions having great power to stir people's imaginations and influence their actions. These inherited tendencies are basic ways of apprehending and responding that are unconscious yet find conscious representation in various potent images and ideas. Jung called these fundamental forms of the collective unconscious archetypes, or primordial images, and investigated how they repeatedly emerge in different guises in dreams, in childhood and adult fantasies, in the delusions of the insane, and in fairy stories, myths, and religions.

Although archetypal images appear in many forms—as supernatural figures, human beings, geometrical shapes, and numbers, for example—Jung held that the archetypes themselves are limited in number. Some major archetypes include birth, death, rebirth, power, magic, unity, the hero, the child, God, the demon, the old wise man, the earth mother, and the animal. For example, the hero archetype is often found in conjunction with imagery of the sun's course and transition from day to night, seared in the human mind from time immemorial. This pattern is found worldwide in various myths of a god-hero born from the sea, who mounts the chariot of the sun; in the west he is awaited by a great mother who devours him as the evening comes; then, in the belly of the night dragon he travels the midnight sea and, after a fight, slays the dragon and is born again.

Jung had a theory about universal human bisexuality. He labeled man's feminine archetype the *anima* and woman's masculine archetype the *animus*. These archetypes not only cause each sex to manifest characteristics of the opposite sex; they also act as collective images that influence the perceptions, misperceptions, and fantasies of one sex regarding the other.

Jung viewed humans as striving for individuation, or self-realization, a psychic wholeness that works to reconcile the tensions of complementary opposites in one's personality. Among the opposed tendencies are: introversion versus extroversion, which direct attention, respectively, to inner and outer worlds; sensing versus intuiting, which are different ways of knowing; and feeling versus thinking, both ways of evaluating. Amplification of any of these psychological orientations in ego-consciousness causes its opposite to become more powerful in the unconscious, and psychic wholeness requires their creative synthesis through personal transformation and self-discovery. This centering process, or full realization and harmonious unification of the self, is integrated in the Jungian system by the transcendent function symbolized by the mandala, an ornamented circular figure divided into four symmetrical sections—a recurrent form in religious art.

Jungian Therapy

Jungian therapy, also known as Jungian analysis, is an in-depth, analytical form of "talk therapy" designed to bring together the conscious and unconscious parts of the mind (or psyche) to help individuals feel balanced and whole. This type of therapy calls for clients to dig deep into their psyches to identify the underlying archetypes and themes that define them in the world. The goal is to discover the "real" self as opposed to the self that one commonly presents to the outside world. Jungian therapy focuses more on the sources of problems than on their manifestations or symptoms. In analysis, one explores the deep-rooted causes of, for example, relationship problems and blocked emotions to achieve "individuation," or wholeness. If one tries simply to address the symptoms alone, the issues will not be resolved and are likely to resurface.

The nature of Jungian analysis requires the client to commit to regularly scheduled sessions and intense work. In addition to talking, the therapist may use a variety of techniques such as dream journaling and interpretation, along with creative modalities like art, music, or dance/movement, in order to foster self-expression and encourage the release of the imagination. Together these represent some of the more popular aspects of Jungian analysis, continuing to draw people to it today. The therapist may also use word association, whereby he or she states a prompt word and records how long it takes for the client to respond with the first thing that comes to mind—and will subsequently explore what the response might mean. A delayed response time can indicate an emotion or subject that is "blocked."

Jungian therapy has been used successfully to assist those with anxiety, depression, family or relationship problems, grief, self-esteem issues, and other emotional problems. It is also appropriate for those who want a deeper understanding of themselves and are willing to make a commitment to the work involved in acquiring that knowledge. Its appeal tends to be greatest among those who are open to a nontraditional view of the world and the importance within it of myth and the life of the spirit. Jungianism enjoyed a resurgence with the rise of the New Age/Alternative Medicine movement in the 1980s but has since faded somewhat as newer, shorter-term therapies have arisen and the culture at large has changed.

Michael Shally-Jensen

See also: Anthroposophic Medicine; Art and Music Therapy; Astrology; Drama Therapy; Dream Interpretation; Gestalt Therapy; Psychoanalysis

Further Reading

Bishop, Paul. 2014. *Carl Jung*. London: Reaktion Books.

Harrison, Judith R., with Tony Woolfson, eds. 2016. *The Quotable Jung*. Princeton, NJ: Princeton University Press.

Jung, C. G., et al. 2012. *Introduction to Jungian Psychology*. Princeton, NJ: Princeton University Press.

Mayes, Clifford. 2016. *An Introduction to the Collected Works of C. G. Jung: Psyche as Spirit*. Lanham, MD: Rowman and Littlefield.

LOBOTOMY AND OTHER "PSYCHOSURGERIES"

The surgical treatment of mental conditions goes back to the time before writing. Fossil skulls from the Neolithic (i.e., late Stone Age) period show that ancient peoples performed a procedure known as *trepanation* (trephination), or trepanning, in which a rectangular opening—a squarish hole—was cut into the skull. Trepanned skulls have been found in Eurasia as well as in the Americas, particularly in the Andes region of what is now Peru. The skulls provide evidence, moreover, in the form of healing at the edges of the incisions, that at least in some cases the patients survived the surgery. One cannot say for certain whether trepanation was performed solely for therapeutic reasons or for magical/religious reasons—or perhaps both. A hundred years ago, however, the influential physician William Osler opined that the procedure "was done for epilepsy, infantile convulsions, headache and various cerebral diseases believed to be caused by confined demons to whom the hole gave a ready method of escape" (quoted in Faria 2013). In other words, it was a crude form of psychosurgery that had the benefit of letting the demons out of a patient's head. You could call it a very physical kind of exorcism. Indeed, the bone that was removed was sometimes worn around the neck of the patient as a talisman to ward off persistent spirits. Whether patients' clinical symptoms improved or their behavior changed following trepanation, again one cannot say. Still, it shows the determination of ancient surgeons to do whatever was needed to restore a person's health.

In ancient Greece and Rome, a variety of medical instruments were developed to penetrate the skull. Hippocrates described the procedure in detail for Greek surgeons. Roman physicians, including Celsus (Aulus Cornelius) and Galen, employed a serrated drill, or burr-hole device, to perforate the cranium and made use of other tools to hold back the skin and remove any fragmented bone. Celsus also wrote about the pros and cons of human (and animal) experimentation, while

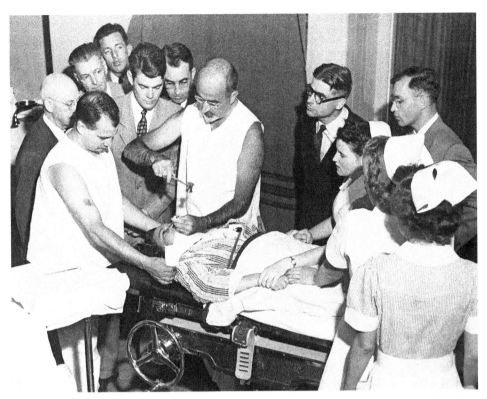

Dr. Walter Freeman performs a lobotomy, in 1949, using an instrument like an ice pick which he invented for the procedure. Inserting the instrument under the upper eyelid of the patient, Freeman cuts nerve connections in the front part of the brain. (Bettmann/Getty Images)

Galen was one of the first to think that there was a physiological basis to mental illness, rather than assuming it was caused by demons, fate, or the like.

During the Middle Ages and the Renaissance, trepanation was performed for head injuries as well as for epilepsy and madness. Well-known works of art from the period depict the surgical procedure in a realistic yet somewhat fanciful way. For example, Hieronymus Bosch's painting *The Extraction of the Stone of Madness* shows an awake patient having his head cut into by an oddly hatted physician using a triangular instrument in an outdoor setting. A similar-looking triangular trepanning instrument designed by Fabricius of Aquapendente (1537–1619) was used to address skull fractures and/or for opening and entering the skull. Fabricius, in fact, is known as the discoverer of the brain structure called the Sylvian fissure (lateral sulcus), which separates different lobes in the brain from each other (specifically, the temporal lobe from the parietal and frontal lobe).

Modern Methods?

As late as the late 19th century, brain science had not progressed very far beyond its medieval antecedents. Anatomy, or description of the brain, had advanced somewhat, but there was still very little understanding regarding the functioning of the brain and its various components. Corelating brain anatomy with behavior was still largely the business of phrenology, a popular pseudoscience at the time. Science-based researchers like J.-M. Charcot, Josef Breuer, and Sigmund Freud had begun to examine psychopathology, or "madness," in new ways, but their methods, if anything, tended to move away from neurology and toward psychology (and psychoanalysis). The classification and diagnosis of mental conditions was quite primitive at the turn of the century, and treatment was even sketchier. Therapies involving water baths, hypnosis, and extended rest and sleep were popular options, as was a rough type of shock therapy in cases of "nervous exhaustion" (neurasthenia), hysteria, and depression.

One American psychiatrist, Henry Cotton (1876–1933), came to believe that serious mental illness resulted from infections in the teeth, tonsils, and bowels. Between 1918 and 1925, Cotton performed over 2,000 surgeries to remove the afflicting organs (or parts thereof). Not only were patients unable to experience eating and defecating as they once had, but hundreds of them died from the surgery or from complications stemming from it. Cotton was soon forced into retirement by a physicians' review board, and his book, *The Defective Delinquent and Insane* (1921), quickly went out of print.

The first modern work in the field of psychosurgery, or surgery on the brain to treat serious mental disorders (e.g., schizophrenia), was done by Egas Moniz (1874–1955) of Portugal. Moniz had learned that destroying the frontal lobes of laboratory monkeys eliminated the animals' aggressive behavior and even made them unafraid of snakes, a traditional (even instinctual) enemy. He believed that the same result might be seen in human mental patients prone to violent outbursts who were given the operation. Thus was frontal lobotomy, as the procedure was called, launched in 1936. Initially, the method required the surgeon to drill two holes in the cranium and use specially designed tools to sever nerve pathways of the frontal lobes. Following the procedure, formerly hard-to-control patients became docile and easy to manage.

In the United States, a doctor named Walter Freeman (1895–1972) refined Moniz's technique and popularized the frontal lobotomy for treating schizophrenia. Freeman performed some 4,000 lobotomies between 1936 and 1958, and as news of his success spread, many other doctors, too, employed the technique. Unlike Moniz, Freeman avoided drilling holes and instead inserted an ice pick–like instrument through the supraorbital foramina, small holes above the eye sockets. From there he passed the instrument through the paper-thin bone separating the eye from the frontal lobes, manipulated the pick, and made the cut. During the years in which Freeman and other lobotomists operated, tens of thousands of patients were given the treatment, not just in the United States but worldwide. Although some patients were able to return to a life resembling a normal one, most of them were left feeling aimless and apathetic, in some cases to the point of being almost completely unresponsive. In addition, from 2 percent to 5 percent of patients died, and another 5 percent or more suffered convulsions. The behavior of many patients became even worse after surgery.

In the 1950s, therefore, lobotomy began to be abandoned in favor of drug therapy involving the use of tranquilizers, antidepressants, antipsychotics, and other medicines. Most psychiatrists today have little or no use for psychosurgery, although in some cases it is recommended that a cingulotomy or capsulotomy, operations that target more specific brain regions, be performed to address conditions such as intractable obsessive-compulsive disorder or severe depression. A procedure known as thalamotomy is sometimes used to reduce tremors in persons with Parkinson's disease.

Legacy and Prospects

Psychosurgery, even when considered successful, does not necessarily eliminate all problems or symptoms. Rather, it generally reduces a patient's reactions to the stimuli causing the symptoms. A person, for example, who hears voices and exhibits paranoia will likely not be completely free of those symptoms after surgery, but he or she will, in the best of cases, feel less threatened by them and will react less violently. Similarly, the repetitive behaviors of an obsessive-compulsive patient may be reduced by psychosurgery, but he or she may show side effects from the treatment that call into question its overall value for the patient. Psychosurgery, then, is usually the treatment of last resort.

One of the latest techniques in brain-behavior science is deep brain stimulation, or DBS. This technique involves the implantation of tiny electrodes deep inside the brain as a means of stimulating specific neuronal groups. Used for certain movement disorders and psychiatric conditions (including posttraumatic stress disorder), DBS has also been used in the treatment of pain, epilepsy, and Tourette's syndrome—not entirely successfully, however. Fortunately, unlike a lobotomy, DBS is not a permanent solution but rather can be stopped or reversed simply by removing the electrodes. It has, nonetheless, raised some ethical questions regarding the potential for brain manipulation and even the control of human perceptions and emotions if, in the future, the technology were to advance far enough for that, together with our own understanding of the complexities of the human brain.

Michael Shally-Jensen

See also: Deep Brain Stimulation; Electroconvulsive Therapy; Hysteria; Mental Hospitals; Mesmerism and Hypnotherapy; Moral Treatment; Neurasthenia, or Nervous Exhaustion; Phrenology

Further Reading

El-Hai, Jack. 2007. *The Lobotomist: A Maverick Medical Genius and His Tragic Quest to Rid the World of Mental Illness*. Hoboken, NJ: Wiley.

Faria, Miguel A., Jr. 2013. "Violence, Mental Illness, and the Brain: A Brief History of Psychosurgery—Part I—From Trephination to Lobotomy." *Surgical Neurology International* 4 (April). https://www.ncbi.nlm.nih.gov/pmc/articles/PMC3640229/

Montgomery, Erwin B., Jr. 2015. *20 Things to Know about Deep Brain Stimulation.* New York: Oxford University Press.

Valenstein, Elliot S. 1986. *Great and Desperate Cures: The Rise and Decline of Psychosurgery and Other Radical Treatments for Mental Illness.* New York: Basic Books.

MENTAL HOSPITALS

People with mental illness have faced many problems from society throughout the ages. In the past, such people were believed to be possessed by demons or the devil and were left in the care of their families or simply abandoned. They were often mistreated. Eventually, society chose to hospitalize people with mental illness, but their circumstances did not always improve. For example, the first mental hospital in Pennsylvania opened in the basement of the general hospital there. Mental health has continued to be the poor stepchild of the wider health care system ever since.

Early Development

Institutional care began in a few Arab countries; asylums were established as early as the eighth and ninth centuries to care for people with mental illness. Somewhat later in Europe, during the Middle Ages, the community began to seek confinement of people who were different. Some monasteries housed the mentally ill, usually treating them well. As societies became more urban and families became less able to care for persons with mental illness, eventually society chose to hospitalize people with mental illness.

In 1828, Horace Mann, an educational reformer, put forward a philosophy of public welfare that called for making the "insane" wards of the state. This philosophy was widely put into effect, and each state assumed responsibility for those with mental illness in that state. States often built their psychiatric hospitals in rural areas. Moral treatment and compassionate care were the main approach at this time, but with rapid urbanization and increased immigration, the state mental health systems began to be overwhelmed. Many elderly people who in rural areas would have been cared for at home could no longer be cared for when their families moved into the cities. Women, as well as men, frequently worked away from home, and there was no one to care for the elderly or see to their safety. Many people with brain-based dementias, probably caused by Alzheimer's or small strokes, became patients in mental institutions for the remainder of their lives. The institutions also had many cases of people in the last stages of syphilis. Many of those suffering from mental retardation, epilepsy, and alcohol abuse were also committed to the institutions; in hard economic times, the number of people admitted to the institutions increased.

By 1861, there were several state mental hospitals, and one federal hospital in Washington, DC. In the second half of the 19th century, attitudes changed and group and treatment practices deteriorated. Massive immigration to the United States led to a growing proportion of foreign-born and poor in the state hospitals. Most psychiatrists, community leaders, and public officials were native-born and generally well off and thus apt to be prejudiced against those who were neither (Rochefort 1993).

The classic asylum of the 1800s and the later mental hospital of the modern era were both designed to insulate the mentally ill from the pressures and community life. Each strove, to a greater or lesser extent, to provide something like a homelike environment in which rest, recreation, education, and religious expression took place alongside work and psychiatric treatment. When such institutions were small and rural, they often provided shelter and reasonably good care. It was as they became large and overcrowded, beginning in the late 19th century, that they became known for their poor conditions. As more and more people were admitted to these institutions, the focus changed from treatment to custodial care. Dangerous and unmanageable individuals increasingly were sent to state hospitals under loosened commitment laws. More patients were alcoholic, chronically disabled, criminally insane, and senile. By the early 20th century, state hospitals were often regarded as places of last resort, with mostly long-term chronic patients.

The present entry provides a kind of snapshot of hospital life for the period extending roughly from the late 1800s to the mid-1900s. Obviously, there were many variations to the basic picture; yet there were strong similarities across institutions as well.

Patient Wakeup

Residential mental institutions imposed schedules on occupants, which—while they varied by time period and patients' diagnoses—varied little by geographical location. Mental hospitals generally had specific times for rising. Friends' Asylum in Pennsylvania, supervised by Thomas Kirkbride (1809–1883) who popularized the linear design for mental hospitals, required residents to rise by 5:00 a.m. (Rothman 1970). At the Texas State Lunatic Asylum in 1861 the timing of the morning bell changed with the seasons, sounding at 4:30 a.m. from May through August, at 5:00 a.m. in March, April, September, and October, and at 5:30 a.m. from November through February (Austin State Hospital 1861).

Proponents of the 19th century "cult of curability" believed that imposing a strict routine on persons with mental illness would result not only in more orderly behavior but also in more orderly thinking (Rothman 1970). In fact, recent research does indicate longer periods between bouts of mania for individuals diagnosed with bipolar disorder when a routine is maintained (Frank et al. 2005). Not coincidentally, adherence to schedules also facilitated the running of institutions that might house several thousand patients.

Grooming

Following the wakeup bell (which later became a whistle), attendants, assisted by better-functioning patients, helped residents comb hair, wash hands and faces, and dress. A diagnosis of mental illness was often partially based on poor grooming, and mental institutions imposed strict standards of personal tidiness. Since longer hair styles for women necessitated more attention, once the "boyish bob" became fashionable in the 1920s, some hospitals required women to adopt this style.

Uniformity of clothing facilitated the identification of any escaped patients. Hospital administrators stressed the need for vigilance in preventing escape, and attendants often personally forfeited the bounty paid to citizens for returning escapees. Most institutions had fences to deter escape, and one enterprising superintendent who could not afford the cost of a fence planted an osage orange hedge instead (Lael, Brazos, and Margo 2007). As institutions became less self-sufficient toward the last third of the 20th century, only the undergarments for large patients were sewn on site.

Medications and Meals

The morning ritual also included dosing of patients. Depending on the time period and the patient's specific diagnosis, medications included sedatives, lithium, or psychotropic drugs such as Thorazine (chlorpromazine).

Dressed for the day, patients went to breakfast, with the men marching to the various dining halls. Women did not march, but followed attendants. A well-balanced diet was part of the treatment regimen. Breakfast typically consisted of oatmeal, fried eggs, biscuits, milk, and coffee (Austin State Hospital 1950).

Following the morning's work, a whistle blew signaling the noon meal, which was generally called dinner. In the 19th and early 20th centuries, most institutions produced most of their own food, which included beef, chicken, mutton, and pork from state hog farms. At this time mental hospitals resembled plantations, slaughtering and curing their own meat and growing and preserving fruits and vegetables. In the time before refrigeration, meat did not keep, and so animals were slaughtered as needed. (Graham 1866, 9).

A population of several thousand necessitated several dining rooms, which varied in quality. Typically, the best dining hall served the doctors and higher-level staff. Meals as well as housing, laundry, and medical care were part of the emoluments the hospitals provided in lieu of higher salaries. Dinner consisted of a main dish, usually meat, although beans and field peas might appear, along with vegetables, bread, iced tea, and dessert. Moving down the hierarchy of dining halls, the next level served attendants, other staff, and the better-functioning patients. At the bottom level seriously disturbed individuals, who in the 19th century were classified as the noisy or filthy insane, had their meals (Dwyer 1987, 17).

The final meal of the day, called tea in the 19th century and supper in the 20, appeared at 6:00 p.m. at the Texas State Lunatic Asylum as it did at Friends'

Asylum in Pennsylvania. A much lighter meal than dinner, it sometimes consisted of only toast and fruit or leftovers from dinner.

Work

Following breakfast many patients reported for work, tending the vegetable gardens or caring for livestock in the 19th and early 20th centuries. Mental institutions of the time strove for self-sufficiency, and most residents, having grown up on farms, knew how to perform these duties. In addition, men worked on carpentry or cement crews, on landscaping teams, or in the woodworking shop. Women performed household chores, cleaning, cooking, washing and ironing clothes, sewing, and even child care. Hospital employees who lived on the grounds in housing provided by the institution usually employed one or more patients.

If a patient had worked at a trade such as blacksmith, brickmason, plumber, or mechanic, he might continue to practice his craft. Many of these men became essential to the daily operation of the institution, and any attempts to discharge them met with opposition from their supervisors, who feared the loss of talented workers. However, patient employment came to an end when the Fair Labor Standards Act of 1973 prohibited unpaid labor in mental institutions. Life on the back wards, reserved for custodial patients or the criminally insane, afforded few opportunities for recreation or treatment. These individuals did not have institutional jobs and rarely left the wards. After dressing and eating breakfast, they often sat all day in the dayroom. Few bothered to interact with others, and as long as they were quiet, the attendants left them alone. They often went to bed immediately after the evening meal instead of the normal bedtime of 9:30 p.m.

Self-Sufficiency

Mental hospitals produced most of the vegetables and fruits consumed on their premises. In addition to fresh produce in season, excess fruits and vegetables were canned or dried for winter use.

Institutions purchased only a few staples, such as coffee beans and flour, from merchants in town. Since agricultural work depended on the labor of horses and mules, hay, fodder, oats, and corn were stored for their feed as well as that of the milk cows and chickens. Pigs received scraps from the dining rooms. The Willard Asylum in New York carried self-sufficiency to even greater extremes, maintaining its own fire department, a small hotel for visitors, and even a local train (Dwyer 1987, 25).

Treatment

Following dinner, patients might participate in various kinds of therapy. Often occupational or vocational therapy coincided with job assignments, so that someone who had expressed an interest in nursing might be placed in the medical facility to perform relatively easy tasks such as wrapping needles. As mental institutions moved toward deinstitutionalization in the 1970s, they began a concentrated effort to provide vocational training so that former patients would be able to support themselves after release.

Another common treatment, recreational therapy, included such sports as bowling, tennis, croquet, and baseball. Other forms of recreation involved walking or simply relaxing on the grounds, talking with other residents and staff, or listening to music. Weekly dances, band concerts, and community sing-songs were common. Art therapy encouraged creative expression, and some patients sold their paintings, which could achieve renown as "outsider art." Ecumenical religious services occurred on Sundays, and holidays might occasion picnics or watermelon feasts.

Most early institutions employed some form of hydrotherapy, which ranged from "needle" showers whose high-intensity spray stimulated lethargic patients, to hot or cold baths for reducing agitation. Many had natatoria, or indoor swimming pools. Patients might also receive enemas or "colonic irrigation."

Sleep therapy, in which patients remained sedated for up to a month, might be prescribed for those diagnosed with mania. While this treatment did reduce manic symptoms temporarily, they soon reappeared. Sedatives such as paraldehyde calmed patients.

Before the development of psychotropic drugs such as Thorazine, not much could be done to reduce the symptoms of schizophrenia. Institutions tried various inventive therapies including spinning therapy in which patients spun in rotation swings until they were dizzy. Many saw electricity as a possible cure and purchased electrostatic shock devices that delivered electric shock to arms or legs. After Cerletti and Bini's observation in 1938 that applying the shock directly to the head improved mental functioning, mental institutions began the widespread use of electroconvulsive shock for treatment of a wide array of mental problems including schizophrenia (Valenstein 1986, 51). Therapeutic convulsions previously had been induced by the use of Metrazol or insulin. The advantage of electroshock was that the patients did not remember the experience as they did with the other methods, serving to lessen fear of the procedures. Electroconvulsive therapy became very controversial and is presently used only in cases of severe depression and risk of suicide.

Psychotherapy, "the talking cure," occurred rarely in mental institutions (Grob 1994, 136). Presently, in-patient care often consists of crisis stabilization and release. Longer stays might be necessary for psychotropic drugs to take effect. Self-help skills and social training may be provided.

Deinstitutionalization

Conditions in mental hospitals changed dramatically after psychotropic drugs became available, with many treated as outpatients or "deflected" to nursing homes. Currently, most institutions admit only the most disturbed or seriously suicidal, and the goal is to release them as soon as they are stable. Institutions for the criminally insane continue to provide long-term care, and these have always resembled prisons more than mental institutions. Prisons themselves now have wings devoted solely to the care of inmates with mental illness, and presently the largest mental institution in the country is the Los Angeles County jail, with an average daily inmate population of about 17,000 and over 10 times that amount processed over the course of a year (Los Angeles County Sheriff's Department 2018).

Sarah C. Sitton and
Donna R. Kemp

See also: Electroconvulsive Therapy; Hysteria; Lobotomy and Other "Psychosurgeries"; Milieu Therapy and Therapeutic Community; Moral Treatment; Neurasthenia, or Nervous Exhaustion; Recovery Movement

Further Reading

Austin State Hospital. Daily Schedule, 7–3 Shift. Austin State Hospital Archive, ca. 1950. *By-Laws, Rules and Regulations for the Government of the Texas State Lunatic Asylum. 1861.* Austin, TX: Intelligencer Book Office.

Dwyer, Ellen. 1987. *Homes for the Mad: Life inside Two Nineteenth-Century Asylums.* New Brunswick, NJ: Rutgers University Press.

Frank, Ellen, et al. 2005. "Two-Year Outcome for Social and Interpersonal Rhythm Therapy for Individuals with Bipolar Disorder." *Archives of General Psychiatry* 62:996–1004.

Graham, Beriah. 1866. *Superintendent's Report from the State Lunatic Asylum.* Austin, TX.

Grob, Gerald. 1994. *The Mad among Us.* New York: Free Press.

Kirkbride, Thomas. 1854. *On the Construction, Organization and General Arrangements of Hospitals for the Insane.* Philadelphia: Lindsay and Blackstone.

Lael, Richard, Barbara Brazos, and Margo Ford. 2007. *Evolution of a Missouri Asylum: Fulton State Hospital, 1851–2006.* New York: Macmillan.

Los Angeles County Sheriff's Department. 2018. Public Data. http://lasd.org/public_data _sharing.html

McGovern, Constance. 1985. *Masters of Madness: Social Origins of the American Psychiatric Association.* Hanover: University of Vermont Press.

Penney, Darby, and Peter Stastny. 2008. *The Lives They Left Behind: Suitcases from a State Hospital Attic.* New York: Bellevue Literary Press.

Perry, John. 1858. *Superintendent's Report for the State Lunatic Asylum.* Austin, TX.

Rochefort, D. A. 1993. *From Poorhouses to Homelessness: Policy Analysis and Mental Health Care.* Westport, CT: Auburn House.

Rothman, David. 1970. *The Discovery of the Asylum.* Boston: Little, Brown.

Sitton, Sarah. 1999. *Life at the Texas State Lunatic Asylum, 1857–1997.* College Station, TX: A&M University Press.

Valenstein, Elliot S. 1986. *Great and Desperate Cures.* New York: Basic Books.

Wallace, David R. 1875. *Superintendent's Report for the State Lunatic Asylum.* Austin, TX: State Lunatic Asylum.

ORGONE THERAPY

Psychoanalysis generated a number of spin-off therapies, each with its own founding figure and special therapeutic emphasis or twist. Undoubtedly the most extraordinary figure from the early generation of therapists, however, was Wilhelm Reich (1897–1957). Reich had been a pupil of Sigmund Freud's in Vienna and was even briefly thought of as a possible successor to the great man, so brilliant was he. Unfortunately, because of his unorthodox views, which developed as his career advanced, Reich ended up being stripped of his membership in the psychoanalytic society and investigated by government authorities. At the same time, he was regarded highly by his friends and clients, who considered him a humanist and a psychological innovator. His most controversial creation by far was the "orgone accumulator," a device designed to relieve its user of pent-up sexual tension.

Character, Tension, and Release

After training with Freud, Reich stayed in Vienna to practice, teach, and write. His specialty was "character analysis," or the examination of individual character or personality. He took character to be the result of a person's *resistance* to his or her own neuroses. Character, in other words, is a kind of "armor" we put on to protect ourselves—from ourselves. Reich wrote a groundbreaking book on the subject (*Charakteranalyse,* 1933; Eng. trans. 1946), which was well received by the psychoanalytic community at the time.

Meanwhile, Reich was also developing an alternative to conventional psychanalysis, which he called *vegetotherapy*. This involved a more direct interaction with patients than was normally allowed, including having them undress down to their underclothes and using hard massage on them to loosen their body armor. The reason it was called vegetotherapy is not exactly clear, but it had to do with prompting "organic reactions," or bodily responses, through aggressive physical (and psychological) treatment. This was needed, Reich said, because

> Every neurotic is muscularly dystonic [i.e., abnormally taut or jerky], and every cure is directly manifested in a "relaxation" or improvement. . . . This process can be observed best in the compulsive character. His muscular rigidity is expressed in awkwardness; unrhythmical movements, particularly in the sexual act, lack of [free] movement, a typically taut facial musculature which often gives him a slightly mask-like expression. . . . The musculature of the buttocks is almost always tense. . . . Muscular rigidity *and* psychic rigidity are a unit, the sign of a disturbance of the vegetative motility of the . . . system as a whole. (quoted in Ehrenwald 1976, 496)

Eventually, then, under Reich's vegetotherapy, the patient begins to relax, ceasing to convulse involuntarily when touched or massaged. Reich saw the result as being on par with reaching a state of orgasmic satisfaction. It was a matter of turning a person's armor plating into a good sack of vegetables.

A paper Reich wrote about the subject, "Psychological Contact and Vegetative Current" (1934), hints at another meaning of vegetotherapy. It had to do with bioelectricity, or energetic currents flowing through the body.

The core of Reich's interest from this time on was sexual orgasm as a therapeutic tool. He saw the freedom to release libidinal energy as the difference between sickness and health. For him, even the scourge of fascism that was then infecting Europe was the product of sexual frustration, a lack of awareness toward sexual responses. Looking to blend psychoanalysis with anti-fascism and Marxism, he argued that repression of all kinds—psychological and social—could be fixed. His surprising philosophy got him kicked out of both the psychoanalytic movement and the Communist Party, which he had joined briefly. His books were burned in Germany, and he fled to Denmark, Sweden, and then to Norway, where he experimented with oscilloscopes in his effort to learn more about bioelectrical activity. Norwegian authorities too, however, soon questioned his methods and pushed him out.

In 1939, therefore, Reich emigrated to the United States, where he would have his greatest impact. At the time, despite the unfolding war, America was a place where the scientific study of sex was beginning to take off. The renowned sex researcher Alfred Kinsey was then launching his work on the sexual behavior of the human male and female, though it wasn't released in final form until the late 1940s and early 1950s. Reich had allegedly already coined the phrase *sexual revolution* by then, at a time when this notion was still unheard of and utterly scandalous (Turner 2011).

Shortly after arriving in America Reich invented his Orgone Energy Accumulator. This was a wooden box or cabinet that stood vertically like a small telephone booth, with a door in front and a seat inside for the user. The unit was lined with sheet iron and insulated with steel wool. The idea behind it, according to Reich, was that it captured an unseen, and hitherto undetected, kind of radiation present in the atmosphere called *orgone energy*. Once concentrated inside the box, with its expectant patient inside, this bioenergetic current recharged the person, in mind and body. (Reich maintained that the box somehow absorbed the orgone energy and the metal lining kept it from escaping.) Ultimately, the device was said by Reich to be capable of curing everything from cancer to mental illness, though he couldn't back up his claim with anything more than a growing body of testimonials from patients who said that they felt better after experiencing the treatment.

Those testimonials came from a notable collection of countercultural figures—William S. Burroughs, Allen Ginsburg, Paul Goodman, Jack Kerouac, Norman Mailer, and J. D. Salinger—as well as ordinary people. Sean Connery, of James Bond fame, is said to have benefitted from the device, and Woody Allen later presented a humorous version of it called the "Orgasmatron" in the film *Sleeper* (1973). Reich called the new field of medical research and treatment he was engaged in *orgonomy*. He once discussed his findings with Albert Einstein in Princeton, but the famous physicist would not condone it. Eventually, as he pressed on with his case, some of Reich's erstwhile colleagues began to question his sanity.

Meanwhile, the government too was getting involved. On the basis of his communist and antifascist background in Europe, Reich drew the attention of the FBI shortly after arriving in the United States; he was briefly detained on suspicion of being a communist (which, by then, he was not) and released, but he continued to be surveilled for years afterward. In 1947, two articles that were critical of him appeared in *Harper's* and *The New Republic*: he was painted as a cult leader who advocated sex and anarchy. These pieces caused the Food and Drug Administration (FDA) to launch an investigation into the use and marketing of the orgone accumulator. Reich was enjoined by a court in 1954 and prevented from leasing or selling his machines. When Reich broke the injunction, he was sentenced to two years in prison. The remaining stock of his accumulators was destroyed along with most of his books and journals, on the grounds that they constituted "false advertising" for his dubious treatment.

When he died of a heart attack in prison, in 1957, Reich was showing clear signs of a psychotic breakdown. Even before his arrest and imprisonment he had been claiming that the world was being invaded by UFOs; he had started producing an "orgone gun" that could be used to defend humanity from an alien invasion. These ideas, of course, were too far out for nearly everyone but Reich to take seriously.

From Orgone to the Organic

It is easy to dismiss Reich as a quack, but in fact he made lasting contributions to the field of psychotherapy. Whereas psychoanalysis was all about the "psychic apparatus" of the patient and the means to resolve psychic conflict, Reich was one of the first proponents, in the West, of a mind–body approach and looking at the somatic ("vegetative") components of neurotic distress. He saw sexual tension, anxiety, and anger as expressed in a variety of bodily symptoms, primarily in the musculoskeletal system. His concept of "armor plating" as an essential element of character (particularly the neurotic character) was novel and played a key part in his development of vegeto/somatic therapy. The principal source of neurotic disturbance for Reich was the blocking of libido, or sexual drive. In all of this, Reich's work had an important impact—spawning a generation of "Reichian" analysts and helping to usher in the sexual revolution of the 1960s and 1970s.

In recent years, moreover, psychotherapists have "rediscovered" the body as an important piece in the overall understanding of neurosis and mental disturbance. The concept of *embodiment* is frequently employed by those in the complementary and alternative health community to refer to the way that the human body "records" or "stores" impacts of psychic conflict, and how it can fuel or "remind" us about them in turn. With the ongoing expansion of mind–body awareness among both patients and doctors, a new field known as *body psychotherapy* has arisen that draws on Reichian concepts and related approaches. However, there seem to be no plans at present to return to the use of the orgone accumulator.

Michael Shally-Jensen

See also: Anxiety and Its Treatment; Biofeedback; Feldenkrais Method; Hydrotherapy; Hysteria; Mind–Body Medicine; Neurasthenia, or Nervous Exhaustion; Psychoanalysis; Rolfing; Sex, Sexology, and Sex Therapy

Further Reading

Ehrenwald, Jan, ed. 1976. *The History of Psychotherapy: From Healing Magic to Encounter.* New York: Jason Aronson.

Pietikäinen, Petteri. 2007. *Alchemists of Human Nature: Psychological Utopianism in Gross, Jung, Reich, and Fromm.* London: Pickering and Chatto.

Totton, Nick. 2003. *Body Psychotherapy: An Introduction.* Philadelphia: Open University Press.

Turner, Christopher. 2011. *Adventures in the Orgasmatron: How the Sexual Revolution Came to America.* New York: Farrar, Straus and Giroux.

OSTEOPATHY

Osteopathy is a branch of medicine that emphasizes the importance of the musculoskeletal system in maintaining health, particularly the integrity and functionality of bones, muscles, and surrounding tissues. It is a field that has evolved greatly over the past 150 years. Originally standing outside the mainstream of American medicine, as currently practiced it has shifted toward conventional medicine (sometimes called allopathic—the type of medicine normally practiced by people with the MD degree). At the same time, other medical professionals and society as a whole have become more receptive to those trained in schools of osteopathic medicine. Around 10 percent of the doctors practicing in the United States have a Doctor of Osteopathic Medicine (DO) degree, with the percentage growing in recent decades. However, outside the United States fewer than 50 countries accept the DO degree for medical practice, while an MD is universally accepted. Nevertheless, osteopathy has come a long way from its origins in unorthodox medicine.

History

Although modern medicine began to emerge in the 19th century, by 21st-century standards many of its practices would be considered barbaric, and the rate of recovery for patients with diseases and injuries was often dependent on factors other than the medical care provided. Dr. Andrew T. Still (1828–1917), who had studied medicine and assisted his father as a medical missionary to Native Americans, worked with the Union Army during the Civil War. Contemporaneous medical techniques seemed a failure in his eyes, not only because of the devastation he witnessed in the field hospitals, but also because four of his own children died from meningitis.

In this period, many physicians around the world were attempting to develop new understandings and treatments of medical conditions. Still was among those who sought to find a better way to deal with the diseases and ailments afflicting people. He came to think that the tissues of the musculoskeletal system, along with those of the adjacent circulatory and nervous systems, played a crucial role in both sustaining health and/or indicating the presence of illness or disease. The results of his investigations became known as osteopathic medicine. Central to Still's practice was the manipulation of the body to address faulty alignments and to ensure structural integrity. (In this, it was not unlike chiropractic, although each evolved differently.) By the mid-1870s, he had developed the basic principles that separated osteopathic medicine from the allopathic (or "regular") branch, and by the late 1880s, he started using the term *osteopathic*. Then living in Missouri, Still opened a school for the study of osteopathic medicine in 1892, hoping to see his approach practiced by others. By the time of his death, osteopathic medicine not only had a school, it had its own academic journals and was recognized by Missouri as a valid way to practice medicine, although legally it was not placed on the same level as an allopathic medicine.

Throughout the first half of the 20th century, the American Medical Association (AMA; the professional association of MDs) rejected the assertion that those with a DO degree had the same level of training as those with an MD. Since the osteopathic schools of medicine did, and still do, have their own accrediting body, the AMA argued that the level of training for a DO was inferior. At the opening of the 20th century, there were substantial differences between MD and DO training, mainly based on Still's advocacy of the manipulation of the musculoskeletal system to correct structural faults and stimulate healing. However, in many other ways, his system of medical practice was more advanced than that practiced by most MDs in that he advocated *preventative* medicine. As the number of individuals earning a DO degree increased, greater pressure was placed on state legislatures to accept this degree as equal to an MD degree, and to have osteopathic doctors certified for various state and federal reimbursement programs. By the 1970s, the DO degree was accepted by all the states. Contributing to this was a shift by schools that trained osteopathic students to a curriculum that was virtually the same as that of an MD, with the addition of the musculoskeletal manipulation, known as osteopathic manipulative medicine. Early this century, the MD and DO schools united in the creation of a single accredited residency program that all graduates enter as their final step to beginning full-time practice.

The Osteopathic Difference

In his early work as a physician, Still began to focus on the body as a unit, rather than on the individual symptoms displayed by a patient. He believed that by manipulating the musculoskeletal system, tissue function could be improved, thereby facilitating healing: bone, muscle, blood vessels, and nerves would be returned to vitality and bring health to the individual. He was also concerned with the overuse of morphine during and after the Civil War, and saw drugs as a palliative measure aimed at relieving symptoms, not addressing the underlying condition. These views marked the major differences between Still's approach and the approach of conventional medicine. During the time that Still was developing his approach, practitioners of conventional medicine began to broaden their understanding of the use and operation of pharmaceutical drugs for pain relief and recovery.

Still taught osteopathic manipulative medicine (OMM) as a central part of the training of new DOs; it was part of his philosophy that the whole patient should be treated. However, sections of the training included many of the same lessons that a person would receive when studying to be an MD, especially a strong focus on anatomy. The outsized role that OMM played in Still's approach was a key factor in osteopathic medicine's initial rejection by the medical establishment. Moreover, even though many 19th-century doctors had been trained via apprenticeship, established medical schools increasingly required longer terms of study than did Still's American School of Osteopathy. By the start of the 20th century, medical researchers had expanded the understanding of germ theory, pharmaceuticals, and immunology, yet Still was hesitant to incorporate these into his core curriculum, preferring to stay focused on the musculoskeletal system. Eventually, however, he made the necessary changes. A 1910 national study of medical schools, known as the *Flexner Report*, had mandated a comprehensive curriculum for all medical teaching institutions, and Still ensured that the osteopathic schools complied.

Over the next few decades, osteopathic schools of medicine gradually expanded the studies required to obtain a DO degree, with the last major area (pharmacology) added in 1929. Although pass rates in states that required DOs and MDs to take the same licensing exam was lower for DOs, the students were studying the same basic curriculum as MDs, with the addition of OMM. Discussions between the AMA and the American Osteopathic Association (AOA) were held on a variety of issues throughout the 20th century, each organization eventually accepting the other's presence and point of view within the wider medical community. (In 1962, the AMA rescinded its statement that consulting a DO was unethical, and in 1969 voted to accept individuals with a DO degree into the AMA, although most osteopathic doctors choose to remain with the AOA.) Indeed, when holistic medicine arrived on the scene in the 1970s as an alternative to conventional practices, osteopathy was in a good position because it already advocated considering the whole body when attending to patients' needs.

Unlike in earlier decades, by the start of the current century most people accepted the idea that individuals holding a DO or MD degree had the same qualifications. Because of the location of osteopathic schools, the distribution of DOs is not even across the United States. Although not everyone accepts DOs as the equal of MDs, DOs have the same professional rights as MDs, including the ability to prescribe medications. All specialties are open to DOs, although a high percentage are in primary care. While the curricula for the two degrees are virtually the same, some have noted that few osteopathic schools are related to major research hospitals or universities, limiting the students' exposure to the opportunities these institutions offer. In addition, as osteopathic doctors have become more mainstream, some surveys have indicated that a smaller percentage of patients are treated with OMM. What was once its primary "alternative" technique is perhaps beginning to recede in importance.

Donald A. Watt

See also: Chiropractic; Feldenkrais Method; Magnet Therapy; Mind–Body Medicine; Reflexology; Shiatsu

Further Reading

American Osteopathic Association. 2018. "What Is a DO?" *American Osteopathic Association.* Chicago: American Osteopathic Association. osteopathic.org/what-is-osteopathic -medicine/what-is-a-do/

Chila, Anthony with the American Osteopathic Association. 2011. *Foundations of Osteopathic Medicine.* 3rd ed. Baltimore: Lippincott Williams & Wilkins.

Mayer, Johannes, and Clive Standen with Patricia Kerslake-Bösch, trans. 2017. *Textbook of Osteopathic Medicine.* Munich: Elsevier.

Parker, Jonathan D. 2014. "Reversing the Paradox: Evidence-Based Medicine and Osteopathic Medicine." *Journal of the American Osteopathic Association.* November. Chicago: American Osteopathic Association. jaoa.org/article.aspx?articleid=2210609

Wu, Patrick, and Jonathan Siu. 2015. *A Brief Guide to Osteopathic Medicine: For Students, By Students.* Chevy Chase, MD: American Association of Colleges of Osteopathic Medicine. www.aacom.org/docs/default-source/cib/bgom.pdf

PSYCHOANALYSIS

Psychoanalysis, or the technique of guiding mental health patients toward emotional insight by having them work through intrapsychic conflicts that originate in childhood experience, was a radical *alternative* therapeutic approach when it first arose at the start of the 20th century. Prior to that, doctors tended to blame the victim for his or her own moral or emotional lapses or sought out organic causes that never could be shown to exist. Psychoanalysis was new not only because of the theory that lay behind it but because of the method of treatment it espoused: the so-called talking cure. So successful was it in treating neurotic conditions—that is, mental disorders that affect only part of the personality rather than the entire persona (as in the case of psychotic conditions)—that it eventually became *the* mainstream method of psychiatry. Then, after a long reign of more than a half century, it faced challenges to its dominance and ultimately became a much smaller force in the field of mental health care.

History and Development

Psychoanalysis is both a theory of personality and mental/emotional development as well as a method for treating neurotic disorders based on the workings of unconscious and conscious forces within the individual. It was founded by the Austrian physician and neurologist Sigmund Freud (1856–1939), whose discoveries grew out of a collaboration with another Austrian physician, Joseph Breuer. Through their work with a number of patients suffering from hysteria, they acquired useful perspectives regarding each patient's symptoms and what might be causing them. Initially, Freud and Breuer employed hypnosis as a technique for getting patients to reveal the nature and meaning of their troubles; but soon they switched to free association—exploratory, uncensored dialogue—to target the hidden content of their patients' minds. The two researchers came to regard neurotic symptoms as the result of unresolved conflicts between instinctual human impulses, on the one hand, and repressive psychic forces, on the other. They became convinced, moreover, that sexuality was singularly important in the development of neurotic symptoms and in personality formation generally.

Freud, who soon broke with Breuer over an intellectual dispute, published his seminal *The Interpretation of Dreams* in 1900. In it, and in later works, he detailed his theories of unconscious mental processes and their effect on conscious thoughts and actions. Freud believed that much of human behavior is irrational, rooted in basic biological drives including sex and aggression. According to psychoanalytic theory, many forbidden impulses and punished behaviors of childhood are repressed (stricken from awareness) but remain in the unconscious and are expressed in dreams, neurotic symptoms, jokes, slips of the tongue, and nervous mannerisms. They also lend themselves to (indirect) expression in art, literature, and religion. Because these unconscious childhood conflicts give rise to anxiety, attempts to uncover them generate resistance. Neurotic symptoms, including phobias, depression, personality disturbances, and sexual dysfunction, are the outcome.

Neuroses, then, are the result of a person's developmental history, particularly of painful experiences in early childhood. According to psychoanalytic theory, childhood development is made up of three broad periods. First, the oral phase encompasses the earliest experiences surrounding a child's close relationships with his or her mother, including feelings of being nurtured and loved. Second, the anal period is characterized by experiences relating to the onset of social demands for orderliness and compliance, epitomized by toilet training. Third, the phallic phase pertains to conflicts arising from erotic wishes toward the parent of the opposite sex: the young boy desires his mother (and resents his father), while the young girl seeks intimacy with her father (and harbors ill will toward her mother). Each period in the child's development presents challenges to him or her that are either successfully overcome or end up producing arrested states that lead to difficulties in achieving mature adulthood.

In addition, according to Freud, every child must learn to adapt to three major components within his or her personality. The *id,* the most primitive and least accessible component, is entirely unconscious and includes instinctive sexual urges and repressed thoughts that seek immediate expression without regard to circumstances. Dreams, impulses, and feelings that may seem strange in normal circumstances can erupt from the id. The *superego,* on the other hand, represents conscience and the rational life. It is composed of ethical and moral principles that the individual acquires early in life. The id and the superego are typically in direct conflict. It is the task of the third major component, the *ego,* to reconcile these conflicting forces and cultivate a sense of independence, autonomy, and self-direction in the individual. This whole area of psychoanalytic theory, including the development of the personality, is known as psychodynamics.

Psychoanalytic Treatment and Later Variants

The treatment provided under psychoanalysis is one of the most systematic and painstaking, if also one of the most time-consuming, forms of psychotherapy. At the peak of its influence in the mid-20th century, psychoanalytic therapy consisted of three or more 50-minute meetings per week with a trained analyst, often extending over a period of years or sometimes even decades. This ideal of lengthy, in-depth treatment continues to inform practice today, albeit not as strongly as in the past.

Based on psychodynamic principles, psychoanalytic treatment seeks to bring about the resolution of intrapsychic conflicts by examining their sources and meanings and working to strengthen the "executive" part of the personality (ego). It is designed to promote emotional insight by helping the patient work through resistances and transference reactions (i.e., the redirection of feelings and desires toward a new "object" or person, such as the analyst). The process is slow, tedious, emotionally laden, and expensive. It relies heavily on the patient's developing ego strength, motivation, commitment, and his or her ability to withstand frustrations and relive painful experiences. It is accomplished by the patient lying on a couch and responding freely and openly to questions or comments posed by the analyst, who sits in a chair located slightly behind and to the side of the patient. The doctor listens and tries to discern the individual's underlying, unconscious thought processes and to help the patient recognize them as well.

As Freudian psychoanalysis developed, it began to attract a circle of followers and psychic explorers, some of whom extended or expanded the master's insights and some of whom ended up developing rival theories and therapeutic techniques of their own. One of Freud's most influential followers, for example, was the Swiss psychiatrist Carl Jung (1875–1961). Jung played an early role in developing psychoanalytic ideas but eventually became estranged from Freud and set out to establish his own system, known as *analytic psychology* or *Jungian analysis*. According to Jung, not only one's past and not only one's psychosexual conflicts go into the making of neurotic behavior, but also one's future strivings and a variety of other determinants as well. Jung examined ancient myths and religions to identify symbols that are commonly reflected in the dreams and neurosis of humanity. He proposed the existence of a *collective unconscious* shared by everyone along with a number of other alternative psychological concepts. Therapy, for Jung and the Jungians, consisted of a deep exploration of patients' dreams and the creative aspects of their lives, looking for revealing symbols. Jung's ideas, initially somewhat on the margins of psychoanalysis, became quite popular later on, particularly in the 1960s as young people began to appreciate non-Western religious traditions and new experiences involving the mind.

Another key early thinker in the Freudian tradition was Alfred Adler, an Austrian physician. According to Adler, who named his system *individual psychology*, the central human motive is a striving for dominance or superiority in the face of feelings of inferiority, rooted in a child's sense of mental and physical inferiority in relation to adults. Neurotic symptoms are failed attempts to deal with such feelings. *Overcompensation* was one of Adler's main contributions to the psychoanalytic lexicon. Humans strive for power over others, he said, and adopt fictitious goals and counterproductive habits in the course of doing so. To be cured, the patient has to develop a sense of community; sociocultural factors were of critical importance to Adler and the Adlerians. The main thing for therapist and patient was to jointly review the latter's style of life and work to overcome any self-defeating neurotic strategies and behaviors.

A subsequent group of thinkers and practitioners, known as the neo-Freudians, placed even greater emphasis on cultural and social-environmental factors. They sought to counter Freud's focus on biological/instinctual components of behavior with a view that stressed humans' adaptive functions and the constructive aims of the individual's efforts to achieve competence, mastery, and self-identity. Therapy, for these practitioners, was designed to build the autonomy and adaptive functions of the ego, and for this reason this school of thought (in at least some of its variants) is also known as *ego psychology*.

Postwar Turn and Decline

During World War II, numerous European psychoanalysts fled the Continent for England and the United States. In these new environments, additional psychoanalytic specialties emerged, such as child and adolescent psychiatry and Gestalt therapy. By the 1950s, psychoanalysis had become a well-accepted approach to psychiatric treatment in the United States and beyond.

It had long been criticized, however, from a scientific viewpoint as advancing vague theories and concepts that were difficult to test empirically. With the rise of ostensibly more rigorous approaches such as behavioral therapy, and advances in biological research in general and biochemical research in particular, psychoanalysis began to lose some of its prestige. More people began to question its high cost and its claims of curative powers, given that treatment lasted for so long and, in some cases, even could become something of an obsession for patients, as they delved into their pasts to figure out their present selves and found it harder and harder to resist continuing the process. (This is known as attachment to therapy.) Still practiced to some extent today, psychoanalysis has declined in both public acceptance and acceptance within the medical community (including the medical insurance industry), as biological psychiatry, cognitive science, and a number of alternative therapies have taken hold.

Nevertheless, many concepts and ideas from psychoanalysis have been absorbed into the thinking of many psychologists and counselors. Among these ideas are the emphasis on the dynamic, adaptive nature of human behavior; the role of strong, often unconscious forces and motives influencing behavior; the recognition of the importance of early experiences vis-à-vis later behavior; and the conflict- and anxiety-reducing functions of various responses. The influence of psychoanalysis has been massive, not only in developmental psychology, personality psychology, and similar areas but in the humanities and Western thought generally.

Michael Shally-Jensen

See also: Client-Centered Therapy; Dream Interpretation; Gestalt Therapy; Hysteria; Jung and Jungian Analysis; Recovered Memory Therapy, "Split Personality," and Satanism

Further Reading

Lieberman, Jeffrey A., with Ogi Ogas. 2015. *Shrinks: The Untold Story of Psychiatry.* New York: Little, Brown.

Pick, Daniel. 2015. *Psychoanalysis: A Very Short Introduction.* New York: Oxford University Press.

Roazen, Paul. 1990. *Encountering Freud: The Politics and Histories of Psychoanalysis.* New Brunswick, NJ: Transaction Publishers.

SEX, SEXOLOGY, AND SEX THERAPY

In the early eras of American history, sex was largely a taboo subject. During the colonial period, for example, the prevailing Puritan strain of Protestantism in the New England region made all considerations of sex outside of procreation a sin. Any deviation from the norm could result in harsh treatments for the participant(s), such as forced placement in stocks, public shaming, and, sometimes, ostracism. All sex acts, and even thoughts of sex, were banned except those that took place in the conjugal bed. And even then strict rules were in place as to what activities could and could not be engaged in. Some other religious sects, such as the Shakers, demanded celibacy in all situations.

Although in the 18th century, under the influence of Enlightenment ideas, a more tolerant attitude toward sex began to emerge, society remained on guard with respect to overt expressions of sexual passion. Romantic attraction was encouraged among social equals, but physical involvement was still thought best limited to marital partners. The fact that married men, particularly members of the elite, sometimes retained mistresses (or enjoyed the company of young men) was kept quiet by social convention. A variety of radical utopian communities, such as the Oneida Community in New York, later experimented with sexual conventions, but most of these were short short-lived. When in the mid-19th century Mormons began to cultivate the practice of polygamy, or "plural marriage," they were roundly condemned by those from other religious denominations and pressured to relocate to Utah Territory.

Well into the 19th century, the thought of nonprocreative sexual activity was considered not only socially anathema but medically harmful. Physicians such as Samuel-Auguste Tissot (1728–1797) in Switzerland and Benjamin Rush (1745–1813) in the United States had earlier laid down the theory that the expenditure of sexual energy, especially (in the case of men) through seminal emission, spelled disaster for the body as a whole, because it depleted needed bodily fluids. One could even go insane from masturbating, Tissot suggested. These ideas persisted through later decades. The U.S. health advocate and cereal developer John Harvey Kellogg (1852–1943) warned against masturbation and promoted his grain products as a means to calm the sexual passions and achieve holistic health. Other observers at the time blamed diseases such as syphilis and gonorrhea on unbridled sexual activity, not, as it later turned out to be the case, on bacterial transmission. The neurologist George M. Beard felt that excessive sex was a key causative agent in the development of the psychosomatic condition known as neurasthenia, or "nervous exhaustion." Groups like the Young Men's Christian Association fought against sexual temptation and for the cultivation of a healthy "body, mind, and spirit."

By the height of the Victorian period, between the 1860s and 1880s, women were pushed toward the role of moral guardian, both within the family and in society at large (even as men continued to enjoy a virtual monopoly on authority). Motherhood was the ideal and childrearing a woman's calling, with nary a hint of the physical body to be recognized in either function. Women's clothing reflected this, with corsets and massive hoopskirts along with high-necked blouses and other accoutrements making it virtually impossible to see the human being behind the garb. The only mention of sex under such conditions was in the form of rules about how to avoid it and public lectures regarding the dangers it posed to society. Contraception, or even the dissemination of information regarding pregnancy or contraception, was essentially off-limits.

Modern Times

Basic sex education for young people began in the early 20th century, but the lessons focused, once again, primarily on abstinence and purity. The risks of venereal disease were emphasized, while anatomy and physiology were given short shrift. In Catholic schools and communities, such topics were largely avoided altogether. With the emergence, however, of "flapper" culture in the 1920s, young (mostly Protestant) women were permitted to go out at night unchaperoned, as sexual mores began to loosen. The increasing presence of the automobile also helped in the area of sexual relations. The first real sexologist, or scholar of human sexuality, Havelock Ellis (1859–1939), published a series of books on the psychology and sociology of sex that helped to change public attitudes. The work of psychoanalyst Sigmund Freud (1856–1939) likewise drew attention to the role of erotic dreams and fantasies in ordinary life. Meanwhile, an old genre of books primarily aimed at women, marriage manuals, was updated to include modest information on romantic experimentation and the pleasures of the bedroom.

The next major breakthrough in the study of human sexuality occurred in 1948, when the American sexologist Alfred Kinsey (1894–1956) published his landmark work *Sexual Behavior in the Human Male,* followed, in 1953, by *Sexual Behavior in the Human Female.* These works, based on statistical data derived from questionnaires, showed that men and women enjoyed engaging in sex and, moreover, pursued a wide range of sexual practices—including homosexuality (then considered illegal). The books had the effect, furthermore, of legitimizing the subject of sex in public discourse: it became okay to be more open about sexuality because, after all, it was a fact of life that touched everyone. Although some of Kinsey's methods and findings would later be questioned, Kinsey undoubtedly gave a boost to the academic discipline of sexology and helped broaden the public's awareness of sexual behavior in many of its specifics.

Behavior is one thing, physiology another. It was the team of William Masters and Virginia Johnson who examined the latter in their landmark *Human Sexual Response* (1963) and other works. Using hundreds of male and female volunteers, Masters and Johnson—themselves eventually married (and later divorced)—did pioneering research on physiological reactions to sexual stimuli, including the first detailed accounts of female sexuality, with scientific confirmation of multiple orgasms. The pair also gained experience in counseling hundreds of couples with sexual problems. They developed a treatment method designed to deal with such complaints, publishing their findings in *Human Sexual Inadequacy* (1966). Their efforts were the first of their kind in the new field of professional sex therapy. The name "Masters and Johnson" became synonymous with advice and counseling in sexual matters.

Kinsey and Masters and Johnson helped open the door to the sexual revolution of the 1960s and early 1970s. That movement, led mostly by youth on college campuses but also by working adults in urban centers, brought nothing less than a complete reformulation of social attitudes toward sexuality and the roles of men and women in society. Two other books of the era, *Our Bodies, Ourselves* (1971), about women's health and sexuality, and *The Joy of Sex* (1974), which illustrated various sex positions and practices, had a great cultural impact, as well. Since then, change has continued to occur but not on so grand a scale. Today, most people view sexual activity between consenting adults and open discussion of sexual functioning as the way of the world (except, of course, among staunchly conservative groups).

Sex Therapy

Even in the context of today's more liberal attitudes, many people are adversely affected by sexual problems, and they require both care and information. Sexual problems can arise from physical conditions, psychological conflicts, or relational difficulties; they can be caused by the use of some prescription drugs or the abuse of alcohol or other substances; they can be aggravated by stress, emotional disorders, or misunderstandings regarding the nature of human sexuality; or they can result from a combination of such factors.

Starting in the 1960s, a number of specialized centers were established to treat people having complaints regarding their sexual functioning. The complaints most commonly presented include male impotence and premature ejaculation, and female nonorgasmic response (anorgasmia) and vaginal pain or difficulties. All such conditions can produce serious dissatisfaction on the part of one or both of the partners involved. Even in the absence of any specific complaint, a general lack of sexual desire can be experienced by both men and women for varying lengths of time—sometimes indefinitely.

A variety of approaches are used in the treatment of sexual dysfunctions. Many sex-therapy programs, for example, specialize in treating couples. Central to this type of treatment is the idea that sexual problems affecting couples demand joint, or dual, therapy. Typically, in about 20 sessions, partners discuss the nature of their sexual distress and are given professional feedback and concrete measures to try in the near term in order to overcome their troubles. In such therapy, the relationship as a whole is usually examined, with the sexual dysfunction issue considered as one aspect of the whole. Communication issues are also often a focus of attention, with partners usually needing to make improvements in that regard.

Michael Shally-Jensen

See also: Aromatherapy and Essential Oils; Behavioral Theories and Therapies; Codependency Counseling; Hysteria; Neurasthenia, or Nervous Exhaustion; Orgone Therapy; Psychoanalysis

Further Reading

Bullough, Vern L. 1994. *Science in the Bedroom: A History of Sex Research.* New York: Basic Books.
Drucker, Donna J. 2014. *The Classification of Sex: Alfred Kinsey and the Organization of Knowledge.* Pittsburgh: University of Pittsburgh Press.
Maier, Thomas. 2009. *Masters of Sex: The Life and Times of William Masters and Virginia Johnson, The Couple Who Taught America How to Love.* New York: Basic Books.
Sadock, Benjamin J., Virginia A. Sadock, and Pedro Ruiz. 2015. *Synopsis of Psychiatry.* 11th ed. Philadelphia: Lippincott Williams and Williams.

12-STEP PROGRAMS

Alcoholism is nothing new in society. As early as the 1700s, Western societies were condemning drunkenness, an "insatiable desire for drink," and the ways that drunkenness affected families and children. Various treatments for alcoholism have existed ever since, but Alcoholics Anonymous (AA) may be the most famous. The group does not keep official records, in accordance with its promise of anonymity; but in 2017, it was estimated that AA had more than 2 million active members and 120,000 active groups.

AA is one of a group of recovery programs referred to as 12-step programs. AA-type programs exist for a variety of other substances and addictions—like gambling—as well. The concept has evolved into a general type of peer support group. While each program differs, the most basic version of a 12-step program lays out 12 steps that, if followed carefully and earnestly, proponents believe can help an addict begin and sustain recovery.

History of Treatment for Alcoholism

The idea that addiction is a disease is new in terms of medical history, but nowhere near as new as people think. In 1784, Dr. Benjamin Rush argued that addiction was a medical illness, not a lack of moral fortitude; he said that addiction must be treated as a disease.

Peer support groups that organize around abstinence aren't a new concept either. In the late 1700s and early 1800s, a leader of the Seneca tribe of Native Americans named Handsome Lake wove antialcoholism messages into tribal beliefs to help reduce drunkenness among members of his tribe.

But these early approaches to treating alcoholism represent the exception rather than the rule. Alcohol use and abuse had a strong presence in many Western countries up to the mid-1600s. During that time period, water in cities simply was not safe to drink. While rural communities could often drink from their local well, city water was often polluted by feces, decomposing food and animals, and much more. Drinking beer or wine was simply safer.

It was in the 1600s, when coffee, tea, and cocoa became common refreshments, and alternatives to alcoholic beverages, that imbibing liquids became a more obvious problem. In the 1880s, when Louis Pasteur proved that germs caused illness, and showed how water carried bacteria, communities began to properly clean their water supplies and ensure the safety of their drinking water. This dramatically reduced instances of diseases like those caused by *e. coli* bacteria and dysentery, for example.

In the intervening years, however, popular attitudes toward drunkenness had it that moral people abstained from gluttony, and those who were gluttonous concerning alcohol were weak and committing a mortal sin. Under those circumstances, there was little that could be done to help people. For the poor, virtually nothing was done to prevent abuse and addiction, and what was done was often dangerous. Common treatments for alcoholism included:

- Injection of chemicals including cocaine, morphine, strychnine, arsenic, and others.

- A belief that alcoholism was somehow passed down from parent to child, and got worse with each successive generation; laws were passed stating that alcoholics could be forcibly sterilized.

- Public drunkenness would often lead to the offender being jailed; continuous drunkenness would often lead to the alcoholic being institutionalized in an asylum.

The Rise of AA

Alcoholics Anonymous was founded in 1935 by two men: Bill Wilson and Dr. Bob Smith. Both men were regular drinkers and had sought treatment, hoping to achieve lasting sobriety. Referred to among AA members as Bill W., the man was at his home in

1934 when he was visited by Ebby T., an old friend and fellow drinker. Ebby had spent time in jail and mental hospitals owing to his drinking, and Bill W. absolutely expected to spend their afternoon and evening drinking and reliving old times. Instead, Ebby T. shared his story of his own sobriety and "a message of hope" with Bill.

In December of 1934, Bill W. entered the Charles Towns Hospital for Drug and Alcohol Addictions in New York City. He had spent time in the hospital three times before, where he would have spent time detoxing from alcohol and receiving various treatments designed to help him stop craving the substance. A few days into his stay, he was visited again by Ebby, who encouraged him to stay sober, assuring him that it was possible. According to Bill W., he never drank again. He regularly said the experience of "one alcoholic talking to another" was what finally changed his perspective; this remains central to 12-step programs and peer support groups.

While, today, various programs (Narcotics Anonymous, Overeaters Anonymous, etc.) have slightly different steps as part of their approach, the original AA 12-step program consists of the following.

1. We admitted we were powerless over alcohol—that our lives had become unmanageable.
2. Came to believe that a Power greater than ourselves could restore us to sanity.
3. Made a decision to turn our will and our lives over to the care of God as we understood him.
4. Made a searching and fearless moral inventory of ourselves.
5. Admitted to God, to ourselves and to another human being the exact nature of our wrongs.
6. Were entirely ready to have God remove all these defects of character.
7. Humbly asked him to remove our shortcomings.
8. Made a list of persons we had harmed, and became willing to make amends to them all.
9. Made direct amends to such people wherever possible, except when to do so would injure them or others.
10. Continued to take personal inventory, and when we were wrong, promptly admitted it.
11. Sought through prayer and meditation to improve our conscious contact with God as we understood him, praying only for knowledge of his will for us and the power to carry that out.
12. Having had a spiritual awakening as the result of these steps, we tried to carry this message to alcoholics and to practice these principles in all our affairs.

Do 12-Step Programs Work?

For many years, 12-step programs were considered the gold standard of programs designed to help alcoholics stop drinking. Recent science, however, has begun to question whether or not such programs really work to support recovery over the long term. Beyond the reliance on concepts of God in the program, which grates on the nerves of many atheists and agnostics, there are questions as to whether people are simply replacing one addiction with another—that is, alcoholism for AA meetings.

The fundamental point that many critics of AA make is simple: AA is not *treatment*. It can provide a great support network, and help those in recovery to find hope that their recovery can be maintained for the long term. Especially in the early years, many people find the strong support of those who have been through similar experiences helpful.

But AA was developed in 1935 by two men who (understandably) did not have a comprehension of modern neurology. We know now that long-term alcohol use fundamentally changes the way the brain works; pleasure-and-rewards systems are altered, and to support long-term change, medical intervention is often needed. There are antidepressants and antianxiety medications that can help manage the mental and emotional distress that caused some people to turn to alcohol or other substances in the first place. Additionally, psychotherapeutic approaches like cognitive-behavior therapy (CBT) and dialectical-behavior therapy (DBT) can offer solid results in changing the thought patterns around alcohol abuse.

AA has only about a 5 to 10 percent success rate—in other words, barely 1 in 10 people who follow the steps of Alcoholics Anonymous stop drinking and maintain recovery. Such results in a treatment population might be acceptable as long as people needing treatment have different options to choose from. In medicine, for example, if one prescription doesn't help, a doctor can prescribe another that might work better for the individual. But in the world of AA, if a member doesn't stop drinking while participating in the program, then that member and his behavior is viewed as the problem, not the program itself. You can't switch up the program, like you can switch up meds, as necessary.

If you or someone you know is experiencing addiction and looking for help, AA or a similar peer support program is one option; these programs can be useful in providing a community of persons who know firsthand the challenge of recovery. Speaking to a doctor about medical support and/or a therapist about behavioral support may, on the other hand, be even more helpful in maintaining long-term recovery.

Kay Tilden Frost

See also: Anger and Anger Management; Anxiety and Its Treatment; Behavioral Theories and Therapies; Depression and Its Treatment; Moral Treatment; Recovery Movement; Self-Help; Stress and Stress Management

Further Reading

"Addiction Treatments: Past and Present." Learn. Genetics. October 29, 2018. https://learn
    .genetics.utah.edu/content/addiction/treatments/

Bill, W. 2014. *Alcoholics Anonymous: The Original Text of the Life-Changing Landmark, Deluxe Edition*. New York: TarcherPerigee.

Dodes, Lance, and Zachary Dodes. 2014. *The Sober Truth: Debunking the Bad Science behind 12-Step Programs and the Rehab Industry*. New York: Random House.

Talcherkar, Anjali. 2018. "Timeline: History of Addiction Treatment." *Recovery*. April 24. https://www.recovery.org/topics/history-of-addiction-treatment/

1960s–1970s

INTRODUCTION

The Mainstream

Medical developments in the decades after World War II followed rapidly one after the other. There was the success of the polio vaccine (1955), which became available a few years later as an oral solution. This was followed by a measles vaccine, soon to be combined with vaccines for rubella and mumps into a single injection (MMR). Additionally, researchers developed more effective antibiotics, cortisone, and drugs for the treatment of hypertension and heart disease. Among the new surgical techniques were coronary bypass, kidney transplants, and heart transplants—including the first (partial) artificial heart in 1966. New medical technology included the CAT scan, and improvements were also made to the heart-lung machine, kidney dialysis, and mechanical ventilation. Significant breakthroughs occurred in biochemistry, molecular genetics, bacteriology, and neurology. As death and disease seemed to come under greater human control, the stature of medicine was raised in the public eye and the influence of the American Medical Association was expanded.

Most regular medical care continued to revolve around the hospital. The symbol of high-tech medicine in the new era was the intensive care unit, which most major hospitals had by the late 1960s or early 1970s. The federal government took an active role in subsidizing medical research and approving drugs and therapies for public use. Congressional funding for the research wing of the National Institutes of Health (NIH), which in 1950 was about $12 million (or approx. $125 million in today's dollars), reached nearly $46 million ($390 million) in 1960 and over $70 million ($455 million) in 1970 (NIH 2015). Publicists promoted medical achievements through professional organizations, magazines, drug advertisements, and national fund drives. All these institutional and political structures came to reinforce for regular doctors the conviction that they were no longer in competition with the "irregulars" of old; rather, they saw the growth in the system as validation of the medical model and proof that alternative conceptions had been put to bed.

At this time, too, medicine became increasingly fragmented into specialties, which had the effect of making medical care more expensive for most Americans. University hospitals in major urban markets became the shining stars of the modern system, attracting high-paid doctors while leaving many rural areas to struggle with maintaining broad-based care. Also contributing to the growth trend in medicine was the passage, in 1965, of Medicare, which provided health insurance for all Americans over age 65; and Medicaid, which provided federal grants to the states to supply medical care to those in financial need regardless of age. These two laws put professional medical care within reach of millions of heretofore underserved citizens, even as some doctors, hospitals, and state governments resisted participation in the programs for financial reasons.

Counterweight

All was not necessarily well in medicine-land, however. It was apparent that much of physicians' resistance to Medicare and similar proposals for increased national health-care coverage was owing to their desire to sustain the high incomes they had lately come to enjoy. This fact was paired, moreover, with a noted *decrease* in patient satisfaction when it came to doctor-patient communication: more and more people found doctors to be aloof and superior. Physicians prescribed drugs and dispatched their patients after brief clinical encounters, barely bothering to listen to what they had to say about their conditions. Patients, on the other hand, desired longer, more detailed discussions about the particularities of their situation; they did not wish to be treated like just another case. Furthermore, when patients did speak with their doctors, they wanted things explained in a meaningful way, not just in terms of test results, measures, and the range of pharmaceuticals available to solve the problem. Critics labeled the medical profession as elitist and self-serving and doctors as unresponsive to their patients and to the needs of the nation's ill as a whole.

By the 1960s and 1970s, overprescribing by physicians was becoming a significant issue. One-time miracle drugs like Miltown and Valium, taken for anxiety, and Lithium, taken for depression, proved hazardous to one's health over the long run. Moreover, these and various other amphetamines and tranquilizers, which were marketed essentially as *lifestyle* drugs to the masses (i.e., drugs that could make you feel better about your life), caused physical dependency and could only be given up under pain of a prolonged withdrawal, usually with little or no personal counseling. Then there was the thalidomide tragedy of the late 1950s and early 1960s. This drug, sold as a sedative or hypnotic, particularly to address the "morning sickness" experienced by pregnant women, was one of the more popular and widely used drugs in the United States and Europe—until it was found to produce serious birth defects. Between it and the other drugs, people began to question the direction of the new medicine. The blockbuster 1966 novel *Valley of the Dolls*, later turned into a popular movie and a TV series, brought wider attention to prescription drug abuse. Another popular novel-film pair, *One Flew over the Cuckoo's Nest* (book 1962, film 1975), brought attention to overprescribing in psychiatric hospitals and to the excessive use of restraints and electroconvulsive (electroshock) therapy by hospital staffs to control patient populations.

The increased expense of medical care and its complexity, size, and technical sophistication thus contrasted markedly with its past organization, types of funding, and forms of delivery. Yet, even in light of the dominance of the medical model, one could ask why certain basic indicators of national health were not showing any dramatic improvement. The United States had the most technically advanced medical system in the world, and yet it continued to fall behind other industrialized nations in measures such as life expectancy, infant mortality, and access to care. All those dollars, it seems, didn't go toward producing the desired results. Critics pointed out, in fact, that what improvements in health indicators that there were might equally be attributed to better nutrition, public sanitation, and smaller family size as to miracle drugs and medical procedures.

By the 1960s, disenchanted and alienated youth were seeking insight through new myths, spiritual movements, and awareness regarding human health, sexuality, and the environment. Discouraged over the nation's unwillingness to fundamentally alter the contemporary state of affairs, despite the best efforts of some, many began to experiment with altered states of consciousness through the use of psychedelic drugs and mind-expanding experiences. They looked for alternatives to Western scientific medicine in the form of traditional health practices from other cultures, such as those of Native Americans, South and East Asians, and Latinos. Some proclaimed the dawn of an age of do-it-yourself medicine, as communes and some college campuses welcomed the arrival of "holistic" health, a term that suggested the rejection of the Cartesian separation of mind and body and the acceptance of the view of human beings as biological, mental, emotional, and spiritual wholes. Practices like acupuncture, meditation, vegetarianism, and naturopathy took off as part of the new counterculture, as did new mental health approaches like group therapy, existential therapy, and even more exotic varieties. Figures such as Thomas Szasz doubted the very existence of mental illness and considered the standard psychiatric approach to be merely a method to label and punish people for not conforming to social norms as dictated by the majority. (This was a radical view then, and so it remains today, though it did force a hard look at psychiatric conventions and must be counted as influential.)

Consider women's health, for example. From the late 1960s feminist critics and others complained of regular medicine's technological orientation, seeing it as intrusive, costly, and insensitive to women's needs. These activists challenged contemporary obstetrical practices and began advocating for home-based alternatives to medically oriented hospital births. They also publicized cautions concerning technologically designed birth-control methods such as oral contraceptives ("the pill") and intrauterine devices. They sought, in short, to preserve women's autonomy against excesses by the male-dominated medical establishment. And in doing so they helped change the context of health care in the later 20th century. The landmark popular book *Our Bodies, Ourselves* (1970) educated women on matters including sexual health, sexual orientation, gender identity, birth control, abortion, pregnancy, childbirth, domestic violence, and menopause. It helped change the narrative from one in which women were regarded as "docile and passive" to one in which they appeared as active agents involved in their own and their family's health and wellness.

Rebirth

Thus, even within the mainstream medical community, a growing number of professional health providers began to become disillusioned with the medical model and with the medical system at large, seeing it as offering only a narrow set of options. At a time when those in the countercultural movement were railing against the federal government (over the Vietnam War), questioning the political economy of science (with its ties to industry and the military), and at odds with authority and the status quo in general, the standard biomedical model of health suddenly appeared limited and constricting. It accounted only for biological variables and their status vis-à-vis the norm. It didn't factor in other variables such as the social, psychological, and behavioral aspects of health and illness. Consequently, interest began to grow, both within the medical community and outside of it, in developing a new, more comprehensive "biopsychosocial" model that would be more sensitive to the human dimensions of sickness and health.

In the early 1970s, several state university medical schools opened programs for training in osteopathic medicine, followed in the 1980s and 1990s by similar programs in other areas. In households across the nation, moreover, people began rediscovering alternative and traditional health systems, such as homeopathy, herbal treatments, and Ayurveda. Interest in health foods, exercise routines, and vitamins and minerals exploded, as new stores, magazines, and television shows supporting these interests emerged as well. For this new generation, holistic/alternative health approaches brought a sense of independence, self-reliance, affordability, and a return to what were seen as valid cultural models, both from the past and from different traditions around the globe. In 1978 the American Holistic Health Association was founded, "dedicated to the concept of medicine of the whole person which emphasizes integration of body, mind, and spirit with the environment" (quoted in Whorton 2002, 255). It began issuing its *Journal of Holistic Medicine* soon thereafter, which dealt with everything from nutrition and psychotherapy to acupuncture and homeopathy. The holistic health movement would prove to be a watershed in the history of medicine and of health care generally in the United States. While there would be excesses and exaggerations in the claims of its promoters, and while the medical establishment would continue to have its doubts, it became common understanding that individuals could find health, wellness, and satisfaction in using the new methods, not as a complete replacement for medical tests and procedures in all cases but as a supplement to them. At least that's how most people approached the prospect of choosing between the two.

Further Reading

Gevitz, Norman. 1988. *Other Healers: Unorthodox Medicine in America.* Baltimore: Johns Hopkins University Press.

National Institutes of Health. 2015. "Appropriations," March 25.

Saks, Mike. 2003. *Orthodox and Alternative Medicine: Politics, Professionalization, and Health Care.* London: Sage.

Whorton, James C. 2002. *Nature Cures: The History of Alternative Medicine in America.* New York: Oxford University Press.

ACUPUNCTURE

Acupuncture has the unique status of being rooted in ancient Asian healing practices while also being recognized in the United States as a beneficial modern form of "complementary" therapy. Even the usually staid and cautious U.S. health insurance industry allows that acupuncture is worth supporting for the good results it brings to patients seeking to relieve pain, to maintain mobility, to stop smoking, or otherwise to improve health. Exactly *how* such positive results are achieved, by nothing more than the insertion of thin needles into specific body points, is not well understood. Most explanations make reference to traditional Chinese conceptions of the body and healing, sometimes in combination with the placebo effect or the power of positive thinking.

Origins and Philosophy

Cases of acupuncture and related forms of therapy are recorded from more than 2,000 years ago, although the ancient Chinese sources in which these reports appear are often unreliable or ambiguous. One such source, *The Yellow Emperor's Inner Canon* (*Huangdi Neijing*), from around 200 BCE, discusses acupuncture theory in some detail. (The Yellow Emperor also wrote an *Outer Canon*, but it has since been lost.) In Chinese philosophy, humans are considered a kind of microcosmic image of the universe. They are prone to the same tensions and disruptions that generally define nature. Nature's immutable course, the Tao, is thought to be expressed in two equal but opposite forces, yin and yang, which are constantly at war with each other. Yin represents that which is cold, dark, feminine, and passive, while yang represents that which is hot, bright, male, and active. (Classical philosophy had its biases.) Under the best of circumstances, there is a balance between yin and yang—both in nature and in the healthy human body. Oftentimes, however, the balance goes awry, and people must take steps to try to restore it.

In addition, according to traditional Chinese medical theory the human body consists of 12 systems, based largely on physiology and function. Each system is associated with a major internal organ and an energy pathway, known as a meridian, tracing itself through the body. Along each meridian flows a vital life force called *chi* (or *qi*), which is thought to function similar to a circadian, or daily, rhythm in keeping the body (and its owner) apprised of processes within. Disruptions in the flow of chi result from disharmonies in the natural forces (Yin and Yang) within the individual. If not corrected, these disruptions can eventually produce a disease condition affecting the organ associated with the meridian or some other point along the meridian where a blockage of the chi has occurred. Acupuncture is designed to address these blockages or imbalances in the flow of the vital life force. More than 365 points have been located along the meridians where patients can be treated via acupuncture's main contribution to medicine: needle therapy. Traditional acupuncture specifies exact locations and details the procedures by which needles are to be inserted and, in some cases, manipulated during treatment. The goal is to reset the energy flow in order to restore the overall balance of yin and yang.

Western Practice

In the West, the most important early advocate of acupuncture was the Dutch doctor and naturalist Willem ten Rhijne (1647–1700). Ten Rhijne visited Japan in 1674, where he observed acupuncture firsthand along with the related practice of moxibustion, or the burning of a substance placed on the skin at one of the meridian points. On his return to Europe, ten Rhijne wrote a detailed account of what he had witnessed, replete with elaborate anatomical drawings. Ten Rhijne, in fact, is responsible for the term *acupuncture*. The problem, though, was that the practice was so alien to Western understandings of medicine that ten Rhijne's treatise barely made an impact upon publication. The idea, in particular, of deliberately penetrating the body with needles was anathema both to Western doctors and their patients, even though the procedure was (and is) quite safe and painless when performed properly. There was a fear, furthermore, that the needles might break off and somehow get "lost" inside the patient's body. As a result, acupuncture did not make inroads into Western culture for more than two centuries. (Moxabustion, on the other hand, found a following because it was similar to a common Western treatment for gout.) Although acupuncture achieved some success in Europe and the United States by the late 19th century as exchanges with China and Japan became more common, it only took off as a popular alternative form of treatment in the 1960s and 1970s, as the youth cultural revolution was unfolding. People then were looking for alternatives to "establishment" medicine, and they found it in acupuncture and other Eastern imports. Further interest during the holistic health revolution in the 1980s expanded acupuncture's reach.

Today, a number of variations on classical acupuncture are available. In some cases, acupuncturists tap needles into place using guide tubes. In others, they apply and manipulate the needles by hand. The needles themselves have become more lightweight (hollow) and disposable, thus reassuring patients—as well as insurers—about hygiene and safety. Sometimes, a small electric current is passed between pairs of needles (electroacupuncture), particularly when treating pain. Acupuncture methods are occasionally combined with Western medical procedures to help address pain associated with surgery, either as an anesthesia beforehand or as a postoperative pain relief measure. Not all of the traditional meridian points are used nowadays, and a few new ones have been added. In most Western applications, the theory of yin and yang is not explicitly drawn on. References to chi and/or "energy," however, are still common enough, depending on the acupuncturist—and on the patient's own background and expectations. Acupuncturists in the United States are expected to have completed a graduate-level training program and be licensed in the state in which they practice. Although widely available, it remains more prominent in areas where there is a significant Asian American population. Customers, on the other hand, range over a variety of demographics.

Modern Understanding

To this day, medical researchers have been unable to identify how or why acupuncture is as effective as it seems to be in helping to relieve pain, increase flexibility/motion, or address other health conditions. All that can be said is that stress, emotion, and other factors play a role in almost any type of pain or illness, and acupuncture, with its theme of managing vital energy flow, seems to serve a therapeutic function in this context. It could be that endorphins—"pleasure" molecules—are released in the brain as the needles are inserted. Or it could be, as those in the acupuncture community are apt to think, that the meridians operate as conduits for electrical signals that have yet to be identified by Western science. Other supporters have suggested that the autonomic nervous system—that is, the nerves that serve the internal organs and glands—may be involved. Some critics have argued that acupuncture is no more than a placebo, or a means to make one feel that a medical solution has been applied and that one's health therefore must be improved. In any case, acupuncture is a relatively inexpensive, harmless treatment that provides a reasonable alternative to standard Western treatments, including drugs.

It should be stated again that acupuncture must be practiced by a qualified, professionally trained therapist in order for it to be safe and effective. Accidents, which happened far more in the past than in today's controlled environments, have nevertheless been documented. These mishaps have included, for example, the piercing of a lung or the heart, or, just as serious, the development of hepatitis or other infections from the use of unsterilized needles. Current safeguards make these outcomes less likely, however. (Among other things, acupuncture needles are regulated by the Food and Drug Administration.) Another point of caution is that, as with most alternative therapies, there is a risk that some patients drawn to this form of treatment could be overlooking symptoms of a condition that might better be addressed by orthodox medicine, or perhaps by a combination of the two.

Michael Shally-Jensen

See also: Chinese Traditional Medicine; Reiki and Therapeutic Touch; Shiatsu; Tai Chi and Qigong

Further Reading

Beinfield, Harriet, and Efrem Korngold. 1992. *Between Heaven and Earth: A Guide to Chinese Medicine.* New York: Ballantine Books.

Bivins, Roberta. 2007. *Alternative Medicine? A History.* New York: Oxford University Press.

U.S. National Institutes of Health, National Center for Complementary and Integrative Health. 2013. "Traditional Chinese Medicine: In Depth." https://nccih.nih.gov/health/whatiscam/chinesemed.htm

Whorton, James C. 2002. *Nature Cures: The History of Alternative Medicine in America.* New York: Oxford University Press.

ALTERNATIVE DIAGNOSTICS

People have sought to know what ails them since time immemorial. Before the advent of modern diagnostic tools like chemoanalysis (lab tests), X-rays, and CT scans, diagnosis was more of an art than a science. In many societies, astrology and dream interpretation played a role. Another common method of diagnosis was use of a medium, or shaman; the medium would enter a state of "possession," or trance, and divine what was wrong with the patient by communicating with the gods. More specific forms of bodily "analysis" also occurred, such as close examination of the pulse, the eyes, the tongue, the breath, the fingernails, and bodily fluids like ear wax and urine. The patient might also be asked *who* could be harming him or her, because illness was thought in many traditional societies to be the result of witchcraft or sorcery.

Modern Western medicine has made great strides, but there are still notable gaps. It does an excellent job of identifying and treating most acute illnesses, including in emergency situations, and of offering life-saving treatments. The ability to treat or cure chronic conditions, such as fibromyalgia, depression, lupus, and others is somewhat more limited, however. In part, these are conditions that medical science has only recently begun to identify and understand. After all, we knew that people died of heart failure for hundreds of years before we were able to try to prevent it. Similarly, understanding that in certain cases the immune system may attack itself is a newer concept that is only beginning to yield results.

But for many people suffering from chronic conditions, waiting for medical science to catch up is painful—literally. Some people may suffer from chronic pain, ongoing stomach or intestinal issues, or mental health disturbances, for example, that Western medicine struggles to diagnose. Alternatively, patients may have diagnosed health conditions, such as allergies, cancer, epilepsy, or fibromyalgia, that Western medicine can diagnose but may not be able to control with traditional therapies.

For many of these conditions, patients may turn to providers like naturopaths, applied kinesiologists, and other alternative medicine practitioners to get help. Many of these providers do not have thorough oversight agencies, and use products like dietary supplements that are also poorly regulated in order to treat conditions. These providers also use alternative diagnostics in order to determine a cause of illness and a treatment. They often uncover conditions that modern medicine has debunked, aren't supported by science, or, sometimes, treatments for which modern medicine has a perfectly sound treatment. We are still, regrettably, a long way off from *Star Trek*–type diagnoses where a simple handheld device can instantly identify all ailments.

Below, though, are a few of the alternative diagnostic options that are currently available.

Homeopathy

Although homeopathic practitioners exist, one of the primary principles of homeopathy is that you don't need formal training to find a homeopathic remedy. You simply look up your family's symptoms in one of many available homeopathic guides and pick one of the different remedies suggested.

Homeopathy was developed in 1796 by Samuel Hahnemann and is based around the idea that "like cures like." If something causes an illness in a healthy person, it can cure the same illness in a sick person. No rigorous scientific studies have found homeopathy to be more than a placebo. This may be because homeopathic treatments are diluted so many times that true homeopathic liquids or pills are nothing more than distilled water or sugar pills. Not even a molecule of the original substance may remain. Most homeopathic treatments are probably harmless, except to your wallet. The problem is, of course, that they do nothing physical to treat the actual condition in question. And if one remedy doesn't work, then you move on to the next one. That is the diagnostic system (because each individual is thought to be unique).

Reiki

Reiki is the most modern version of the ancient practice of "laying on hands." A Reiki practitioner studies and develops the ability to feel the "life force energy" that surrounds all beings. By manipulating this energy, Reiki masters state that they can cure all manner of ailments, from physical pain to emotional distress through removing blocks and impediments to proper energy flow. The theory is somewhat similar to acupuncture and acupressure. To diagnose a patient, the practitioner uses his or her hands to sense these energy "blockages" and then treats them by "channeling" energies through and around them until proper flow is restored.

There isn't any science that backs up Reiki, but it certainly can be stress relieving. Many Reiki practitioners also engage in a sort of guided meditation technique that can help their "patient" feel more relaxed, in touch with their breathing, and experience a sort of mindfulness. Gwyncth Paltrow, Naomi Watts, and Angelina Jolie are all said to be big fans of Reiki; and Jennifer Aniston supposedly has Reiki performed on her dog regularly.

Biofeedback

Certain things your body does—like raising your arm and waving to a friend—are voluntary actions. Certain other things are involuntary. You don't directly control your heartbeat or your blood pressure or your skin temperature. When certain things happen, your body just reacts in certain ways.

Biofeedback proposes that you can change the way these functions of your body work. You can work to treat migraines, blood pressure problems, chronic pain, and other illnesses in this way, with a little training.

During a biofeedback session, sensors are attached to your body that measure these involuntary functions. A monitor is placed so that you can see all the different functions as they're occurring. You can see the immediate feedback as stress responses happen in your body, and therapists work to assist you in trying to change these automatic responses. You may also use guided breathing, mindfulness exercises, and progressive muscle relaxation to help calm your body's automatic responses to stress.

Depending on the condition you're trying to treat, biofeedback can actually be effective. Many of the exercises used during the session are commonly used to reduce anxiety, for example, and seeing the physiological proof that the body is calming down can encourage a patient to continue to practice the exercises. Biofeedback isn't likely to be harmful, either.

Applied Kinesiology

Kinesiology studies the mechanics of how the body moves. While there isn't a specific medical profession called a kinesiologist, a practitioner who focused on this treatment would probably be something like a physical therapist. PTs certainly use a lot of kinesiology in their work.

Applied kinesiology (AK) is something different, however. This methodology suggests that different glands and organs are linked to different muscle groups throughout the body. By finding muscle weakness in the various muscle groups, therefore, a practitioner can diagnose chemical imbalance, nerve damage, or other conditions in distant parts of the body. They use the theory of "energy pathways"—similar to meridians in traditional Chinese medicine.

Given its base in body mechanics, applied kinesiology may be useful in finding nerve damage or in uncovering sources of problems that most patients wouldn't expect. For example, an AK practitioner might recommend hip stretches to treat tension headaches—but so might a physical therapist! Tightness in the hips can affect posture, which can cause shoulder tension, which can cause headaches.

It is when AK is used to treat diabetes or learning disabilities that many doctors get concerned. At that point, AK goes from being a kind of physical therapy to being a pseudoscience that may be risky or dangerous. Practitioners often recommend high-priced supplements and vitamins—which, conveniently, they often sell—in order to treat conditions that are diagnosed by testing muscle groups, while certain substances are held in the hand or under the tongue. These supplements are generally unregulated, and can often do more harm than good.

In Sum

When patients are unable to get treatment from modern medicine, it makes sense that they seek alternative avenues for treatment. Some patients also seek what is called complementary or integrative medicine, where alternative doctors work closely with traditional doctors to get the best benefits for a patient. They might work together to manage the nausea from chemotherapy, for example.

All too often, unfortunately, alternative diagnostics are about placebos and untested supplements, and less often about the long-term health of the patient.

Still, the field of integrative medicine is advancing through a combination of testing procedures and assessments of patient health and satisfaction.

Kay Tilden Frost and
Michael Shally-Jensen

See also: Astrology; Ayurvedic Medicine; Biofeedback; Chinese Traditional Medicine; Craniosacral Therapy; Dream Interpretation; Homeopathy; Mind–Body Medicine; Phrenology; Reflexology; Reiki and Therapeutic Touch; Shamanism and Neo-Shamanism; Witch Trials and Exorcisms

Further Reading

Arden, John. 2010. *Rewire Your Brain: Think Your Way to a Better Life.*
"Complementary and Alternative Medicine (CAM)." 2018. *MedicineNet.* November 5. https://www.medicinenet.com/alternative_medicine/article.htm#tocb
Frazier, Karen. 2018. *Reiki Healing for Beginners.* San Antonio, TX: Althea Press, July 24.

AROMATHERAPY AND ESSENTIAL OILS

Aromatherapy is the practice of using fragrant oils from various plants to treat illness and promote health. The oils are often used as massage oils or else vaporized and inhaled. Proponents of aromatherapy believe that compounds in the oils

---

How We Ended Up Ingesting Aromatherapy Oils

As far back as ancient Egypt, we believed that the practice of putting certain oils on our skin, inhaling them, or using them in perfumes could prevent or cure various illnesses and ailments. That practice carried through the Greeks and Romans, through medieval Europe, and into modern day. But when did we start ingesting essential oils?

Essential oils are highly concentrated versions of extractions from plants, flowers, herbs, and more. Several high-profile companies have started selling their versions of essential oils through representatives on Facebook. One company in particular was famous for claiming that their oil was the only one safe enough and pure enough to ingest.

Some natural medicine practitioners argue that it can be safe to ingest certain essential oils, but it's absolutely necessary that this be done under the care of a physician. Essential oils are much more concentrated than the versions used in teas or tinctures. For some of these oils, a very small amount can result in serious burns, health problems, or even death.

Some essential oils also market themselves with language like "therapeutic grade" or "100% pure." It's important to understand that these are marketing terms; there is no external, unbiased agency responsible for verifying these claims.

So, should you ingest the kinds of essential oils that are used in aromatherapy? Probably not, unless you're working with a trained and trusted natural medicine professional.

activate certain parts of the brain and/or endocrine system, thus releasing chemicals in the body that may have a beneficial effect. About 40 oils are commonly used in aromatherapy, in settings ranging from the home to the private massage room to the yoga studio. Oils may be added to one's bathwater, burned in aromatic candles or diffusers, or smelled in diluted form from a bowl or container holding a base mixture such as vegetable oil or alcohol. Aromatherapy is said to help pain, depression, stress, and other conditions and to promote positive mood changes.

That scents activate the olfactory system, thereby causing the brain to respond, is an undisputed fact of science. Some oils may also be absorbed through the skin. The question that remains is whether these effects lead to health benefits, and, if so, what kind?

Background

Plants and plant oils have played a fundamental role in human society since its beginning. In addition to providing food, fiber, dwelling materials, and ornamental elements, plants provide spices such as pepper and turmeric, drinks such as tea and coffee, medicines such as quinine, digitalis, and various antibiotics, and addictive and/or narcotic products such as tobacco and opium. There are also many poisonous and allergenic plants. People interested in aromatherapy must be careful if they suffer from allergies or sensitivities to specific plants or plant-based substances.

Plant oils featured prominently in several ancient cultures, including the Chinese, Indian, Egyptian, Greek, and Roman. In these cultures they were used in spiritual and ritualistic contexts as well as in perfumes, cosmetics, and drugs. The Hebrew Bible contains numerous references to frankincense (a tree resin) as an altar offering and to its use with various oils in "anointing" newborns and others seeking spiritual assurance. In medieval times, Arabic physicians explored the use of essential oils.

The birth of modern aromatherapy is attributed to René-Maurice Gattefossé, a French chemist who in the 1930s burned his hand while working in the laboratory and proceeded to treat the wound with lavender oil. To his surprise, the wound healed promptly and did not leave a scar. The favorable result inspired him to study the medicinal uses of essential oils, which he recorded in his 1937 book *Aromathérapie: Les huiles essentielles, hormones végétales* (Aromatherapy: Essential oils, plant hormones). In it, Gattefossé asks a series of questions:

> Are aromatic substances similar to vitamins? Is not their role in the plant world the same as that of hormones in the animal kingdom? Are they not consequentially indispensable to plant life and valuable to human life? ([1937] 1993, xii)

In fact, the parallel that Gettefossé draws between animal and plant fluids might have more accurately referred to fats, or fatty acids, in the case of animals, because both animal fat and plant oils contain fatty acids as a basic building block. In that sense both are indeed "indispensable" to the maintenance of the health—indeed, the life—of the organism. The parallel to vitamins is perhaps more of a stretch. And yet vitamins are nothing more than a group of organic substances that, in minute quantities, play a key role in nutrition. So, yes, they are essential substances, but, no, they don't really operate like fats or oils.

Organic oils are a basic component of all forms of plant life. Virtually every species of plant produces some quantity of oil during its life cycle. However, only relatively few plants produce oils in sufficient quantity to become useful in commerce or other applications. Among the most common in this category are soybean oil, corn oil, peanut oil, olive oil, palm oil, coconut oil, and a variety of others. One key difference between these oils and essential oils is that the latter require much greater amounts of plant material from which to extract a comparatively small amount of oil. (This process generally involves distillation using steam and condensation.) Hence the term "essential," suggesting a concentration of the "essence" of the plant. Common essential oils include lavender, tea tree oil, peppermint, eucalyptus, clove, rosemary, and frankincense oil (a distillation of the resin). In making such oils, different parts of a plant may be used: bark, berries, flowers, leaves, roots, seeds, and so on.

The current interest in essential oils is tied to the rise of holistic health and wellness consciousness beginning in the 1980s, gaining much steam in the 1990s, and continuing today. Whereas at one time consumers could find essential oils only in specialty shops catering to complementary and alternative medicine users, nowadays the little vials of liquid essence are widely available in grocery stores and elsewhere. There are also distribution firms that rely on multilevel marketing schemes, or "pyramid selling," to reach consumers—in the manner of Avon, Herbalife, or the Pampered Chef. (Some of these companies have faced legal challenges.)

Claims and Cautions

Claims of the beneficial uses of essential oils include the following:

- Frankincense—apply to scalp for hair loss or to skin to keep it young
- Clove, rosemary, eucalyptus solution—imbibe as an immune-system booster
- Nutmeg and/or spearmint—inhale to sharpen focus
- Citrus blend—add to water in order to detox
- Rosemary—supports healthy digestion and internal organ function; also, respiratory health
- Eucalyptus—for bronchitis or colds
- Cypress—for mononucleosis
- Tea tree oil—acne, fungal infections, and/or general purification
- Vetiver (bunch grass)—mental imbalances
- Peppermint or chamomile—teeth grinding (bruxism)
- Bergamot—cough

- Ylang ylang—stress, anxiety
- Sweet orange—depression
- Rose geranium—digestion issues or dry skin

This small sampling, of course, cannot do justice to the full range of applications claimed for aromatherapy. Moreover, different professional therapists will prescribe different substances for different conditions. In fact, consumers of aromatherapy often find this "mix-and-match" aspect of the system to be one of its more appealing aspects: one can *explore* the use of different oils/aromas to see what works best in one's own case. Obviously, this type of thinking goes directly against orthodox medical science, with its rigorous tests and trials. Many professional aromatherapists would not recommend free exploration, either. Yet, there appears to be no clear consensus as to the appropriate applications of specific essential oils, and both traditionally and today there was and is an openness to using aromatherapeutic remedies broadly to address any number of conditions, or simply to make one feel better.

Few "double-blind" scientific studies have been done on essential oils' effects in humans, and those that have been published have offered only modest results. It appears that lavender oil may have some effect in relieving anxiety and improving sleep. The scent of lavender is thought to have a calming effect on the nervous system. Peppermint, too, may alleviate symptoms of headache and irritable bowels. Tea tree oil is known to have some minor antimicrobial effects. Beyond that, there is not a great deal of scientific evidence.

On the other hand, if combined with a massage, or experienced in a warm bath, aromatherapy is definitely relaxing. But it is unclear whether the effect is caused by the oil, the massage, the bath, or some combination of these. An initial meeting with an aromatherapist may last an hour or more, during which time the therapist takes a brief medical history and possibly examines the client. This is often followed by massaging a diluted essential oil into the skin of the client. The process is generally relaxing and enjoyable, owing both to the massage and to the pleasant aroma. In the case of chronic or recurring conditions like anxiety, headache, or stiffness and pain, aromatherapists usually suggest regular sessions to address the symptoms and keep them at bay.

The risks in using essential oils may not be great, but they are present in many cases. Undiluted oils should never be taken orally, as some of them may be carcinogenic. And yet the practice occurs. As one expert has stated: "You hear about completely untrained housewives [i.e., home-based distributors] telling people to ingest up to fifty drops. That is insanity. That is medically dangerous. It's a crazy situation" (quoted in Monroe 2017, 37). Adverse effects can include allergic reactions, phototoxicity (or rendering the skin susceptible to damage by light), nausea, headache, respiratory reactions, and so on. Although the U.S. Food and Drug Administration is charged with preventing sellers of alternative-health products from making unfounded medical claims, the essential oil industry—particularly the home-based distribution sector—is prone to relying on such words as "vitality" and "balance" to get around these strictures. At selling seminars, which are a key part of this industry sector, one can often hear much bolder, and patently false, claims.

For the casual or occasional consumer, however, aromatherapy can offer short-term destressing effects that contribute to an overall sense of well-being. It is generally sound, therefore, to employ it as a simple therapy for relieving feelings of anxiety and improving the quality of life. Other applications will vary depending on the characteristics and mindset of the individual.

Michael Shally-Jensen

See also: Antioxidants; Ayurvedic Medicine; Chinese Traditional Medicine; Detox Diets; Folk Medicine; Herbal Remedies; Meditation and Mindfulness; Patent Medicines; Spas and Mineral Waters; Vitamins and Minerals

Further Reading

Gattefossé, René-Maurice. [1937] 1993. *Gattefossé's Aromatherapy*. Edited by Robert B. Tisserand, translated by Louise Davies. Saffron Walden, UK: C. W. Daniel Co.

Homes, Peter. 2016. *Aromatica: A Clinical Guide to Essential Oil Therapeutics*. London: Singing Dragon.

Monroe, Rachel. 2017. "Something in the Air: Essential Oils Have Become Big Business—But Are They Medicine or Marketing?" *New Yorker,* October 9, 32–37.

Singh, Simon, and Edzrd Ernst. 2008. *Trick or Treatment: The Undeniable Facts about Alternative Medicine*. New York: W. W. Norton.

ASTROLOGY

Astrology is a kind of divination based on the belief that the celestial bodies influence human affairs. It is practiced both to predict and to affect the course of human events, at both the individual level and at the level of the wider group. Astrology's central premise is that the position of the sun in relation to other heavenly bodies determines the auspiciousness of certain days and the character and fortunes of persons based on their date and time of birth. Various characterizations of individuals and their prospects—including health decisions—can be made according to the occult science of astrology. While astrology has no standing in the mainstream medical community, it is sometimes used as part of an overall complementary and alternative healthcare strategy.

History and Method

Astrology seems to have originated in Mesopotamia some 4,000 years ago. Not yet a fully developed system, it was made up of a mix of astronomical observations and mathematical calculations aimed at assisting in decision making in areas such as planting/harvesting and war making. The movements of the sun, moon, stars, and planets had long been a key indicator in the agricultural cycle for the Mesopotamians and other settled peoples. Astrology was simply an attempt to systemize, by way of a calendar, the flow of seasons, the rains, and the growth cycles of plants. As such, it was not distinct from astronomy, which would only much later, after the Middle Ages, hive off from astrology. The Chaldeans and Babylonians, in particular, established the foundations of early astrology. Under them, the movements of the heavenly bodies were traced and were linked to a complex mythology and cosmology.

The Egyptians too contributed. Seeking to employ the star system as a clock, the Egyptians identified a series of 36 bright stars whose annual first-risings on the horizon were separated by 10 days. Each star was thought of as a spirit or minor deity having control over the period of time in which it reigned. Later, under the Hellenistic Greeks, each spirit came to be associated with a part of the chart of the heavens, the zodiac, based on the arrangement of constellations.

It was the Greeks of the Hellenistic period who really formalized Western astrology/astronomy. Under them, an astrological view of causation pervaded scientific thought, especially in medicine. They came to develop the horoscope, or map showing the relative positions of the heavenly bodies and the different sectors, each dominated by a constellation with its particular zodiacal sign. For the Greeks, the zodiac was a "circle of animals," or animal spirits such as Aries (Ram), Taurus (Bull), Gemini (Twins), Cancer (Crab), and so on. The horoscope, used to establish information about the present and predict events to come, makes use of the standard arrangement of the celestial bodies and their mythological characters. The degree of influence on an individual of each body and/or character is modified by its geometric relationship with the other celestial bodies and/or characters, depending on the day and time of the person's birth and the present arrangement of planets and stars. The heavens as a whole are represented by a circle of 12 zodiacal sections, called houses. Each of these houses is assigned sets of qualities relating to human life, such as learning, marriage, and career.

An older form of astrology spread to India and was elaborated according to Indian tradition. There, the gods, most of which are anthropomorphic figures, serve as benevolent forces aligned against malevolent demons; the *dharma*, or fundamental principle ordering the universe, is represented by a wheel symbol. The *dharmachakra* wheel serves, in addition, the Buddhist tradition, where it marks the Four Noble Truths and the Eightfold Path to enlightenment. Thus, very different meanings are loaded onto these South Asian symbols and traditions as compared to Western astrology.

In ancient China, too, a system developed that related the observable cosmic order with natural phenomenon, human activities, and fate. The Chinese zodiac is built on a 12-year cycle with an animal attribute for each year: the Rat, the Ox, the Tiger, the Rabbit, the Dragon, and so on. The Chinese system, while again distinct from the Western, shares more similarities with it than the Indian.

Additionally, by the first millennium CE, Islamic science drew on parts of the Hellenistic Greek tradition to develop its own understanding of astrology, which in turn influenced both European civilization and, via the Mongol expansion and after, China and India. Celestial bodies in Islam are not separate spiritual presences but rather illuminating lights of the Prophet and his truth, a different conception altogether.

In the Americas, too, astrological and calendrical systems were developed by the Mayas and used to predict events and regulate social activity. As recently as 2012 fears erupted over the purported end of the world based on the termination of the Mayan calendar in that year. Needless to say, humanity survived the event.

In medieval Europe, Christian leaders typically condemned astrology as a pagan holdover while privately drawing on it as a source of counsel and allowing it to flourish among the populace. Most of the top European universities had chairs of astrology. The unseating of the astrological worldview came about only through the scientific work of Nicolaus Copernicus, Tycho Brahe, and Johannes Kepler in the 16th and 17th centuries. Even then, astrology remained a popular approach to understanding the meaning of things beyond the limits of scientific rationality or church dogma.

Medicinal and Predictive Aspects

Well into the 18th century in Europe and America, astrology remained an integral part of medicine. Few medical practitioners at the time had university degrees or received formal training. Most, in fact, were folk healers, midwives, or nominally apprenticed medical men operating from a set of beliefs going back to the Renaissance or earlier, including the notion of the four humors (choler, blood, melancholy, and phlegm). Astrology was considered a useful tool in both the diagnosis and treatment of illness. Medical texts such as Nicholas Culpeper's (1616–1654) *Astrological Judgment of Diseases* were reprinted frequently and remained in wide use for over a century. Culpeper also published an "herbal," or book of herbal treatments, that made use of astrological data. Almanacs, too, which were bestsellers in the largely rural North American continent, typically included astrological information and provided medical advice about bloodletting. The latter might be based, for example, on connections between parts of the body and the positions of celestial bodies. With the advent of modern medicine in the late 19th and early 20th centuries, some of the older assumptions and methods began to fall away.

Still, contemporary astrology is a popular and lucrative art. Media organizations around the world publish daily astrological forecasts, which are read by millions (billions?). Books and magazines devoted to astrology and the occult arts are in wide circulation; and professional astrologers everywhere routinely prepare detailed predictions for millions of paying believers. In East Asia, using astrologers to pick auspicious days for important functions is an essential activity, and the practice has begun to migrate to Western countries as well. Nancy Reagan famously relied on an astrologer to help arrange her and her husband President Ronald Reagan's social calendar, much to the consternation of more rational actors in the Reagan administration.

The horoscope is the key tool in such applications. It shows the relative positions of the sun, moon, stars, and planets at a given time. To make an individual's horoscope, the astrologer must have the exact time and place of his or her birth. Each of the 12 signs of the zodiac is associated with different aspects of character, temperament, physiology, aptitude, and the like. Once the necessary information is known, the astrologer can then predict the person's future or counsel him or her regarding pending decisions or actions. Although most of the time clients walk away satisfied, questions have been raised recently about when an astrologer or other psychic practitioner might cross the line and become liable for malpractice, or even criminally responsible for deceptive advertising and the like (George-Parkin 2014).

In addition to aiding individuals, astrology has been used to address collective concerns. Astronomical events such as comets, eclipses, and other phenomena are often seen as portents of wars, calamities, or even positive developments. The prophecies of Nostradamus, a 16th-century physician-astrologer, continue to sell well, particularly in times of crisis. People today still consult Nostradamus and claim that he accurately foretold events. Some modern researchers have examined the astrological significance of such major events as the French Revolution and 9/11 (Tarnas 2006). In today's marketplace, astrological handbooks, or "how-tos," remain bestsellers. There are also a number of more specialized works on medical astrology available. And street-front psychics, who draw on astrology and other techniques, continue to do a lively business.

Michael Shally-Jensen

See also: Anthroposophic Medicine; Chinese Traditional Medicine; Crystals; Folk Medicine; Herbal Remedies; Jung and Jungian Analysis; Spiritualism

Further Reading

Bobrick, Benson. 2006. *The Fated Sky: Astrology in History.* New York: Simon and Schuster.

George-Parkin, Hilary. 2014. "When Is Fortune-Telling a Crime?" *Atlantic,* November 14. https://www.theatlantic.com/business/archive/2014/11/when-is-fortunetelling-a-crime/382738/

Goldschneider, Gary, and Joost Elffers. 2013. *The Secret Language of Birthdays: Your Complete Personology Guide for Each Day of the Year.* New York: Viking Studio.

Hill, Judith. 2004. *Medical Astrology: A Guide to Planetary Pathology.* Portland, OR: Stellium Press.

Tarnas, Richard. 2006. *Cosmos and Psyche: Intimations of a New World View.* New York: Viking Penguin.

AYURVEDIC MEDICINE

The traditional medical system of India is called *Ayurveda,* "science of longevity," or "knowledge of healthy life." Like many systems of its type, it has religious-philosophical roots as well as various empirical elements arrived at through practice and explained on the basis of cultural conventions. In other words, it is a kind of "folk medicine" that nevertheless serves the needs of millions and has drawn much attention in the West.

Historical Development

India is a vast area displaying great regional differences in terrain and climate, albeit much of it semitropical. It also has long been marked by a high population density and continuing contact with neighboring countries and overseas merchants. As such, throughout India's history its populace has faced serious infectious diseases such as smallpox, dysentery, and yellow fever along with the full array of other human illnesses. The earliest medical writings date to circa 1500–1800 BCE (the Vedic period). They are part of a song cycle named Atharva-Veda, which contains a mix of magical spells, medicinal knowledge, and spiritual advice. By about 600 BCE, the subcontinent had become home to a rational system of healing known as Ayurveda; accompanying it were various metaphysical systems that aimed to explain human nature and fate. During the so-called Classical Period (800 BCE–700 CE),

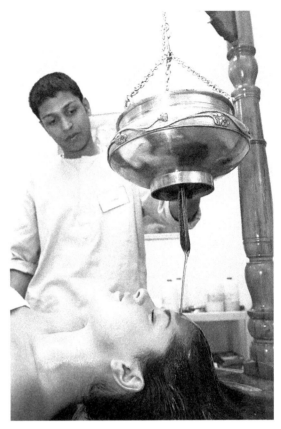

Shirodhara is an Ayurvedic purifying treatment involving pouring warm liquids, like oil or milk, over the forehead. It is used to treat a variety of physical ailments as well as some mental conditions. In Ayurveda, the distinction between the two is not firm. (Valery Kraynov/Dreamstime.com)

Ayurveda was developed into a practical art designed to express religious and philosophical principles as well as to heal individual sufferers. By advancing the restoration and maintenance of health, Hindu physicians sought equally to help persons achieve greater longevity and to guide them toward moral-spiritual perfection.

The bulk of classical Ayurvedic medicine was described in the *Charaka,* a medical textbook, of sorts, written around 120 CE. It was supplemented by the *Suśruta* and the *Astanghrdaya.* Each represents a compilation of teachings by one or more master healers combined with transmitted knowledge from other (unknown) ancient sources. In general, health is viewed in these texts as a balance of bodily energies (*doshas*) and a healthy mental state (*prasana*). Disruptions in this equilibrium are said to bring on illness and require an investigation, by a healer, into the cause. The healer uses three sources in making a determination: observation, inference or interpretation, and the wisdom of the medical sages (also referred to as "case histories"). Three pulse points are taken to read the flow of vital forces. In the end, a rational judgment is reached and a solution or "adjustment" (*yukti*) provided.

According to traditional Ayurvedic theory, the body consists of five "tissues" or materials: earth (muscle and bone), wind (breath), fire (bile), water (phlegm), and space (hollow areas). They are energized by the flow of doshas, three of which—*vata* (air), *pitta* (fire), and *kapha* (earth)—are key and correspond to the major tissue centers as well as to a trio of human bodily and psychological types (*vata:* slender and alert; *pitta:* medium and aggressive; *kapha:* heavy and stubborn). When the three doshas work together harmoniously, good health is produced. If, however, there are any excesses or deficiencies with these energies, illness results. Hence the reason they are referred to as the "three troubles" (*tridosha*). In addition, breath, or *prana,* relates not only to respiration but also to a systemwide circulatory operation made up of channels running throughout the body. It (prana) distributes the life forces (doshas) and produces movement—in part by igniting or stoking the internal fire (pitta). The goal of Hindu medicine is to restore the balance of elements through diet and drugs while also reducing any emotional disturbance associated with an illness.

Classical Applications

In Ayurveda, a good deal of attention is paid to the causes of a disease and to prescriptions of a hygienic, or "cleansing," nature. A direct anatomical review is sometimes necessary and may involve inspection of the flesh (particularly the tongue), muscle, bone, fat, chyle (lymph), blood, and sperm along with the sense organs and other bodily parts. Treatments are developed on the basis not only of symptoms but according to the determination of causes and the physiological "type" of the person. To address a fever, for example, the healer may provide "cooling" or antithermic drugs; yet he or she may also prescribe measures such as detoxification followed by medication to restore the balance of doshas. To eliminate stress, to take another example, the *vata* dosha, which governs actions and the nervous system, might be adjusted for by keeping oneself warm, sticking to a routine schedule, using calming oils, listening to music, performing yoga, enjoying sweet aromas and warm colors, and consuming ginger tea and warm milk, among other recommendations.

Classical Ayurvedic medicine also included surgical treatments, when needed, as described in the *Suśruta.* Such treatments often involved wounds and fractures of the limbs, but the text addressed other matters as well. The ancient text describes obstetrical procedures, the extraction of cysts, the suturing of the gut, skin grafting, and the removal of cataracts. Indian pharmaceuticals, too, were quite well developed, with numerous substances explored not only for alchemical purposes but for the preparation of mineral drugs.

Influence

Some scholars believe that traces of Indian traditional medicine are present in the works of the Greek physician Hippocrates and in the Platonic dialogue *Timaeus.*

Indian cyclical concepts (*yugas*) are referred to by both Heraclitus and a third-century BCE Babylonian priest named Berossus. Classical Indian medical practices were adopted, in part, in Tibet and eventually spread, in modified form, into central and eastern Asia. Ayurvedic medicine continues to be widely used in India, particularly in rural areas where the majority of the population lives.

During the late 1960s and early 1970s, Ayurvedic medicine became popular with young people in the United and other Western countries as people sought alternatives to mainstream or "establishment" practices—medical or otherwise. Waves of hippie venturers traveled to India to experience firsthand the beauty and uniqueness of the land and learn about the country's rich cultural heritage. Many visitors stayed on for extended periods of time or even ended up taking up residence in the subcontinent. Those who returned to their countries of origin brought back components of Ayurveda together with other treasures. At the same time, Indian citizens, including a variety of gurus and healers specializing in Ayurveda, traveled to Western countries, spreading their cultural knowledge and expanding people's horizons. By the 1980s, when the Holistic or New Age era spawned further intercultural exchanges, Ayurvedic medicine had already begun to establish itself as a compelling alternative/complementary form of medicine in the West.

Among the contributions of Ayurvedic medicine to Western medicine is reserpine, a drug derived from the Indian snakeroot plant and used today to treat hypertension and to control psychotic symptoms. For inflammatory conditions, Ayurvedic practitioners use turmeric, an herb of the ginger family. Modern clinical trials of turmeric show that it may help with arthritis and certain digestive disorders, but the research is limited. A type of frankincense, or aromatic tree resin, is used traditionally to address immune conditions and inflammation. Some recent clinical studies have shown that osteoarthritis patients treated with this resin experienced a reduction in pain.

Nevertheless, one must also be cautious. Some Ayurvedic products are known to have the potential to be toxic. A 2008 U.S government study, for example, examined the content of 193 Ayurvedic products manufactured in either the United States or India and purchased over the Internet. The researchers found that 21 percent of the products contained levels of lead, mercury, and/or arsenic that exceeded the standards for daily intake accepted by the medical community in the United States (National Center for Complementary and Integrative Health, 2015). Various other substances in common use by Ayurvedic practitioners have not been adequately studied for safety, but increasingly they are made in controlled conditions in the West and in India. Ayurvedic products are marketed in the United States as dietary supplements; therefore, they are not subject to the safety and effectiveness standards that conventional medicines are.

Michael Shally-Jensen

See also: Aromatherapy and Essential Oils; Chinese Traditional Medicine; Folk Medicine; Herbal Remedies; Meditation and Mindfulness; Naturopathic Medicine; Yoga

Further Reading

Filliozat, Jean. 1991. *Religion, Philosophy, Yoga.* Delhi: Motilal Banarsidass Publishers.
National Center for Complementary and Integrative Health. 2015. "Ayurvedic Medicine: In Depth." nccih.nih.gov/health/ayurveda/introduction.htm
Ninivaggi, Frank John. 2008. *Ayurveda: A Comprehensive Guide to Traditional Indian Medicine for the West.* Westport, CT: Praeger.
Oliver, Paul. 2014. *Hinduism and the 1960s: The Rise of a Counter-Culture.* London: Bloomsbury Academic.
Wujastyk, Dominik, trans. and ed. 2003. *The Roots of Ayurveda: Selections from Sanskrit Medical Writings.* New York: Penguin.

BIOFEEDBACK

Biofeedback is exactly what the word says it is: a technique for making bodily processes that are normally unconscious or involuntary *perceptible* to the individual, so that they can be consciously controlled or manipulated—at least to a degree. The way such processes are made perceptible is through the use of an electronic monitoring device attached to the person by means of surface electrodes (or similar) and featuring signals or a screen readout of some kind, which the user learns to react to as a way of controlling his or her bodily functions. Using biofeedback, individuals become adept at controlling key physiological responses—like heart rate, muscle tension, brain activity, sweat—in order to address underlying problems like stress, bad bodily "habits" or reactions, certain injuries, and other conditions.

Thus, biofeedback works in the same way that a room thermostat does. If an indicator, which can be a line on a graph, a blinking light, or a tone, goes above or below a certain point, the "system" kicks in to correct the room temperature—or, in the case of biofeedback, to adjust the person's physiological reaction—thus lowering or raising the indicator to the preferred level. In working to control the indicator, the person also controls the underlying physiological processes that are being monitored.

NASA has used biofeedback to train astronauts to avoid succumbing to motion sickness in extreme conditions. Biofeedback has been used successfully to control a variety of medical and psychiatric conditions, including tension headaches, gastrointestinal problems, high blood pressure, anxiety disorders, poor circulation, teeth grinding, and substance abuse, among others.

The key to the technique is learning to control the autonomic nervous system, also known as the involuntary nervous system. This includes the smooth muscles, but not the striated or "action/movement" muscles. The autonomic system is essential to the regulation of digestion, respiration, circulation of the blood, and so on. This system is not normally under voluntary control. Through biofeedback, however, the individual can be conditioned to control his or autonomic system voluntarily—within limits. People will not be able to "heal" themselves spontaneously through sheer force of will or to perform superhero-like feats of physical daring by controlling their bodily systems. They will, though, be able to

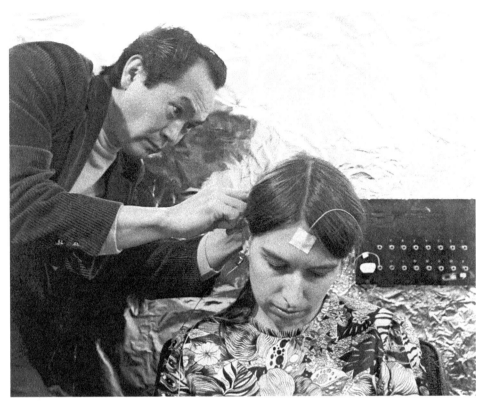

Pioneering researcher Joe Kamiya of the Langley-Porter Institute in San Francisco puts electrodes on a subject for an alpha-wave biofeedback experiment in the 1960s. Learning to maintain "alpha states" had the potential to reduce stress. (Ted Streshinsky Photographic Archive/Getty Images)

benefit from an expanded awareness of the mind–body connection—with a little help from technology.

Learning to Learn

As with many medical advances, biofeedback started out as an experimental technique but is today accepted as a conventional treatment option. Its origins lie in the 1950s and early 1960s, when both behavioral science and cybernetics, or the study of communication and control systems, were becoming prominent. In the latter field, Gregory Bateson applied cybernetic theory to human beings and other "living systems," noting that what is transmitted in a neuron is not a direct "impulse" from its source (e.g., heat from a hot surface) but rather "news of a difference" between one state (normal temperature) and another (heat); such, in fact, is the nature of *information* (Bateson 2000, 490). Bateson also explored the phenomenon of "learning to learn," whereby our bodies and our minds become progressively more adept at receiving and interpreting signals from our environment. Meanwhile, in psychology, B. F. Skinner was advancing the idea of behavior modification through operant conditioning, showing that old habits or other unwanted behaviors could be altered by homing in on stimuli and responses and using a system of rewards and punishments to steer behavior in the desired direction. Another, less stringent behaviorist, Edward Tolman, employed the notion of "latent learning" to suggest how learning could occur without the presence of an explicit reinforcement or reward; it appears, that is, that we take in more about our world than we need for our own good—and know more than we think.

Numerous other researchers worked on developing or improving the technology of biofeedback: the electromyograph (EMG), which measures electrical activity in the muscles; the electrodermograph (EDG), which measures skin conductance levels based on changes in amounts of sweat; the temperature sensors, which monitor body temperature and indicate changes in blood flow; the electroencephalograph (EEG), which measures the electrical activity of the brain (brain waves); the electrocardiogram (ECG) and various pulse monitors to measure heart rate and electrical activity; the pneumograph, to measure respiration rate; and others devices used to measure blood flow and pressure, oxygen-CO_2 exchange, and so on. In modern biofeedback sessions, which are usually conducted in quiet and relaxed settings, patients will be connected to one or more of these sensors and have their baseline data recorded before moving on to learning the control techniques needed to produce the preferred levels of activity.

One of the first research areas where human subjects were used was that of epilepsy research. Patients were taught to recognize the behavioral "triggers" that led to seizures and to avoid them using biofeedback techniques. Stress and the tools needed to achieve relaxation as a way to ameliorate the damaging effects of stress was another early area of success. Biofeedback has been used since the 1970s to treat tension headaches, Reynaud's syndrome (a circulatory disorder), cardiac arrythmia, incontinence, irritable bowel syndrome, migraine, and a host of other conditions. The Biofeedback Research Society was founded in 1969, later transitioning to the organization it is today, the Association for Applied Psychophysiology and Biofeedback (AAPB), which identifies itself as an international society "for mind–body research, health care, and education."

Most biofeedback professionals practice a range of therapies, though specialization is becoming more common. For patients, the first session may last an hour and usually includes a medical history and the creation of some baseline data. Subsequent sessions may be only 30 minutes, particularly after the patient has become familiar with the technique and the equipment and has been taught how to gain control over the responses monitored by the machines. Biofeedback is often not the sole treatment but typically is used in conjunction with others. Treatments may continue for anywhere between one and three months. The goal is to be able to produce the beneficial responses on one's own, outside the therapist's office and without the help of technology. Meanwhile, over-the-counter biofeedback devices are increasingly available.

Learning and Gaming

One of the newer areas into which biofeedback is expanding is called brain-computer interface training (AAPB). If not quite the Bionic Man or Bionic Woman of 1970s television fame, this area of research could end up paving the way for people who are at home with human-computer interactions at levels not seen before. There could indeed be some cyborg applications on the horizon. (Note that *cyborg* is short for "cybernetic organism.") And as humans adjust themselves to feedback from machines, so too do machines adjust themselves to feedback from humans. Certain computer games and other apps already make use of simple biofeedback data from users to adjust their speeds, responsiveness, and so forth.

In the 1970s a game called Will Ball, produced by Charles Wehrenberg, styled itself as a competitive relaxation game. Players hooked themselves up to an electromechanical "ball" or disk that tracked across a gaming table in one direction or the other depending on which player had attained the highest level of relaxation. A digital version was created in the 1980s. The gaming industry produced little else in this area other than a version of Tetris 64 in the 1990s that changed speeds based on user reactions. Then, in 2011, a horror-themed game called Nevermind was presented by Erin Reynolds. Players witness ugly, uncomfortable scenarios resembling memories from a trauma patient. If they exhibit signs of stress, the gaming environment reacts by becoming more difficult; if they remain unperturbed, the environment reverts to its default easy state. A new version of Nevermind from 2016 makes use of a webcam and a biometric app that reads facial expressions to determine the state of the player and adjust the game accordingly (Reynolds 2016).

Another vision of the future is presented in the 2013 film *Her,* by Spike Jonze (and featuring Joaquin Phoenix and Scarlett Johansson). In this story, computer operating systems (OSs) have developed to the point where they can sense a user's mood and thought processes and respond as any thoughtful, caring, loving human being would respond—at least with words and advice. The degree of understanding and connection can be so close that some users fall in love with their OSs. If not in the near future, then in the somewhat more distant future such a scenario many not be so fanciful.

Michael Shally-Jensen

See also: Alternative Diagnostics; Anger and Anger Management; Anxiety and Its Treatment; Behavioral Theories and Therapies; Breathwork; Depression and Its Treatment; Meditation and Mindfulness; Mind–Body Medicine; Self-Help; Stress and Stress Management

Further Reading

Association for Applied Psychophysiology and Biofeedback. www.aapb.org

Bateson, Gregory. 2000. *Steps to an Ecology of Mind: Collected Essays in Anthropology, Psychiatry, Evolution, and Epistemology.* Chicago: University of Chicago Press.

Reynolds, Erin. 2016. "Biofeedback and Gaming: The Future Is upon Us (Seriously)." www
.gamasutra.com/blogs/ErinReynolds/20160511/272295/Biofeedback_and_Gaming
_The_Future_Is_Upon_Us_Seriously.php

Robbins, Jim. 2008. *A Symphony in the Brain: The Evolution of the New Brain Wave Biofeed-back*. New York: Grove Press.

Thompson, Michael, and Lynda Thompson. 2015. *The Neurofeedback Book*. 2nd ed. Wheat
Ridge, CO: Association for Applied Psychophysiology and Biofeedback.

CRANIOSACRAL THERAPY

As the word *craniosacral* suggests, this form of therapy focuses on a bodily system made up of the cranium, or braincase; the sacrum, or lower part of the spine (located in the pelvic region); and the cerebrospinal fluid that connects them. The system also includes the nerves, tissues, and membranes of the area between the top of the skull and the tip of the spine (coccyx). Craniosacral therapy is designed to ensure, by the use of a hands-on procedure involving light touch, optimal flow of the cerebrospinal fluid and any "subtle energies" associated with it. Although it focuses on this system, its range of treatment is quite comprehensive. As one of the field's founders puts it,

> CranioSacral Therapy (CST) is a gentle, hands-on method of whole-body evaluation and treatment that may have a positive impact on nearly every system of the body. Whether used alone or with more traditional healthcare methods, it has proven . . . effective in facilitating the body's ability to self-heal. CST helps normalize the environment of the craniosacral system, a core physiological body system only recently scientifically defined. (Upledger 2008, 1)

Origins and Modern Practice

Craniosacral therapy emerged from osteopathic techniques developed by the U.S. physician William G. Sutherland (1873–1954) in the early 1900s. As an osteopath, Sutherland already specialized in the musculoskeletal system, the soft tissue around bones and joints, and the flow of blood and lymph. In his work, he became particularly interested in the cranium and the sacrum. They and the spinal cord are enclosed in a membrane called the *dura*. The cranial and sacral structures consist of many distinct bones that are flexible at their joints in infancy and childhood but tend to become more rigid or fuse together later on. Sutherland maintained that his research had shown that subtle movement of these bones continued to exist throughout an individual's life, and moreover these movements reflected the pulsing of the cerebrospinal fluid. This rhythmic activity, which Sutherland termed the *primary respiratory impulse*, was seen by him as essential to the self-healing processes of the body. Sutherland's writings include *The Cranial Bowl* (1939). His wife wrote a biography of him, entitled *With Thinking Fingers* (1962).

A number of Sutherland's followers refined and enhanced his approach over the years. All generally focused, however, on restoring the craniosacral rhythm when it became restricted. Therapists today generally use this same approach, although in recent decades more attention has begun to be paid to natural "energy flows" and the intangible element of the "spirit" of the body as well as ordinary physiological matters.

A therapist may begin a session with a client by lightly touching the base of the skull and/or the sacrum and then moving on to examine other areas in order to gauge the state of the craniosacral system and the health of the person overall. One area of focus is the detection of "energy cysts," or blockages to the natural flow of fluids and connections. Through the use of gentle touch, the therapist identifies these cysts and disperses them in order to restore proper functioning. Another, similar technique involves correcting the direction or strength of flows when these have been identified as issues.

A second technique is that of myofascial release. This entails getting at connective tissues that surround the muscles through the use of manipulative bodywork, a somewhat heavier hands-on method. The goal in this case is to restore effective functioning to the muscular fascia (*myo*- means "muscle"; *fascia* refers to fibrous connective tissue), thus relaxing the muscles themselves and improving the circulation of blood and lymph in the area. Through such targeted optimization, an area should better be able to heal on its own.

A third technique is concerned with addressing the effects of injury or trauma. This technique, called somatoemotional release, can be applied to certain cases of mental and emotional dysfunction as well as physiological dysfunctions. In this case, the therapist and client work together to place the body into a position that reflects the state of affairs obtaining when the problem first arose. In other words, the body's memory is being tapped into. One of the technique's lead developers, John Upledger, states that when he and his colleagues were first developing it, they learned to rely on a client's "inner intelligence or wisdom" to guide them to the correct position (Upledger 2010, 375). When the level of activity of the craniosacral system suddenly drops, the therapist knows that he or she has located the problem and the "energy" surrounding it has been released. Soon afterward, the baseline potential of the client's craniosacral rhythm will resume and health should be improved (or restored).

With somatoemotional therapy, words, images, or thoughts can be used in place of body placement or in addition to it. As Upledger explains, "intentional touch was a powerful method of helping the patient to liberate suppressed emotions, memories and experiences. It also became clear that . . . when a significant word was spoken [or] a significant thought was brought forward," the patient's craniosacral system's activity dropped off and then restarted, indicating a healthful psychophysiological response (ibid.). Ultimately, Upledger notes, he and his colleagues used what he calls "consciousness energy fields" to establish connections between patients and therapists.

Beyond the Body

Craniosacral therapy, then, can be and often is more than just healing touch and bodily manipulation. The titles of some of the popular books in the field reflect this: *Wisdom in the Body*; *Your Inner Physician and You*; *The Heart of Listening*; and *Engaging the Movement of Life*. Its adherents hold that it can be used to treat a wide range of conditions, including birth trauma, attention-deficit disorder, autism, rheumatoid arthritis, cerebral palsy, chronic fatigue syndrome, fibromyalgia, head-aches, depression, gastroenteritis, asthma, and many others. It remains a compelling and flourishing treatment option among those working in the complementary and alternative health field, and it has been endorsed by the American Holistic Nurses Association, among other bodies.

Its status among practitioners of conventional medicine, on the other hand, is not particularly high. For the most part, researchers from the latter group find that there is insufficient evidence to support its effectiveness beyond what it may offer in terms of the relaxation effects of gentle touch and the positive impact of care and attentiveness being shown a client by a good therapist (Singh and Ernst 2008).

Michael Shally-Jensen

See also: Acupuncture; Alternative Diagnostics; Aromatherapy and Essential Oils; Ayurvedic Medicine; Chiropractic; Crystals; Cupping; Magnet Therapy; Mind–Body Medicine; Naturopathic Medicine; Phrenology; Reflexology; Reiki and Therapeutic Touch; Shiatsu

Further Reading

Ackerman, Diane. 2003. "Cranial Sacral." www.poetryfoundation.org/poetrymagazine/browse?contentId=41927

Kalinowska, Liz, and Daška Hatton. *Every Body Tells a Story: A Craniosacral Journey*. London: Singing Dragon.

Singh, Simon, and Edzard Ernst. 2008. *Trick or Treatment: The Undeniable Facts about Alternative Medicine*. New York: Simon and Schuster.

Upledger, John E. 2008. *Craniosacral Therapy: What It Is, How It Works*. Berkeley, CA: North Atlantic Books.

Upledger, John E. 2010. *Cell Talk: Transmitting Mind into DNA*. Berkeley, CA: North Atlantic Books.

DANCE THERAPY

Dance, along with music, has long held a position of honor in human society. It serves to mark life's cycles, to establish the place of the individual or the group in the larger universe, to communicate with the gods, to express collective emotions at particular times and places, to prepare the community for war or the hunt, and, of course, to facilitate the healing of individuals through curative ecstatic dances or similar means. Traditional cultures supported dance virtually from cradle to grave. Life and dance were closely integrated—as indeed they still are in some societies.

Curative dances came in a variety of forms. One such form was mystic trance, induced by drumming or whirling. Dancers engaged in "superhuman" acrobatic feats and found mystic communion with divine forces—sometimes induced by

---

The "Female Charlie Chaplin" of Dance Therapy

One notable contributor to the development of dance therapy was the Swiss American comedy dancer Trudi Schoop (1904–1999), known as the "female Charlie Chaplin." Cutting a striking figure, Schoop was known to bring "great gusto and good humor" to her Chaplinesque performances onstage and onscreen (Anderson 1999). She did anti-Fascist cabaret shows in (neutral) Switzerland during World War II, bringing her work to New York both before and after the war. Eventually, she settled in Los Angeles and came to work with another early Swiss-U.S. import, Tina Keller-Jenny, in helping people with schizophrenia to deal with their illness through dance and movement therapy. Schoop referred to the form of treatment she provided as the body-ego technique, which encouraged patients to express their feelings of isolation and interact with others. People responded well to her warmth and humor, thus putting movement/dance therapy on solid footing in its early years.

Source

Jack Anderson. 1999. "Trudi Schoop, 95, Pioneer in Therapy Using Dance," *New York Times,* July 23.

---

intoxication or the use of narcotics. The dance helped to produce magic powers, including immunity to pain or self-mutilation by fire or sword. Such a dance could be participated in by the "patient" or, as was more common, be carried out by a shamanic figure on behalf of the patient.

A related form was the exorcistic dance performed to frighten away demons and evil spirits. There is overlap here with trance dancing, but the focus in this case was less on communion and power building and more on eliminating malign forces possessing the individual patient. In this variety of dance as psychotherapy, an imagined "journey" was often conjured in the form of recited myths and stories, the shaman-healer symbolically venturing into the "badlands" of the other world to capture the evil demon and cast it out from the patient. The common result was a feeling of relief and a sense of healing.

Western societies, too, employed dancing to maintain the health and well-being of the community. Members of the Shaker religious sect would, during worship services in meetinghouses, march, sing, dance, and engage in symbolic gestures like shaking the hands to rid themselves of evil; they also sometimes twitched or jerked about. Similarly, some Pentecostal churches and those of the Holiness movement encourage members to pray, sing, move, dance, speak in tongues, and lay hands on the sick. The idea is that in doing so they are invoking and/or responding to the presence of the Lord, who is there to take care of them. In one famous historic case from the Alsatian city of Strasbourg in 1518, hundreds of citizens got wrapped up in a wave of hysterical dancing in the streets in the wake of a serious famine and drought. Dozens died from heatstroke, heart attacks, or exhaustion as a result of the dance mania. Unfortunately, it doesn't seem that their efforts proved fruitful in ending the tortuous environmental conditions (Backman 1977).

Dance Therapy

Dance therapy is a form of psychotherapy that uses the healing power of dance to promote wellness, usually in group settings but sometimes in one-on-one sessions between client and therapist. It is designed to help advance the social, emotional, cognitive, and physical well-being of those needing support in these areas. It draws on the nexus of body, mind, and movement to produce positive responses and cultivate feelings of confidence, control, emotional release, and satisfaction. As such, it is an expressive form of therapy allied with other such forms like art therapy and drama therapy. Dance therapy is commonly used with those experiencing emotional problems, cognitive/intellectual disabilities, age-related illnesses (e.g., Alzheimer's, Parkinson's), and even some physical impairments. It is widely used in psychiatric hospitals, mental health centers, day-care centers, private practices, and special schools for disabled students. The goal in most cases is to facilitate nonverbal communication, enhance emotional stability, and build a positive self-image.

Some attribute the origins of dance/movement therapy to the Swiss psychoanalyst Carl Jung (1875–1961) and his associate Toni Wolff (1888–1953), who together suggested that movement was a form of "active imagination." The concept was explored therapeutically by another Jungian, Tina Keller-Jenny (1887–1985) in the 1930s and 1940s. Modern dance therapy, however, really only developed in the 1950s and 1960s through the work of the American Marian Chace (1896–1970), who both danced and taught (modern) dance before becoming more interested in its use as an expressive medium in therapeutic settings. Chace, influenced by Jung, worked at St. Elizabeth's Psychiatric Hospital in Washington, DC, helping emotionally troubled patients; she later obtained psychiatric certification and treated her own patients using dance. She was a principal in the founding of the American Dance Therapy Association in 1966.

Another early contributor, likewise a dancer and a Jungian, was Mary Starks Whitehouse (1911–1979). After studying with the modern dance pioneers Mary Wigman and Martha Graham, Whitehouse became a psychoanalyst. Employing dance in her practice, she helped establish the practice known as "authentic movement," which she explained as follows:

> When the movement was simple and inevitable, not to be changed no matter how limited or partial, it became what I called "authentic"—it could be recognized as genuine, belonging to that person . . . [a] truth of a kind unlearned, but there to be seen. (quoted in Karkou, Oliver, and Lycouris 2016, 152)

In this way, to use current parlance, the patient became "empowered" as an individual, someone whose body and soul, as it were, had been unified through movement.

At a less esoteric, more pragmatic level, people are helped by means of dance/movement therapy every day. Survivors of sexual abuse or other forms of trauma can be assisted to work out troubling emotional associations and bodily fears.

People dealing with stress, grief, or anxiety can be led to relax and redirect their energies toward more productive thoughts and actions—or simply to forget, for a moment, their problems and enjoy being human. Those with intellectual or physical disabilities can be guided to develop improved awareness, coordination, strength, and balance. And those suffering from Alzheimer's can be helped to reconnect with loved ones and/or their better selves by listening and moving to old favorites or other musical sounds. In most cases, the larger group plays an essential role by sharing in the experience and providing collective support. Dance has always been, and remains, a social phenomenon.

Professional training of dance/movement therapists takes place at the graduate level, with a master's degree and state licensing or certification usually required. In recent years the field has been treated as part of the larger field of "body psychotherapy and somatic psychology," itself a part of the general mind–body approach to health and wellness. That the field is as broad and deep as it is, is a reflection of the appeal, and success, of dance therapy and the significance of the mind–body connection.

Michael Shally-Jensen

See also: Aging Prevention, or "Successful Aging"; Art and Music Therapy; Drama Therapy; Jung and Jungian Analysis; Meditation and Mindfulness; Mind–Body Medicine; Yoga

Further Reading

Backman, E. Louis. 1977. *Religious Dances in the Christian Church and in Popular Medicine.* Westport, CT: Greenwood Press.
Karkau, Vicky, Sue Oliver, and Sophia Lycouris, eds. 2017. *The Oxford Handbook of Dance and Wellbeing.* New York: Oxford University Press.
Meekums, B. 2002. *Dance Movement Therapy: A Creative Psychotherapeutic Approach.* Thousand Oaks, CA: SAGE.

ENCOUNTER GROUPS

In the opening scene of one 1969's most popular movies, *Bob and Carol and Ted and Alice* (directed by Paul Mazursky), an aerial tracking shot follows a sport convertible winding its way through the forests, mountains, and cliffs of the California coast to a remote New Age retreat modeled on the real-life Esalen Institute of Big Sur, California. Upon arriving, husband and wife Bob and Carol pass by a number of people immersed in the new therapeutic practices of the late 1960s: one group is practicing tai chi; some kneeling women are facing the sun, naked and as if in prayer; two men are letting out primordial screams in a forest; and a young couple with their eyes closed are exploring each other's faces with their hands.

Next, Bob and Carol find themselves in a 24-hour marathon "encounter group" session with a dozen other residents of different ages. Led by a trained guide, the group goes through a number of practices designed to tear away their social personas and put them in touch with their "authentic" inner selves. They first circle the room, silently stopping in front of one, then another, person to look deeply into his or her eyes. Subsequent scenes have them challenging one another to confront buried fears that are preventing them from fulfilling their true potential in life. Laughter alternates with crying, small group circles are formed and then rearranged, the individuals cluster in and out of group hugs, and the guide encourages them to speak only in "I feel" and not "I think" statements.

After the grueling 24-hour session and a series of tense confrontations and personal breakthroughs, Bob and Carol emerge from their encounter-group weekend feeling closer, as if reborn, and communicating more honestly than ever before. With missionary zeal they seek to bring their friends Ted and Alice into this new world of openness and unbridled honesty, which ultimately includes experimenting with open sexual relationships.

Encounters with Esalen

Bob and Carol and Ted and Alice introduced many Americans to one manifestation of the new Human Potential Movement pioneered largely at the Esalen Institute. Founded in 1962 by two former Stanford University psychology students, Michael Murphy and Richard Price, and named after the ancient Native American people who had lived on the land, Esalen sought to bring together Eastern meditational practices with Western humanist psychology. Various practices such a yoga, meditation, alternative medicine, therapeutic message, hot tubs, psychedelic drug exploration, and the new encounter-group marathon were popularized at Esalen. Guest residents included the eclectic anthropological thinker Gregory Bateson, the humanist psychologist Abraham Maslow, the myth researcher and theorist Joseph Campbell, the U.S. Buddhism pioneer Alan Watts, the Gestalt therapist Fritz Perls, the founder of the Rolfing method Ida Rolf, and the psychologist of alternative consciousness Stanislav Grof.

The underlying goal behind all of the various approaches and practices was to shed the socially accrued personas that kept people from living in the moment and experiencing their authentic selves and to encourage them to connect instead with the "universal soul" of which we are presumed to be a part. More specifically, the encounter groups were designed to help individuals to remove their social "masks" and have them become conscious of their defense mechanisms and "cop-outs" (excuses, rationalizations), as those things keep people from fulfilling their true potential and finding happiness in life. Uncompromising honesty with others and with oneself was seen as the key to unlocking one's true selfhood.

Esalen was popular with many figures from Hollywood's entertainment industry and other middle-class, predominantly white, Americans inspired by the youth-driven counterculture movement sweeping the nation in the late 1960s and early 1970s. In his seminal 1976 article for *New York* magazine, "The Me Decade and the Third Great Awakening," journalist Tom Wolfe included Esalen with several other movements as evidence of an U.S. obsession with the self bordering on narcissism.

In his unflattering portrait of an encounter-group session, Wolfe writes, "Encounter sessions . . . were often wild events. Such aggression! Such sobs! Tears! Moans! Hysteria!, vile recriminations, shocking revelations, such explosions of hostility between husbands and wives, such mud balls of profanity from previously mousy mommies and workadaddies, such red-mad attacks! Only physical assault was prohibited" (Wolfe 1976, 146).

The encounter group approach was also adopted by other movements such as Scientology (with its Dianetics system), the Arica School, and Primal Scream therapy. All of these movements or approaches (some of them were accused of being cults) were rooted in the 1960s and 1970s revolt against technology, commercialism, middle-class hypocrisy, the Protestant work ethic, and the sense of isolation captured in works such as the David Riesman's book *The Lonely Crowd* and Simon and Garfunkel's hit song "The Sound of Silence."

Roots and Remnants

Despite rising to prominence with the counterculture ethos of the 1960s and 1970s, encounter sessions can be traced back much further, to 1914 when the German psychologist J. C. Moreno wrote *Invitation to an Encounter.* The work pioneered experimental theater, role reversal, and role playing—all techniques that would become familiar decades later.

In the years after World War II, "sensitivity training" ("T-groups") was developed; it used small-group dynamics as a means to encourage corporate employees to open up and make managers aware of workers' needs in the interest of improving company morale (and productivity). Less extreme than the encounter groups, these sensitivity or T-groups were occasionally used with veterans from World War II suffering from what a later generation would term posttraumatic stress disorder, or PTSD.

Moreno's ideas overlapped with the humanist psychology promoted in the mid-20th century by Carl Rogers and Abraham Maslow as well as with Aldous Huxley's 1950s work on "human potentialities," which paved the way for the Human Potential Movement of the 1960s. Murphy and Price sought to integrate these Western trends in psychology with the secular spiritualism they had been exposed to from the East when they founded Esalen in 1962.

The confrontational techniques used in encounter groups began to fall out of favor by the 1980s and were increasingly criticized as potentially abusive and even dangerous. Contemporary concern with "triggering" and sensitivity to past trauma has made the anarchic and confrontational explorations of encounter groups, by and large, a practice associated with a unique, albeit bygone, era in American history.

Nevertheless, the age of the encounter group has not been forgotten by popular culture. In the 2015 finale of the popular TV series *Madmen* (about Madison Avenue advertising executives in the 1960s), the show's protagonist, Don Draper, goes to an institute clearly meant to be Esalen. It is 1970. There, in the final scene of the seven-season show, Draper, whose whole life has been devoted to the highest form of artificiality, advertising, is pushed silently by another resident at the institute until he finally has a breakthrough that puts him in touch, for the first time in his life, with his true self. The final shot is of Don radiating a smile of discovery and inner peace.

Robert Surbrug

See also: Codependency Counseling; Dianetics; Drama Therapy; Est and Other "Human Potential" Therapies; Existential Psychotherapy; Health and Wellness Gurus; Narrative Therapy and Writing Therapy; Primal Therapy and Feeling Therapy; Self-Help

Further Reading

Kripal, Jeffrey J. 2007. *Esalen: America and the Religion of No Religion.* Chicago: University of Chicago Press.

Lattin, Don. 2004. *Following Our Bliss: How the Spiritual Values of the Sixties Shape Our Lives Today.* New York: HarperOne.

Mazursky, Paul, dir. 1969. *Bob and Carol and Ted and Alice.* Columbia Pictures.

Moreno, Jonathan D. 2014. *Impromptu Man: J. L. Moreno and the Origins of Psychodrama, Encounter Culture, and the Social Network.* New York: Bellevue Literary Press.

Wolfe, Tom. 1976. "The Me Decade and the Third Great Awakening." In *Mauve Gloves and Madmen, Clutter and Vine.* New York: Farrar, Strauss and Giroux.

EST AND OTHER "HUMAN POTENTIAL" THERAPIES

If there is one phenomenon that could be said to symbolize the 1970s-era "Human Potential Movement," it would be "est," or Erhard Seminar Training. (*Est* also means "to be" in Latin.) The creation of a former car salesman named Jack Rosenberg, who had abandoned his first wife and four children and changed his name to Werner Erhard, est was established in 1971 and would run through 1984, riding a wave of popularity and celebrity endorsements. It would also spark controversy because of its rather coercive, cultlike techniques and because it looked to some like a repackaging of self-help approaches ranging from Dale Carnegie's *How to Win Friends and Influence People* to L. Ron Hubbard's Scientology, with a little existentialism and Eastern meditation added to the mix (Erhard had studied for a time with the U.S. Buddhism pioneer Alan Watts in the 1960s).

Therapy in Public

Est sessions typically took place at rented hotel ballrooms and were attended on average by 200 participants. The seminars would take place over two weekends, for a total of approximately 60 hours, with marathon sessions that required participants to remove watches, not speak unless spoken to by the leader, and to refrain from using the restroom except during designated break times. Often the marathon weekend sessions ran from 9:00 a.m. through midnight, and were sometimes accompanied by short evening weekday sessions. Nor was attending the seminars inexpensive.

The goal of the est sessions was to foment a personal breakthrough in each participant, leading to transformation of the kind that would enable him or her to take control of his or her lives. (Or at least this was the premise.) Participants would then be free to live "authentically" on their own terms rather than living to meet social expectations or falling back on defense mechanisms developed earlier in life; these were both considered self-defeating. In working toward these ends, est sessions often became confrontational as the group leader sought to strip away the supposed artifices, excuses ("cop-outs"), and false beliefs about oneself, all of which inhibited personal growth. Selected audience members would line up in the front and be asked to discuss their goals in life; then they faced group criticism aimed at stripping the individuals of any false beliefs and negative behaviors that were holding them back. Erhard, in the existentialist vein, emphasized the need for individuals to take personal responsibility for their happiness. As with another popular form of group therapy at the time, encounter groups, unremitting self-revelation and merciless honesty were demanded of each participant. Profanity and name-calling were sometimes part of the group leader's arsenal in the effort to strip away falseness. The self-revelations were seen as the gateway through which, unshackled by past behavior patterns and denials, a person could achieve self-directed growth and improvement.

An est session was in some ways like a military boot camp in that it sought to break down, then build up and remake, the individual. The final breakthrough moment was called "getting it." Testimonials from many who had "got it" by attending an est seminar spoke of life-changing personal transformations. These included celebrities like the former 1960s Yippie activist Jerry Ruben, the singer-songwriter John Denver, and two costars of television's popular *Mary Tyler Moore Show*, Cloris Leachman and Valerie Harper. One thing that made est sessions different from the more esoteric practices of encounter groups and personal growth retreats like the Esalen Institute in Big Sur, California, was its lack of counterculture associations. Trainers and attendees dressed in the conventional, casual clothing of the workaday world; hippie attire and slang were the exception rather than the norm. Thus, est might be seen as an example of how the spiritualism and inner explorations of the 1960s counterculture had migrated, to some extent, into the mainstream, predominantly white, middle-class culture of 1970s America.

Controversy

By the second half of the 1970s, however, a backlash against est had occurred. Est seminars were Exhibit A in the journalist Tom Wolfe's iconic 1976 *New York* magazine article, "The Me Decade and the Third Great Awakening." The central thesis of Wolfe's piece was that the 1970s was defined by an obsessive preoccupation with the self, and that the search for one's true self was carried out through intense, irrational, emotional experiences (drug-induced or otherwise) that severed the individual from the past and the future and served only him- or herself. Wolfe's article began by describing an est session at the Ambassador Hotel in Los Angeles, participants taking turns describing the one thing in their life they wished they could get rid of. Wolfe summed up the responses: "My husband! My wife! My homosexuality! My inability to communicate, my self-hatred, self-destructiveness, craven fears, puling ["whining"] weaknesses, primordial horrors, premature ejaculation, impotence, frigidity, rigidity, subservience, laziness, alcoholism . . ."—not to mention "My hemorrhoids" (Wolfe 1976, 132). Wolfe also described participants removing the folding chairs from the ballroom floor, lying on their bellies and releasing all their negative emotions in long primordial screams and moans. Wolfe writes, "Each soul is concentrated on its own burning item . . . and yet each unique item has been raised to a cosmic level and united with every other until there is but one piercing moment of release and liberation—a whole world of anguish set free" (ibid).

The skepticism toward est continued in 1977 with a ruthless parody in the Burt Reynolds's movie *Semi-Tough*, which portrayed a fictional group called B.E.A.T. as a cultish, abusive scam. Est soldiered on, however, until 1984, after which Werner Erhard would periodically repackage it in more low-intensity seminars designed primarily for individuals in the corporate workplace. In 1991 CBS's *60 Minutes* aired a scandalous piece on Erhard that accused him of, among other things, molesting one of his daughters (a charge it later retracted). Erhard fled the United States for a number of years, charging that the source for the *60 Minutes* segment was the leadership of the Church of Scientology, an organization believed by many to be a cult and that had a long-standing gripe against Erhard on the basis of his allegedly having appropriated some of Scientology's ideas. Journalists that have explored the matter have concluded that Erhard's accusations against Scientology were well founded; the church had planted and/or encouraged. the negative *60 Minutes* report. For his part, Erhard eventually returned to the United States and, in his eighties, continued his professional and personal growth seminars.

Robert Surbrug

See also: Codependency Counseling; Dianetics; Drama Therapy; Encounter Groups; Existential Psychotherapy; Health and Wellness Gurus; Narrative Therapy and Writing Therapy; Primal Therapy and Feeling Therapy; Self-Help

Further Reading
Bartley, William Warren, III. 1978. *Werner Erhard The Transformation of a Man: The Founding of EST*. New York: Clarkson N. Potter.
Fenwick, Sheridan. 1976. *Getting It: The Psychology of EST*. Philadelphia: J. B. Lippincott Company.
Moreno, Jonathan D. 2014. *Impromptu Man: J. L. Moreno and the Origins of Psychodrama, Encounter Culture, and the Social Network*. New York: Bellevue Literary Press.
Pressman, Steven. 1993. *Outrageous Betrayal: The Dark Journey of Werner Erhard from EST to Exile*. New York: St. Martin's Press.
Wolfe, Tom. 1976. "The Me Decade and the Third Great Awakening." In *Mauve Gloves and Madmen, Clutter and Vine*. New York: Farrar, Straus and Giroux.

EXISTENTIAL PSYCHOTHERAPY   205

EXISTENTIAL PSYCHOTHERAPY

Existential therapy is a humanistic form of psychotherapy that emerged in the mid-20th century from out of the phenomenological and existential strains of philosophy and psychology. According to the *phenomenological* perspective, a person's perception of reality or an event is more important than the event itself. An *existential* perspective maintains, in addition, that people form their lives by the choices they make. A fundamental idea behind existential psychology is free will, the freedom to choose. Existentialists and others representing the humanistic approach argued that neither Freudianism nor behaviorism made allowances for free will; according to Freudians, human behavior is largely controlled by unconscious factors, and according to behaviorists, much of human behavior is caused by external circumstances. From an existentialist point of view, however, humans are constrained neither by the unconscious nor by external factors but rather are free to choose both what they think and how they will behave. Existentialist *psychotherapy* therefore insists that human will and intentionality are fundamental for the understanding and healing of personality.

From Philosophy to Psychology

Existential psychology is rooted in existential philosophy, particularly the writings of Søren Kierkegaard (1813–1855), Martin Heidegger (1889–1976), and Jean-Paul Sartre (1905–1980), among others. A number of basic assumptions and principles form the foundation of existential philosophy. As noted, one principle is that humans have free will. Along with free will comes responsibility. A bad childhood does not excuse bad adult behavior; the individual has chosen the effects that the bad childhood has had on him or her. Another assumption is that life has no intrinsic meaning. Thus life puts people in a position where they must search for their own meaning. Life may be experienced as meaningful through many, diverse routes, and each person chooses unique meaning, which may transform from moment to moment. Another assumption is the importance of phenomenology, an individual's particular perception or experience. Each person has his or her own way of viewing experiences. In a family with children of similar age who sit together with their siblings and parents at dinner and who all ride together in a car as they go on vacation, the children may nonetheless, despite that they may seem objectively similar in a number of ways, have very different perspectives on events—the parents' argument during dinner or the hysterical laughing that occurred in the car while on vacation. These differences in perspective are each child's unique phenomenology. To completely understand one another, people must be aware that life is experienced by each individual through his or her own, unique, selective filter. Understanding others requires an open-minded, nonjudgmental attitude. Each person's individual essence or "true" nature, moreover, is not fixed in advance but rather is established through the choices that he or she has made and continues to make in life.

Karl Jaspers (1883–1969), whose career moved through medicine and psychiatry to philosophy, had a scientific orientation not present in most existentialists.

Yet he maintained the existentialist credo, drawn from Kierkegaard and Friedrich Nietzsche, that all fundamental thinking depends on self-comprehension, self-awareness. Although avoiding religious orthodoxies, which he found limiting, Jaspers nevertheless stressed the importance of what he called "transcendence"—meaning a kind of leap past ordinary experience to human freedom and "authentic" existence.

The first actual existential psychotherapist was Swiss psychiatrist Ludwig Binswanger (1881–1966), a student of Carl Jung and close friend of Sigmund Freud. In his book *Foundations and Knowledge of Human Existence*, published in 1942, Binswanger described different levels of existence and modes of interpersonal relations. The highest level is *Eigenwelt* (literally, "own world"). Individuals operating at this level are self-aware and self-actualizing. They experience life in relation to their own personal meanings; the norms of society and opinions and judgments of others are secondary to the individual's own values and perspectives. Binswanger believed that most people crave purpose in their lives, but many do not know their purpose. Many people, in their search for meaning and direction, make decisions without thinking such as following an organized religion or joining a political cause. This lack of authenticity causes suffering.

Other existential therapists came after Binswanger, including Austrian psychiatrist Viktor Frankl (1905–1997), famous for inventing his own form of psychotherapy, logotherapy (*logos* means "meaning" in Greek). In logotherapy, the client is encouraged to find his own meaning in life. Frankl describes a number of ways that people experience meaning, including creating or accomplishing something, giving to others, and loving another. In logotherapy, the therapist presents the client with alternative ways of looking at events, in an attempt to reveal the client's unique meaning or purpose in life. Frankl eloquently describes his philosophy, in addition to his experience as a captive in a number of concentration camps in World War II, in his book *Man's Search for Meaning* (1962).

Probably the most controversial existential therapist was the Scottish/British psychiatrist R. D. Laing (1927–1989). A critic of the psychiatric profession and of the standard medical model of mental illness, Laing helped inspire the skeptical "antipsychiatry" movement. He is noted for his view that schizophrenia is a kind of healing response—a sane reaction to an insane environment. In *The Divided Self* (1961), he proposed that insecurity about one's existence prompts a defensive reaction in which the self splits into separate components, producing psychotic symptoms (as those associated with schizophrenia). Laing rejected treatment in the form of hospitalization and electroshock and instead helped create therapeutic centers where patients and therapists lived together. In these supportive group situations, a patient's thoughts, feelings, and behaviors were accepted as efforts to cope with a difficult world. Laing also explored the use of mind-altering drugs and meditative practices to uncover hidden aspects of the mind and human experience. In doing so, he and his followers opened themselves up to the criticism that they tended to romanticize psychosis as a spiritual journey of discovery or self-actualization. Laing later modified some of his more controversial positions, going on to publish dialogues with children and works of prose poetry.

Another noteworthy existential psychotherapist is U.S. psychiatrist Irvin Yalom (1931–). Yalom sees existential anxiety as the root of most neurosis. In his book *Existential Psychotherapy*, published in 1980, he describes four causes of existential anxiety: fear of death, human freedom (which means that we are responsible for our choices), isolation (humans enter and exit this existence alone), and meaninglessness. Unlike Laing, Yalom argues that the individual can respond to these factors, or "givens," in either a functional or a dysfunctional way. The object is to work through them in a beneficial way, including, perhaps, by writing about the therapeutic experience in collaboration with the therapist. Yalom is also well known as a group psychotherapist and applies his existential principles to both individual and group therapy. He has written a variety of novels and stories as well as works about humanistic psychiatry and overcoming the fear of death. One historically based fictional work, *When Nietzsche Wept* (1992), was turned into a motion picture in 2007. Yalom's *Becoming Myself: A Psychiatrist's Memoir* was published in 2017.

Existential psychotherapy exists in the present day; however, it is not nearly as popular as other forms of psychotherapy such as cognitive-behavioral or behavioral psychotherapy. Additionally, existential psychotherapy is difficult to test empirically for a number of reasons, including that it assumes individual meanings rather than general laws of human nature. However, some research lends support to fundamental principles of existential psychology or psychotherapy. For instance, research shows that most people value meaning in life—as much as or more than they value wealth. Additionally, it is widely understood that therapy is more effective if the therapist recognizes the client's unique perceptions and experiences, along with what he or she has to say about them in the "here and now." More generally, existentialism has demonstrated that interest in human existence, in finding human meaning in life, is something that touches all of us. Similarly, existentialism's affirmation of freedom and its rejection of abstract concepts or dehumanizing social institutions has left a positive impact, overall, on the culture. Existential psychotherapy, like other humanistic therapies, played a role in the emergence of the *recovery movement* in the 1980s and 1990s.

Michael Shally-Jensen and
Gretchen Reevy

See also: Client-Centered Therapy; Codependency Counseling; Drama Therapy; Encounter Groups; Gestalt Therapy; Meditation and Mindfulness; Milieu Therapy and Therapeutic Community; Mind–Body Medicine; Psychedelic Drugs; Recovery Movement

Further Reading

Frankl, Victor. 2010. *The Feeling of Meaninglessness: A Challenge to Psychotherapy and Philosophy.* Edited by Alexander Batthyány. Milwaukee, WI: Marquette University Press.

Schneider, Kirk J., and Orah T. Krug. 2017. *Existential-Humanistic Therapy.* 2nd ed. Washington, DC: American Psychological Association.
Van Deurzen, Emmy. 2010. *Everyday Mysteries: A Handbook of Existential Psychotherapy.* 2nd ed. New York: Routledge.

FELDENKRAIS METHOD

The Feldenkrais method is a type of movement therapy based on the twin ideas that posture is important and the body and the mind form a unitary whole. Its founder, Moshe Feldenkrais (1904–1984), was an Israeli engineer and physicist who suffered from severe, chronic knee pain. Nothing he tried seemed to help his condition, so he decided to develop his own therapy, as he outlined in his 1949 book, *Body and Mature Behavior: A Study of Anxiety, Sex, Gravitation, and Learning.* Feldenkrais was also a judo instructor, so it made sense that his method incorporated body mechanics. The anxiety and sex part belonged to his larger view of health, motion, and development.

Philosophy and Development

The crux of the Feldenkrais method, according to the standard description provided by Feldenkrais Guild members, is "somatic education," or a form of physical training that

> uses gentle movement and directed attention to improve movement and enhance human functioning. Through this Method, you can increase your ease and range of motion, improve your flexibility and coordination, and rediscover your innate capacity for graceful, efficient movement. These improvements will often generalize to enhance functioning in other aspects of your life. (Mester 2018)

Thus, besides improving movement, Feldenkrais is intended to expand one's "self-image" by means of sequences of movement. These movements help "bring attention to parts of the self that are out of awareness" (ibid.). This refers to the way in which we fall into patterned movements, or "false" behaviors, performed more out of habit than out of awareness. Such habitual motions are thought by Feldenkrais practitioners to leave the neuromuscular components in the areas involved somewhat atrophied and inefficient—and to leave the mind that operates them rather dulled and uncreative. Through prescribed movement exercises, therefore, one can change one's body and change one's mind, or sense of self.

Feldenkrais trained therapists in his method in San Francisco in 1975–1978, and in Amherst, Massachusetts, in 1980–1984. It spread from there to a larger community in the Americas, Europe, Australia, and New Zealand. In *The Potent Self: A Study of Spontaneity and Compulsion* (1980), he explored the relationship between faulty posture, pain, and the emotional mechanisms that both produce habitual behavior and can lead to healthy change. Feldenkrais also noted the influence of the Russian mystic and spiritual teacher G. I. Gurdjieff on the development

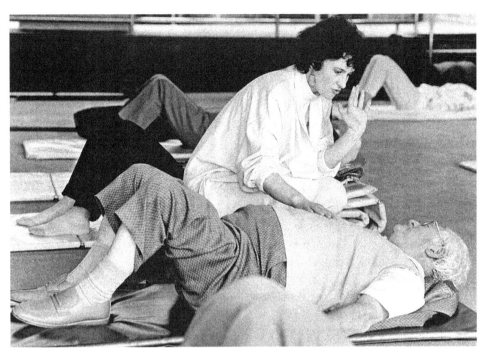

A Feldenkrais instructor works with seniors to teach them gentle movements and exercises that will allow them to move efficiently and with greater ease. (Dick Loek/Toronto Star via Getty Images)

of his method, particularly Gurdjieff's notions of "automaton" thinking/behaving and the "sacred dances" he used as a means to break the cycle of habit. According to Feldenkrais's biographer, the movement expert eschewed the concept of "energy therapy" as unscientific and worked to make his own method acceptable to the medical community (Reese 2015).

The Method in Action

The therapy is carried out in two steps: "functional integration" and "awareness through movement." Both are designed to identify how one "carries" oneself and to reeducate the body so as to eliminate harmful habitual movements and allow the individual to achieve his or her highest potential, mentally and physically. The therapy is traditionally carried out in small groups, though individualized treatment is also often available. Once the lessons are learned, the patient is expected to practice the techniques continuously at home. The conditions treated include musculoskeletal problems and psychosomatic problems. Athletes and performance artists sometimes use Feldenkrais to improve their movement. Older people and those with disabilities also seek benefits in using the method.

During the first, "functional" phase, the practitioner uses touch and gentle manipulation to determine the range of motion a patient has in specific areas of the body (hips, shoulders, arms, back, etc.). Points where limitations are evident and improvements might be made are noted. Much of this takes place with the patient lying down, clothed, on a padded surface. In the course of the session, the patient is directed to be attentive to his or her movements and to report any pain or discomfort that may arise from them. There might be a particular activity or motion that the person performs every day, for example, that causes discomfort, and this can be identified during the introductory session. (Pain, in fact, is the most common complaint that sends people to Feldenkrais therapists.)

The theory is this: most people who experience pain or discomfort while going about their daily routines compensate for it by adjusting their motions—and this is often done in a semiconscious way. A feeling of pain or distress in one foot, for example, will be compensated for by shifting one's weight to the other foot. Or a pang of discomfort in the shoulder, say, while reaching up may be compensated for by turning or tilting the body in some way in order to make use of a different set of muscles and nerves. This is a very common phenomenon and is understood well by physical therapists, whose job it is to help patients move better and in comfort. Feldenkrais is similar except that it goes beyond the specific complaint to appreciate overall integration of functions, including how the brain and body interact to perpetuate habitual movements.

During the second, "awareness through movement" phase, the practitioner teaches the patient to correct any so-called false movements. Patients are taught to become aware of problem areas and of their bodily movements in general, so that they can "see" and understand their self-image and make adjustments as necessary. Patients are encouraged to observe and learn about themselves and practice discipline in performing their exercises at home to achieve maximum benefit. Of course, the body should not be forced to do anything that might cause serious pain or discomfort. If pain does already exists, however, the idea is to work around it initially and then gradually bring improvement to the troubled area through movement that increases circulation and builds healthy tissue and flexibility. This is not so different from physical therapy, except that Feldenkrais incorporates a kind of Gestalt perspective that looks at bodily motion as a whole, together with personal awareness, flexibility, coordination, breathing, and so on. In some ways it is closer to yoga than to PT.

Another aspect of Feldenkrais is that it is able, within the scope of its method, to address some psychosomatic disorders. These involve psychic or emotional traumas that have been "embodied," or incorporated into physical symptoms. Because of the method's interest in mind–body connections, it seeks to explore such symptoms with the patient through the use of movement and awareness. The goal, once again, is to reeducate the neuromuscular system and, along the way, open up new "channels" of thinking and understanding about one's posture, movement, and health.

Does It Work?

The Feldenkrais Guild of North America states that there is a growing body of research conducted by health researchers and Feldenkrais practitioners exploring all aspects of the Feldenkrais method, including its application, theoretical basis, and efficacy. These are not all rigorous clinical trials in top medical journals, but the work to which the Guild points does suggest patient benefits in such areas as back pain, range of motion, balance, hypertension, breathing, mood, "healthy aging," and more. The technique also may help those with physical disabilities, including children, the elderly, and adults. The results are not uniform across all populations, but they suggest the utility of the Feldenkrais method overall.

Of note too is that the Feldenkrais method does not carry with it any serious risks. Most consumers can feel comfortable giving it a try, as long as it serves their purposes. Celebrities who have done so include Whoopi Goldberg, Yo Yo Ma, Neil Young, Andrew Weil, Julius Erving, and, of a previous generation, Yehudi Menuhin, Helen Hays, and Margaret Mead.

Michael Shally-Jensen

See also: Aging Prevention, or "Successful Aging"; Dance Therapy; Gestalt Therapy; Meditation and Mindfulness; Mind–Body Medicine; Rolfing; Walking and Jogging; Yoga

Further Reading

Feldenkrais, Moshe. 2010. *Embodied Wisdom: The Collected Papers of Moshe Feldenkrais.* San Diego, CA: Somatic Resources/North Atlantic Books.
Feldenkrais Guild of North America. 2018. www.feldenkraisguild.com
Mester, Uwe. 2018. "The Feldenkrais Method with Uwe Mester." www.vermontfeldenkrais .com/index.php/about-feldenkrais
Reese, Mark. 2015. *Moshe Feldenkrais: A Life in Movement.* San Rafael, CA: ReeseKress Somatics Press.

HERBAL REMEDIES

We sometimes think that knowledge of anatomy and bodily functions is a recent development in human history. Leonardo da Vinci's diagram of human anatomy is taken by many people as an illustration of the first time humans understood accurately the various parts of the body. Actually, of course, knowledge of anatomy goes back much farther than Leonardo. The ancient Egyptians, Greeks, Chinese, and Indians all have a demonstrable history of anatomical research—even in India, where it was forbidden to cut a corpse open with a knife. (The Indians followed the gruesome practice of soaking a corpse in water for days, until it was so putrefied that it would fall apart.)

The ancients knew the various parts of the body and had theories as to how and why things worked. Some of these theories we might scoff at today—such as the Egyptians' idea that the brain was fairly useless and could be disposed of before mummification. It took the work of Herophilus (335–280 BCE), in Greece, to propose that the brain, not the heart, was the seat of intellect. In other times and places, it was thought that what passed through the circulatory system was air, not blood. The ancient Chinese lacked a specific word for "muscle" and were far more preoccupied with energy flows and the pulse.

Herbalism across Time

Thus, people knew something about the body, although they knew about it in different ways and approached the healing arts in accordance with their understanding. For many ailments, knowing the layout of the body and having some theories about how it might work was useless without also knowing how to *treat* a patient. And for eons in human history, virtually the only available treatments were herbal or botanical medicines. We have records of herbal treatments dating back to ancient Sumer. A type of medical practice known as the Empiric school arose in Greece based on its members' use of herbal and other remedies and their belief in the idea that if something worked, that is all that mattered; you didn't have to know how or why it did so. Traditional folk remedies in the Americas, which were also heavily herbal based, operated on much the same principle. In many cultures that had writing, from Egypt to China and beyond, large works called "herbals" were prepared that listed common ailments and the various herbal "recipes" that addressed them.

In Europe, during the Middle Ages, most areas would have a wise man or wise woman who would treat illnesses with different herbs, often made into drinkable solutions and tinctures to increase their potency and make them palatable, more or less. Over time, these individuals were recast as potion makers and witches. While there are some debates about whether or not witches were routinely burned at the stake, and how many may have suffered this fate, it is clear that over time the role of the wise person of the village was transformed—downgraded, as it were—by monks and doctors who promoted bleeding, prayer, and other treatments that were probably less effective.

During the Renaissance, there was both renewed interest in Greek and Roman medical writings as well as in the creation of new, European "herbals" that drew on local resources along with more modern concepts. One of the most popular, and enduring (though there were many), was Nicholas Culpeper's *Complete Herbal* (1653), which also employed an elaborate astrological system of correspondence between diseases, remedies, and planetary motions. For this reason, Culpeper was known as an "astrological botanist." Nevertheless, his herbal continued to be used well into the 18th century in America.

In the early 19th century, in the United States, a popular collection of home herbal remedies was promoted under the name of Thomsonian medicine, named after its founder, Samuel Thomson (1769–1843). His system relied heavily on the emetic *lobelia* ("puke weed"), steam baths, and hot cayenne pepper; the idea was to clear the body of toxins while also keeping it very warm (blankets were used as well). Thomson's motto was "Every man his own physician," meaning that anyone should be able to cure his or her illness at home by using his methods—and by buying the products he sold.

Modern doctors have found that many herbal remedies actually work. Here are a few modern medicines that have their roots in ancient herbal or botanical treatments.

- The Chinese used the ephedra shrub in their medicine, which has been refined to the medicine ephedrine (used for asthma, narcolepsy, and other conditions).

- Chaulmoogra seed oil is another Chinese remedy, and was one of the first effective treatments for leprosy.

- St. John's Wort is a plant used by the ancient Greeks that is still sold as a treatment for mild depression.

- Plants and herbs containing salicylic acid, most famously willow bark, have been used for thousands of years. Eventually, these herbs were refined into aspirin, which is still a cornerstone of modern medicine.

Modern Herbalists

Herbalism is still practiced in various forms today, both by amateur herbalists who have perhaps read a book or two on the subject and by trained, experienced herbalists who work with clients and may even write books or articles about their practice. Traditional Chinese medicine and Ayurveda both continue to use herbal remedies to rebalance energies and treat illness. Herbal supplements, like other dietary supplements, are not subject to oversight by the Food and Drug Administration (FDA); this means that there is no guarantee of potency or purity.

Some shops continue to sell herb that can be made into medicinal teas, but it is not always clear how often their stock is rotated; customers may be buying old product with whatever potency it might originally have had aged out of it. Many different companies also make prepared herbal teas (technically tisanes) that are said to help with everything from weight loss and insomnia to flu or cold symptoms and general well-being. There are teas and tinctures for insomnia, stress, menstrual cramps—you name it.

Most dietary supplements (apart from vitamins and minerals) are derived from plants or herbs. People take supplements because they believe they can help prevent or treat various chronic conditions, such as arthritis, migraine, osteoporosis, and immune-related conditions as well as more acute conditions like an infection or an upset stomach. Herbal supplements are also popular because they are perceived as being *natural* and therefore safe and healthy. But "natural" does not invariably mean "safe." Any remedy that is strong enough to have a beneficial health effect is also potentially strong enough to be damaging. Tobacco, for example, is a natural herbal product, and yet smoking it is obviously harmful. Some plants such as nightshade and hemlock can be extremely toxic when ingested, even causing death. Clearly, consumers are advised to approach herbalism with the right amount of caution and awareness. Still, naturopathic medicine, which includes herbal remedies, has been immensely popular since the 1980s and the New Age movement.

Essential Oils

For many years now, essential oils have been used in aromatherapy. Oils may be heated, which causes them to boil off and release their fragrance into the air. This has not been shown to have very much, if any, medical benefit. Pleasant smells can be relaxing, and are often used in spas and during massages. Certain smells can sometimes help someone to meditate or lessen anxiety, especially if they practice associating the scent with the experience of a calmer body.

But recently, multilevel marketing companies have begun selling essential oils that are used for specific medicinal purposes. Many of these oils have been shown to be dangerous, especially if they are ingested or used directly on the skin. They can result in burns, allergic reactions, or poisoning.

Essential oils, like other herbal/botanical products, have no government agency overseeing them for quality. This means that there is no guarantee that the oil one purchases is safe or effective; it may not even carry a significant amount of the herb that it claims to feature.

Some studies have shown that essential oils may benefit anxiety when used as a complementary medicine, but other health claims have not been backed up by science. Most of these oils are supplied by one particular company that sells through Facebook parties and individual consultants. In 2014, the company was told by the FDA that it had to stop making medical claims about its products. Samples submitted to independent labs showed that the company's purity claims were not supported by the evidence.

Celebrity Interest

Many of Hollywood's stars turn to essential oils and other herbal preparations for various benefits. There are those who have endorsed traditional (i.e., premodern) medicine in one way or another and have spoken with particular passion about herbalism. Elle McPherson, a supermodel, has said that she makes use of traditional Chinese medicine, and has often spoken about the benefits of treating ailments with herbal remedies. Olivia Newton-John, singer and actress most famous for her role as Sandy in *Grease*, fought cancer with modern medicine, but also used complementary medicine that her doctor endorsed, including herbs and other treatments.

Dr. Andrew Weil may be one of the most famous alternative medicine practitioners due to his commonsense approach to complementary medicine. He famously said that if he was in a car crash, take him to the emergency room, and if he had a bacterial infection, then give him antibiotics. But, as he also noted, combining natural and modern treatments is the best way to support the body's natural healing potential. Among his hugely popular works are those that promote the use of herbal remedies to boost the immune system and prevent illness. Scientific research regarding such claims, however, is still in process.

Kay Tilden Frost and
Michael Shally-Jensen

See also: Antioxidants; Aromatherapy and Essential Oils; Ayurvedic Medicine; Chinese Traditional Medicine; Eating Organic; Folk Medicine; Juice and Juicing; Naturopathic Medicine; Purgatives and Emetics; Stress and Stress Management; Vitamins and Minerals; Witch Trials and Exorcisms

Further Reading

Griggs, Barbara. 1997. *Green Pharmacy: The History and Evolution of Western Herbal Medicine*. 3rd ed. Rochester, VT: Healing Arts Press.

Midura, Ryn, and Katya Swift. 2018. *Herbal Medicine for Beginners*. Berkeley, CA: Althea Press.

St. Claire, Debra, et al. 2016. "Herbalism." In *Natural Healing: Wisdom and Know-How*, edited by Amy Rost, 53–186. New York: Black Dog and Leventhal.

Weil, Andrew. 2008. *8 Weeks to Optimum Health*. Rev ed. New York: Knopf.

MACROBIOTICS

Macrobiotics is a philosophical system relating to a manner of living, but especially to what and how one eats. While it is possible to eat according to a macrobiotic diet without accepting the ideas from which it is derived, most people who follow this diet also accept at least part of the related philosophy. In fact, the types of foods that are included in a macrobiotic diet are generally very healthy and follow many of the suggested guidelines developed by conventional nutritionists. However, nutritionists warn that some vitamins and minerals are not readily available in certain versions of the diet. In addition to recommendations regarding food, the philosophical system also encourages exercise and mindfulness.

History

Although it was the 1960s when macrobiotics started to become known by more than a just small group of people in the United States, its Japanese foundations stretch back several decades. A few individuals can be seen as contributing to the macrobiotic movement prior to the 1890s there, but Sagen Ishizuka (1850–1909) is generally seen as the person who developed the basic theories that became macrobiotics. Trained as an army doctor, Ishizuka became disenchanted with Western medicine and began to teach that eating whole grains as well as balancing sodium and potassium in the diet produced good health and helped heal diseases. He also advocated eating locally produced food and foods that are in season.

In 1911, George Ohsawa (1893–1966; his birth name was Nyoichi Sakurazawa) read one of Ishizuka's books and followed its advice on diet. He had had symptoms of tuberculosis, which was the cause of death in both his mother and brother. Ohsawa claimed that his change in diet saved his life. As a result, he became the leading advocate for this lifestyle, to which he applied the term *macrobiotics* in 1949. In 1960, Ohsawa traveled to New York and began giving public lectures on the new lifestyle and philosophy. He quickly wrote the first edition of the book he named *Zen Macrobiotics*, although macrobiotics had nothing specifically to do with Zen Buddhism. Shortly after these lectures, newsletters, macrobiotic restaurants, and study groups began to form. Macrobiotics' nontraditional approach to life and diet appealed to young people of the emerging counterculture in the 1960s, causing it to grow rapidly (although few completely adopted the lifestyle). With the 1965 second edition of *Zen Macrobiotics*, the general public became more aware of the movement, and more people tried out or adopted the diet plan without necessarily accepting all the tenets of the philosophy.

Unrelated to the movement, many food co-ops offered the types of products needed to maintain a macrobiotic diet. Michio and Aveline Kushi (1926–2014; 1923–2001) began to emerge as leaders of the macrobiotic movement, eventually establishing the Kushi Institute, which provided numerous programs on macrobiotics as well as training for those seeking to adopt the lifestyle. Although the Kushi Institute closed its physical campus in 2018, it left a legacy of individuals and organizations that pursue to the macrobiotic philosophy of life. Some of the groups based on macrobiotic principles are seen by authorities as similar to religious cults in their dogmatic approach to food and health, while other, less fervent organizations' teachings are seen by some to have potential health benefits.

Macrobiotic Diet and Lifestyle

While the book that has been the foundation of macrobiotics is entitled *Zen Macrobiotics*, the only relationship between macrobiotics and Zen is an uncluttered approach to life, which results in a simplified lifestyle with a strong tie to the traditional Japanese way of life. The dietary philosophy that George Ohsawa, as a young man, found to be beneficial, is a high-fiber, low-fat diet. Many aspects of such a diet have been shown, of course, to be healthy, but the claims made for macrobiotics go well beyond anything that science has verified. The founders, and many current advocates of macrobiotics, believe that the diet and lifestyle reduce the risk of certain diseases, and moreover that it can cure certain forms of cancer and other diseases. The idea is that by paying attention to one's body, being mindful of one's lifestyle, having a positive outlook on life, and balancing the traditional forces of yin and the yang, one can live an optimal life. Although not specifically against modern scientific knowledge, advocates of the macrobiotic lifestyle believe that the traditional teachings should be adhered to as one strives to live the best possible life.

The foundation for living a life in accordance with macrobiotic ideals is the macrobiotic diet. The primary ingredients in this diet are whole grains, such as brown rice, oats, corn, and barley. By weight, the recommended allowance would comprise 40 to 60 percent of one's food. Vegetables—local, organic vegetables if available—would make up another 20 to 30 percent. Not all vegetables are recommended, however, with potatoes, tomatoes, peppers, spinach, beets, and zucchini being off the menu. Beans, including bean-based products, and sea vegetables are another 5 to 10 percent of the diet.

Those three categories, along with any necessary vegetable cooking oils and a limited range of condiments, represent the bulk of the daily diet. Other items, such as seafood, are generally acceptable a few times a week, as are fruits, seeds, and nuts. According to those who follow the strictest macrobiotic guidelines, fruit is to be eaten only when it is from the climate in which one lives; thus, for people in the northern United States, apples are fine but pineapple is not, while for those living in Hawaii the opposite would be true. Foods to be phased out of one's diet include meat, dairy, eggs, and poultry. In addition to water, various teas are recommended, although strongly caffeinated tea (the type most people drink) is not. Highly processed, artificially enhanced, and chemically treated foods are prohibited, as are hot spices, whether natural or artificial. Modern nutritionists warn that following this diet makes it difficult to get enough of certain nutrients, such as calcium and vitamin D.

In preparing the food, you are supposed to use a gas or wood stove, not an electric stove or a microwave oven. Traditional cooking vessels, such as cast iron, earthenware, or stainless steel are acceptable to use, but no Teflon-coated items. You should eat or drink only when hungry or thirsty, and then in moderation. You should be relaxed when eating and chew each mouthful about fifty times. You are not restricted in the number of meals you can take, but no food is to be consumed within a few hours of retiring to bed. You should not starve yourself, but at the same time, you should stop eating when you are satisfied, not only when you feel completely full or satiated.

The key to the system is avoiding foods that are considered either strongly yin (e.g., alcohol, mushrooms, soy, dates) or strongly yang (pickles, miso, certain teas, certain fish) and relying on "neutral" foods such as grains for the bulk of the diet. There are elaborate ways to try and balance a dish through varying proportions of yin and yang elements, including the way the food is prepared (e.g., steamed vs. stir-fried). The macrobiotic approach holds that there is no uniform way to address the dietary (or other) needs of the individual; rather, each person is unique and must experiment to discover his or her ideal balance.

In addition to the food aspects of macrobiotics, a simple lifestyle is recommended. The preferred clothes are cotton, nothing made of wool or synthetics; and only limited accessories, of natural material, should be worn. Cleanliness is emphasized, with a daily scrubbing of the body with a hot towel being best. Long showers or baths are not. Cleaning agents, for both the person and the home, should be natural and nontoxic. Fresh air should be part of each day, ideally by exposure to the outdoors for at least a half hour but also by having windows open when at home. Exercise, such as yoga or martial arts, should be practiced. Electronic devices should be used on a limited basis, with protection from electromagnetic fields. In addition, a positive outlook on life is to be cultivated.

So, does macrobiotics work? It is impossible to say, really, because there are no consistent scientific findings to compare it against—particularly in the area of the lifestyle as opposed to the diet. It is true that avoiding the harmful additives in processed foods and instead eating fresh, locally grown food is better for one's health, but it is apparent, too, that certain nutritional deficits can show up if one keeps a strict macrobiotic diet—deficits that must be made up for in some other way. (Adding eggs and dairy products might fill the gap in some cases.)

Donald A. Watt

See also: Antioxidants; Chinese Traditional Medicine; Detox Diets; Diet and Exercise; Eating Organic; Juice and Juicing; Paleo Diet; Vegetarianism; Vitamins and Minerals

Further Reading

Kushi, Michio, with Alex Jack. 2013. *The Book of Macrobiotics: The Universal Way of Health, Happiness and Peace.* Garden City Park, NY: Square One Publishers.

Kushi Institute. 2018. "What Is Macrobiotic Diet?" Becket, MA: Kushi Institute. www.kushiinstitute.org/what-is-macrobiotics/

Ohsawa, George, and Carl Ferre, eds. 2013. *Zen Macrobiotics: The Art of Rejuvenation and Longevity.* 5th ed. Chico, CA: George Ohsawa Macrobiotic Foundation.

Raso, Jack. [1990] 2015. "A Kushi Seminar for Professionals." *Quackwatch* (print: *Nutrition Forum*). Chapel Hill, NC: Quackwatch. www.quackwatch.org/01QuackeryRelated Topics/kushi.html

Ratini, Melinda. 2018. "Macrobiotic Diet." *WebMD.* New York: WebMD LLC. www.webmd.com/diet/a-z/macrobiotic-diet

Waxman, Denny, and Susan Waxman. Introduction by Michio Kushi. 2015. *The Complete Macrobiotic Diet: 7 Steps to Feel Fabulous, Look Vibrant, and Think Clearly.* New York: Pegasus.

MAGNET THERAPY

Magnets have long been promoted as devices for relieving pain and addressing other medical conditions. Advocates claim that they improve circulation, relax tense muscles, reduce inflammation, and boost levels of the "feel-good" hormones called endorphins in the central nervous system.

A variety of sophisticated magnetic devices are employed today in conventional medicine, mainly in the field of medical imaging (e.g., magnetic resonance imaging, or MRI). These devices make use of electromagnets, which employ a series of electric charges to produce a fluctuating magnetic field. Most magnets used in alternative medicine, on the other hand—in wristbands, leg wraps, shoe inserts, and mattress pad covers—are static magnets, conventional magnets, which have a permanent magnetic field.

A typical magnet has two ends, of course, a negative ("north") pole and a positive ("south") pole. (In some magnets the negative end has a small indentation in it, while the positive end is unmarked.) Two magnets attract or repel each other, depending on which ends are brought together. Opposite poles—north and south—attract each other, while identical poles repel each other. A compass needle is a magnetized object that aligns its negative end with the earth's North Pole and its positive end with the South Pole. All magnets have this same "compass" property; it can only be observed, however, if a magnet is suspended or otherwise can turn on its axis.

Modern magnetic healing is based on the qualities that static magnets have as part of their basic makeup. The magnetic field is considered to interact with the body in specific ways, either aligning or deflecting various bodily substances and generating energy flows in one direction or another. The negative pole of a magnet is thought to be "deflective" or "dispersing": it works to clear out accumulations or buildups such as those associated with inflammation, infections, hypertension, headaches, arthritis, skin ailments, cataracts, and bodily pain (Tierra 2016).

The positive pole, in contrast, is regarded as "augmentative" or "consolidating": it addresses weaknesses or deficiencies such as those involved with poor digestion, compromised immune systems, general weakness, asthma, hair loss, nerve damage, faulty metabolism, and stiffness or paralysis (ibid.).

Other theories about their health effects state that magnets (1) produce a slight electric current and thus stimulate the nerves to produce beneficial effects or (2) disrupt chemical bonds in such a way as to increase the rate and amount of communication between cells or (3) attract or repel charged particles in the tissue and bloodstream (including so-called free radicals), serving to increase oxygen and improve prospects for healing (Micozzi 2015, 226–27). Most researchers, however, admit that the precise mechanism of magnetotherapy is little understood.

In standard practice, magnets are taped or wrapped to the body to bring them into contact with the affected area. A magnetized stone ("lodestone") or a regular static magnet may simply be laid on a part of the body, as in the treatment of lower-back pain. People also use magnetized shoe inserts to alleviate foot pain or simply to "ground" themselves as they go about their daily lives; and they use magnetized mattresses to improve sleep at night or to "draw out" the stresses and conflicting energies that have accumulated during the day. In short, magnets are an easy and inexpensive way to address health concerns according to the methods and techniques of modern complementary and alternative medicine (CAM). Whether they work has not been proved.

Magnetism in the Flux of History

Healers in ancient China, India, and Greece are thought to have used lodestones on the body to address imbalances in the flows of natural energies or forces. During the Middle Ages, magnets were used by alchemists and healers alike to explore the physical and physiological universe. One of the earliest "modern" studies of magnetism was by William Gilbert (1544–1603), who determined that the Earth was magnetic and argued, provably, that magnetism and static electricity were not the same thing. Gilbert demonstrated his experiments before Queen Elizabeth I and may even have used magnets on her to alleviate her joint pain. (Elizabeth suffered from rheumatism.)

In the late 1700s the German physician Franz Anton Mesmer (1734–1815) used magnets over the bodies of patients to demonstrate his theory about celestial forces governing the flow of fluids and energies in the human body. Mesmer later concluded that the magnets were not necessary and he could produce the same results by merely passing his hands over his patients and making forceful eye contact—he called his new method "animal magnetism," and it became a popular sensation. He opened a clinic in Vienna, Austria, and attracted all the best clients. Later, he went on to perform additional studies in Paris, combining magnetism with hypnosis. A scientific board there, however, identified Mesmer as a quack and he was forced to leave the country. His medical practice never recovered.

Many folk doctors in the United States practiced magnetic healing, as did some trained physicians—whose "training," however, often consisted of no more than serving as an apprentice for a few months. One such doctor, Andrew Taylor Still (1828–1917), began in the 1870s to develop a theory of human health based on the musculoskeletal system and the flow of energetic (and spiritual) forces within it. Still came to combine magnetism with the manual manipulation of bones, eventually calling his hybrid science Osteopathy. Osteopathic medicine, after experiencing a period of controversy and undergoing further refinement of its theories, proved to be a worthy complement to mainstream medicine and today is generally accepted.

Another noted figure, Daniel David Palmer (1845–1913), established a magnetic healing clinic in Davenport, Iowa, in 1887. Palmer, like Mesmer before him, soon was convinced that he could control a patient's "vital magnetism" by the use of his hands alone, and, like Mesmer and Still, began adding other components. After conceiving the idea of an "innate intelligence" circulating through the nervous system, Palmer focused on blockages to the flow of energy and the means to unblock the flow. The result was the new science of chiropractic, or skeletal manipulation and bone "resetting." Chiropractic was further developed by Palmer's son and others and eventually became a major complementary and alternative technique in its own right.

Magnetism's Virtues and Vices

Besides being used in medical imaging, pulsating electromagnets are now used to help promote the healing of bone fractures, particularly a kind of fracture known as a nonunion fracture, where the natural healing process has not taken place. Additionally, electromagnets have been studied for use in treating joint pain, bone and tissue problems, migraines, and fibromyalgia. While some of the results have been promising, more work needs to be done. Magnets are not a panacea, though some natural healers think them so.

One type of electromagnetic therapy that has been approved by the U.S. Food and Drug Administration (FDA) is a high-tech procedure called transcranial magnetic stimulation (TMS). TMS entails the passing of electromagnets across a patient's head in order to interrupt the brain's own magnetic field. Like electroconvulsive therapy, the precise mechanism of TMS's operation is not well understood, and yet the technique has been used successfully to treat depression, especially mild depression.

Meanwhile, *static* magnets, too, continue to be researched and widely used within the CAM community. There too, however, the results that have been achieved have not invariably proved to be better than results obtained from using a placebo (e.g., a nonmagnet). The use of static magnets, then, is generally not accepted by the mainstream medical community. Nevertheless, magnets remain very popular and the marketing of magnets and magnetic wraps has become a big business. Animal wraps, as well, are now available—including magnetic shin wraps for horses, which are promoted as a treatment for tendon and bone injuries.

The bottom line is that magnets are cool and interesting and tap into a popular concept of "energy flows," and control of same, yet many questions remain.

Michael Shally-Jensen

See also: Acupuncture; Biofeedback; Chiropractic; Cupping; Deep Brain Stimulation; Electroconvulsive Therapy; Mesmerism and Hypnotherapy; Mind–Body Medicine; Osteopathy; Reiki and Therapeutic Touch

Further Reading

Kahn, Sherry. 2000. *Healing Magnets: A Guide for Pain Relief, Speeding Recovery, and Restoring Balance.* New York: Three Rivers Press.
Micozzi, Marc S. 2015. *Fundamentals of Complementary and Alternative Medicine.* 5th ed. St. Louis, MO: Elsevier Saunders.
National Center for Complementary and Integrative Health (NCCIH). 2013. *Magnets.* Washington, DC: NCCIH.
Tierra, Lesley. 2016. "Home Therapies: Magnets." In *Natural Healing: Wisdom and Know-How,* edited by Amy Rost, 863–64. New York: Black Dog and Leventhal Publishers.

MEDITATION AND MINDFULNESS

Meditation, broadly speaking, is a way of achieving wholeness. Traditionally a spiritual pursuit, it has been practiced in recent decades as a means of "recentering" one's core being amid the flurry of daily activities. It is by its nature a healing maneuver, a way to integrate oneself with the wider cosmos and, in some ways, bridge the gap between the way things are and the way they ought to be. Meditation is, then, both a method of contemplation and a kind of end in itself, a way of perceiving what is true and real and attaining it on a spiritual or mental plane. It entails concentration and abstraction, and is intended to produce heightened awareness and bodily calm.

Historic Varieties

Meditation in one form or another has been associated with most of the great world religions. In the Hindu philosophical tradition, the school of *yoga* concerns more than just bodily postures but in fact represents an elaborate system for purifying the mind, the soul, *and* the body. By tapping into energies residing both within oneself and outside the limits of the body, the meditator is said to leave the world of surface impressions to reach a deeper, silent level of pure consciousness. This sense of transcendence goes by different names in different traditions: enlightenment, Nirvana, the Infinite, the One. In a number of religions, spiritual purification is sought through the verbal or visual repetition of a particular sound or image—for example, the mantra in Eastern thought; Christ or Mary in Christian tradition; the prayer recitation, or rhythmic *davening*, in Jewish tradition; the ritual "remembrance" (*dhikr*) in mystical Islam. In both the West and the Middle East, emphasis is traditionally placed on the content of meditation—that is, on the image, word,

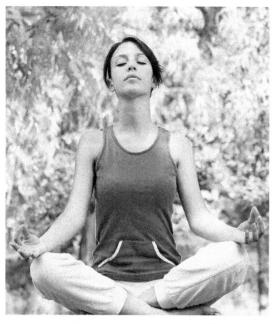

A woman meditates in a natural setting. (Marco Lensi/Dreamstime.com)

or text and its sacred meaning. This idealized content is held up for personal consideration. This may mean learning by heart a passage from the Bible or the Koran that serves to focus attention away from the self and toward the object. The goal is not to interpret or understand the object but rather to allow *it* to take over the will, the being, of the meditator and move him or her to another plane of experience. The icon (sacred image) in the Orthodox Church serves this purpose, as does, in the Roman Catholic Church, reciting the rosary, with its accompanying handling of threaded beads and its meditation on the events of the life of Christ and his mother, Mary.

In the Far East, in contrast, greater emphasis is placed on "contentless" meditation, or the striving toward openness and receptivity in connection with the unfolding cosmic order. In Tibetan Buddhism, for example, the *mandala* ("circle," or cosmic diagram) is a visual device for concentrating one's attention on universal forces. In Zen Buddhism, a koan—a meditative paradox—is used as a focal point. ("What is the sound of one hand clapping?") The intent is to empty the mind, to wear down the reasoning mind and experience pure being ("no mind"). In effect, the "mindlessness" of the meditative effort brings about a new "mindfulness," a different kind of awareness or sensitivity.

In Zen, the student meditator is guided through a series of steps designed to produce a deepening perspective. Breathing methods are altered in the early phase of meditation, followed, typically, by intense meditation on a challenging koan. In other forms of Buddhist meditation, the koan may be replaced by some other object of concentration, including ordinary things (e.g., a primal sound or mantra) and more abstract qualities (color, light) or concepts (death, life). The *zazen,* or characteristic meditative position in Zen, is assumed throughout. Various meditative exercises are intended to help one break through to the true nature of reality and thus develop insight and wisdom (*prajñā*). At the end of a session, the *roshi,* or master, will usually dialogue with students to review their experience and assess their progress.

Different cultural and religious traditions have developed different postures and motions to assist the mind in shedding its connection to daily affairs and entering into the meditative framework. The many *asanas,* or yogic "poses," represent perhaps the most extensive of such systems. From Taoism comes *Tai Chi,* a system that involves rhythmically precise movements designed to optimize the flow of natural vital energy within the body and connect with broader forces in the environment. One goal in Tai Chi is to have the student become sufficiently adept in the movements as to permit him or her to integrate them into daily activities, so that a sense of harmonizing one's actions with the cosmos is developed. A somewhat similar practical effect is evident in the Native American tradition of treating ordinary activities such as hunting game or harvesting plants as meditative moments reflective of a wider set of spiritual forces at work.

Transcendental Meditation and After

Although based on ancient Hindu tradition, Transcendental Meditation (TM) was developed by Maharishi Mahesh Yogi (1918–2008) in the 1950s and introduced to the West by him in 1958. TM, like the other meditative traditions, is premised on the idea that people can transcend the daily kaleidoscope of thoughts and impressions in their heads to reach a deeper, richer level of consciousness. ("I am therefore I think.") The trancelike state of transcendence is regarded as a source of unlimited energy and "creative intelligence." It has the power, according to TM theory, not only to eliminate the stresses of modern living but also to help people realize their full potential and help humanity improve the world.

Maharishi Mahesh Yogi was a graduate (1942) in physics at Allahabad University in Uttar Pradesh (northeastern India). A student of one Guru Dev, Maharishi spent two years in the Himalayas and then began to teach TM in India. Subsequently, he traveled abroad to promote his "World Plan" for spreading TM and the science of Creative Intelligence. He lectured, wrote books, and made recordings and videotapes of teachings. After founding the International Meditation Society, Maharishi and his supporters established Maharishi International University in Switzerland and Fairfield, Iowa. (It is now the Maharishi University of Management.) Especially active in the United States, Canada, and (then) West Germany, Maharishi often appeared on television talk shows where he earned the epithet "the Giggling Guru" because of the way he laughed during conversations.

The Maharishi became particularly famous for an encounter he had with the Beatles in 1967. After meeting with the "fab four" in the United Kingdom, Maharishi became the group's official spiritual adviser, or guru. In early 1968 the Beatles and several other celebrities arranged for an extended stay in India for the purpose of learning fully the methods of TM and the philosophy of the Maharishi. Confusion arose, however, over the matter of sexual boundaries and allegations of misconduct involving the Maharishi, although no clear light was ever shed on the incident. The various parties simply ceased their association and went their separate ways. Despite the kerfuffle, TM continued to gain adherents in the West. The Maharishi's 1963 book, *The Science of Being and the Art of Living,* became a bestseller and was translated into 15 languages.

Avoiding the special postures, lengthy contemplative exercises, and other techniques associated with traditional meditation, TM claims to be a powerful yet effortless technique that anyone can learn in a few hours. Best learned from a professional teacher, TM requires only one or two 20-minute meditation periods a day. During these periods the meditator repeats a mantra that is assigned to him or her by the teacher according to a proprietary formula, one that takes account of the individual's makeup and mental outlook. Reciting the mantra, the meditator achieves a state of rest deeper than sleep, accompanied by slowed breathing and a lessened heartbeat. Such rest helps to erase daily thoughts and feelings and is thought to bring renewed energy to the meditator. As a result, his or her health may generally improve, and such self-destructive activities as the use of drugs and alcohol may decline. In the waking state, the TM practitioner's mind is believed to be more aware of its surroundings, and the person's work may improve as a consequence. Social relations, too, may become richer and more harmonious. Indeed, Maharishi believed that improved harmony at the social level would lead to significant changes at the level of international politics, perhaps even bringing world peace.

In the late 1960s, a Harvard medical researcher, Herbert Benson, carried out studies of TM and determined that it had beneficial effects. Mainly, it helped to bring about a state of relaxation, which in turn helped decrease the responsiveness of the sympathetic nervous system, lower one's heart and respiration rate, reduce the levels of cortisol (a steroid hormone) in the bloodstream, and boosted the presence of alpha waves in the brain (indicating a wakeful yet relaxed state). Benson went on to develop a relaxation method of his own, called the "relaxation response." It can be used by persons facing stressful situations in their daily life—without the need, necessarily, to "pull over" and meditate. So successful was Benson's relaxation response that a number of hospitals soon adopted it to work with patients who experienced stress or anxiety regarding their medical condition and/or hospitalization.

A spin-off, of sorts, of both TM and the relaxation response later emerged in the form of so-called mindfulness meditation, or the process of achieving a state of mindful awareness through meditation. Dr. Jon Kabat-Zinn, of the University of Massachusetts Medical School, is a key figure here. The idea with mindfulness meditation is to maintain awareness of bodily sensations and thoughts without becoming critical or judgmental regarding them. The mindful person, rather, lets go of his or her worries and ongoing mental attachments in order to focus on inner resources and the elimination of anxiety. The concept of mindfulness has since become part of the general culture, as more and more people strive to maintain awareness of their actions in everyday life and their effects on both themselves and others around them.

Michael Shally-Jensen

See also: Aromatherapy and Essential Oils; Biofeedback; Faith Healing and Prayer; Health and Wellness Gurus; Mesmerism and Hypnotherapy; Mind–Body Medicine; Tai Chi and Qigong; Yoga

Further Reading

Benson, Herbert, with Miriam Z. Klipper. 2000. *The Relaxation Response*. Updated and expanded ed. New York: Quill/HarperCollins.

Kabat-Zinn, Jon. 2005. *Wherever You Go, There You Are: Mindfulness Meditation in Everyday Life*. 10th anniv. ed. New York: Hachette.

Maharishi Mahesh Yogi. 2001. *Science of Being and Art of Living: Transcendental Meditation*. New York: Meridian.

Monaghan, Patricia, and Eleanor G. Viereck. 2011. *Meditation: The Complete Guide*. Rev. ed. Novato, CA: New World Library.

MILIEU THERAPY AND THERAPEUTIC COMMUNITY

Milieu therapy refers to a situation where a number of individuals being seen for mental health reasons receive treatment, and the interactions between them (and with their environment) become the focus of the therapy. Until the later part of the 20th century, the usual setting was the ward of a psychiatric hospital. But, as the closing of large state psychiatric hospitals occurred, beginning in the mid-1950s, milieu therapy moved along with patients to shorter-term units of smaller, local and private hospitals, group homes, and day programs. It became, essentially, a form of treatment called therapeutic community.

Milieu therapy first emerged in the World War II era in military hospitals in Great Britain. It went on to become an important influence in U.S. psychiatry during the mid- to later 20th century, particularly as therapeutic community. Although therapeutic community has faded somewhat from the U.S. psychiatric scene, it continues to be drawn on in group settings in which many people with mental illness are treated. It has, lately, in fact, experienced a resurgence, of sorts, at least in the case of a few selected institutions operating today.

A Brief History of Therapeutic Community in the United States

As noted, modern therapeutic community began during World War II in Great Britain in military hospitals treating men found unfit for military service, and later, traumatized soldiers returning from the front. Psychoanalysis, particularly as practiced at the Tavistock Institute in London, was an influence, as was the social psychology and "action research" (group dynamics) of Kurt Lewin (1890–1947). Psychodynamic group therapy was being developed simultaneously with the therapeutic community, and S. H. Foulkes (1898–1976), one of group therapy's founders, was an officer in one of the first military therapeutic communities.

The U.S. psychiatrist Karl Menninger (1893–1990), whose family founded the influential Menninger Clinic, was an officer in the U.S. military during World War II and visited the military therapeutic communities in Great Britain late in the war. He brought back the new treatment ideas to the United States. Another U.S. military officer and psychiatrist, Harry Wilmer, also visited British hospitals and returned to start his own therapeutic communities for men with psychiatric casualties from the Pacific and Korea. Wilmer discussed his work in his 1958 book *Social Psychiatry in Action*. Maxwell Jones also came to the United States on several extended occasions and was influential in the growing acceptance of therapeutic community as a treatment for mental illness, starting communities in prisons and community mental health centers. Robert Rapoport, a U.S. anthropologist, researched one of Jones's communities in Great Britain, with the resulting influential book *Community as Doctor* (1960). Loren Mosher (1933–2004), also influenced by the work in Great Britain, especially that of the existential psychiatrist R. D. Laing (1927–1989), initiated Soteria House in the early 1970s for young patients experiencing their first psychotic episode. Mosher and his Soteria House experiment went on to influence similar projects in other parts of the United States and in Switzerland. During several decades following World War II, therapeutic community flourished and became widespread in the United States.

Although people with mental illness continued to be treated in milieu settings, therapeutic community per se eventually faded from the professional dialogue. One reason why was the late20th century's emphasis on pharmacological treatments and its fascination with the new findings of neuroscience, culminating in the Decade of the Brain (1990s). This trend deemphasized all sorts of psychosocial treatments, including therapeutic community, as the bulk of funding and professional research centered on neuroscience and psychopharmacology.

The philosophy of therapeutic community also contributed to its disappearance from the professional dialogue. It was a central value of therapeutic community not to define itself too strictly but rather to keep evolving. This was done in order to give members/patients the opportunity to develop independence and responsibility through their own interactions. It was fully expected that each community would be unique to some extent.

Therapeutic community may have also been a victim of its own success because it was the accepted psychiatric canon for several decades of the mid- to late 20th century, to the point where almost all groups were called by the name therapeutic community, even when they provided no more than the old hierarchic way of doing business.

Another factor in the fading influence of therapeutic community is that it is a difficult method or approach to research given its many variables, and it developed at a time when researching the effectiveness of treatments was considered less crucial than it is currently. Nowadays, for example, evidence-based care has become the standard.

Contemporary Therapeutic Community

A few therapeutic communities, consciously identifying themselves as such, continue today. These include Austen Riggs Center in Stockbridge, Massachusetts, and the small farm-based communities of Spring Lake Ranch in Vermont and Gould Farm in Massachusetts. Cooper-Riis is a newer, private community in North Carolina, while Fountain House, in New York City, also makes use of therapeutic community. As a *practice* combining self-reflective principles of psychotherapy and community living, therapeutic community continues to be re-created in many settings, especially in areas where staff are still influenced by psychoanalytic or social psychology principles. It is also operative in some cases in substance abuse treatment settings (see Clark 2017).

The Sanctuary model of Sandra Bloom (1997) is a contemporary, conscious elaboration of therapeutic community. The model both draws on therapeutic community's roots of treating traumatized soldiers returning from war and enhances the earlier paradigm through the addition of recent research on trauma. Bloom has instituted this work in community settings ranging from psychiatric hospitals to children's residential treatment facilities. She has found, as did therapeutic community practitioners before her, that the use of community meetings, giving clients the skills to talk about their feelings, and sharing the responsibility for the daily life and safety of the group/milieu has led to a much-decreased incidence of assaults and to a secure environment in which healing can take place.

Looking Ahead

Although therapeutic community may have lost some of its earlier luster in the overall landscape of mental health treatment, people with mental illness continue to be treated in milieu settings that are influenced by its legacy. Therapeutic community provides both a theory and a means of increasing the effectiveness of treatment; it also addresses the inevitable problems and crises that arise when groups of people are thrown together.

In contemporary settings for people with mental illness, evidence-based practices (e.g., supported employment; treatment of substance abuse and mental illness concurrently; and teaching skills of wellness self-management) are dominant. While there is research to support such practices, the setting in which they are delivered has not been addressed, and it is often in large outpatient day treatment programs, rehabilitation programs, or vocational programs, where clients attend several days a week, several hours a day. Therapeutic community can and does provide a healthy milieu in which these evidenced-based methods are carried out successfully.

Mental illness continues to be a heartbreaking, draining problem, without easy solutions. Gerald Grob, a historian of U.S. psychiatry, has reflected on the "sobering . . . cyclical pattern alternating between enthusiastic optimism and fatalistic pessimism" (2000, 253) as popular treatments have been exalted and then abandoned in disappointment. "Rhetorical claims to the contrary, little is known about the etiology of serious mental disorders. Treatment—whether biological or psychosocial—does not necessarily eliminate the disorder. . . . For too long, mental health policy has embodied an elusive dream of magical cures for age-old maladies" (254–55). Therapeutic community is not a magical cure, although it may have been exalted as such by some in its heyday. It is, however, a valid treatment that can still contribute vitally to milieu treatment and related practices. It is a once popular treatment that has returned, on a limited basis, as an alternative to mainstream medicine, representing a different—and effective—approach to mental illness.

Julie Kipp and
Michael Shally-Jensen

See also: Encounter Groups; Existential Psychotherapy; Gestalt Therapy; Mental Hospitals; Moral Treatment; Psychoanalysis; Recovery Movement

Further Reading

Bloom, Sandra. 1997. *Creating Sanctuary: Toward the Evolution of Sane Societies.* New York: Routledge.

Clark, Claire D. 2017. *The Recovery Revolution: The Battle over Addiction Treatment in the United States.* New York: Columbia University Press.

Clark, David. 1964. *Administrative Therapy: The Role of the Doctor in the Therapeutic Community.* London: Tavistock.

Grob, Gerald. 2000. "Mental Health Policy in Late Twentieth-Century America." In *American Psychiatry after World War II (1944–1994),* edited by R. W. Menninger and J. C. Nemiah, 232–58. Washington, DC: American Psychiatric Press.

Jones, Maxwell. 1968. *Beyond the Therapeutic Community: Social Learning and Social Psychiatry.* New Haven, CT: Yale University Press.

Kennard, David. 1998. *An Introduction to Therapeutic Communities.* 2nd ed. Philadelphia: Jessica Kingsley.

Mosher, Loren. 1996. "Soteria: A Therapeutic Community for Psychotic Persons." In *Psychosocial Approaches to Deeply Disturbed Persons,* edited by Peter Breggin and E. M. Stern, 43–58. New York: Haworth.

PRIMAL THERAPY AND FEELING THERAPY

Primal Therapy

After developing the therapeutic system known as *primal therapy* in the late 1960s, and publishing his first book, *The Primal Scream*, in 1970, Arthur Janov felt himself to be a visionary in the mold of major thinkers of the past. Janov maintained that his primal therapy could cure neurosis and its symptoms, depression and anxiety disorders, alcoholism and drug use, and even epilepsy and asthma. Although at its height in the 1970s, primal therapy indeed drew masses of followers, including big-name celebrities like John Lennon and Yoko Ono, by the 1980s Janov's work was considered of marginal interest within the field of clinical psychology. Still, the story of the "primal scream" is worth knowing for what it tells us about the human condition—as it was understood in the midcentury United States.

Janov (1924–2017) was born and raised in a lower-middle-class neighborhood of Los Angeles. At the University of California, Los Angeles, he earned a bachelor's degree in psychology and a master's in psychiatric social work, or the providing of assistance and counseling to mental health patients. He operated as a mainstream

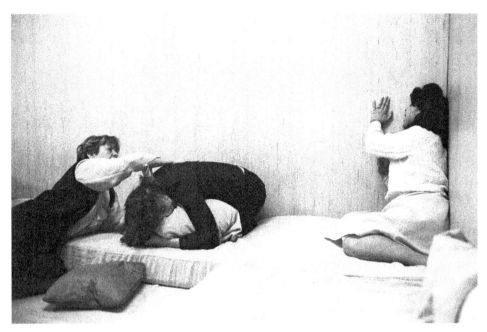

A primal therapy session for a group of patients at a hospital in 1981. One patient curls around a pillow, while another cries and calls out while huddled in a corner of the room. (Manuel Litran/Paris Match via Getty Images)

therapist/counselor for about 20 years, first in hospital settings and later in private practice. In the course of doing so, he earned a PhD in psychology at the Claremont Graduate School (one of the Claremont Colleges).

While working with one of his patients in the late 1960s, Janov encouraged the patient not simply to talk about his parents but to try seeing them, experiencing them, even to cry out to them. Soon, the patient was writhing around on the floor in a sort of agonized regression to his past, attempting to communicate with his parents. As Janov continued the story in *The Primal Scream*: "Finally, he [the patient] released a piercing, deathlike scream that rattled the walls of my office. . . . All he could say afterward was, 'I made it! I don't know what, but I can *feel!*'" (Fox 2017). Here was the origin of primal therapy.

The premise of primal therapy is this: Adult neuroses are rooted in early childhood, even infant, traumas. But whereas Freudian and other classical psychotherapies tend to focus on the "symbolic" import of experience, grounded in a child's overall psychosexual development, Janov and other primal therapists looked to identify so-called primal pain in the life history of the child. Children, that is, have a need for love. Calming a baby when it is crying, feeding it when it is hungry, comforting it when it is unsettled, and so on, are expressions of that love. As the child grows up, it is important for the parent to continue satisfying the child's needs and to let him or her be who he or she is. When this does not happen, the child experiences pain, and the most common way to deal with that pain is to repress it, to push it into the unconscious. There it remains "stored," along with a buried need for love; from there it gives rise to neurotic behaviors, sleep disorders, sexual problems, drug and alcohol use, depression, and more.

Much of this sounds rather like conventional psychoanalytic thinking, but Janov and his colleagues were accused by their critics of simplifying human psychodynamics and coming up with a questionable therapeutic solution, namely, working to restore the patient's access to his or her childhood pain. This, according to primal theory, allows the patient to feel that pain once again and to release it from the unconscious. In experiencing the primal scream, the patient is thought to break through his or her mental defenses, thereby causing all neurotic behaviors and other ailments and symptoms to dissipate completely. The patient is said to be cured and able now to live his or her "real" life.

In later years, Janov pushed back the time envelope for experiencing primal pain to one's departure from the womb at birth and even to time spent inside the uterus. Janov's therapy rooms were supplied with teddy bears, dolls, baby rattles, playpens, cribs, and other nursery items to help his patients regress to the primal moment. His books, *The Primal Scream, The Primal Revolution* (1972), *Prisoners of Pain* (1980), and others, sold in the millions and were translated into numerous foreign languages. John Lennon and Yoko Ono recorded their Plastic Ono Band albums (1970)—albums with lots of screaming on them—while in treatment with Janov. Other famous clients included the actor James Earl Jones and the pianist Roger Williams. Apple cofounder Steve Jobs tried it but didn't like it.

Janov's work was considered by many mainstream psychologists and psychiatrists to be at once too elementary in its theoretical framework and too absolute in its belief about "curing" patients by reconnecting them to their childhood pain. There was never any proof offered by Janov of the supposedly near universal existence of primal pain, the burying of that pain, the value of reexperiencing it, or the long-term effectiveness of the methods used in primal therapy. The main proof was that feeling of "breaking free" that many patients reported—this, at a time in the 1970s when breaking free of social constraints and the repressive habits of one's parents was highly valued. As one observer has noted, "Janov's primal therapy is a classic instance of being the right charismatic therapist at the right time" (quoted in Fox 2017). After a wave of excitement in its early years, primal therapy faded in popularity and today is practiced by a dwindling few.

Feeling Therapy

An offshoot of primal therapy in the 1970s was "feeling therapy." Although its impact was less significant, its beliefs and practices were even more controversial. It mostly attracted people who were familiar with Janov's books or had heard about the primal scream. The founders of feeling therapy, Joseph Hart and Richard Corriere, distinguished their system from Janov's by arguing that theirs was newer and better. They stated that the notion of a definitive "cure" as claimed by the primalists was false and misleading, and that the proper goal of psychotherapy was to work perpetually toward recovery—as in the case of alcoholics. Hart and Corriere also adopted the premise of "therapeutic community," or milieu, in which fellow patients interact with each other and/or cohabit a space in order—hopefully—to get better together. Since there is no end to the disorder and pain one suffers in life, said feeling therapy's founders, people needed ongoing assistance. They needed "community" in which to share their experiences. A Center for Feeling Therapy opened in Los Angles in 1971, and there therapists and clients lived, worked, and played together.

The first thing a patient undergoing feeling therapy needed to know was that there was not going to be any "primal moment," no blast from the past that was supposed to clear out the debris of one's life and make oneself whole. Instead, the focus was on the *present*—especially on how one is feeling in the present—and on making behavioral changes to adjust one's feelings. Initially, the Center's program required a patient to isolate him- or herself for 24 hours before starting a three-week course of intensive therapy. Later, this practice was changed, just as other methods and theories were changed as the Center's practice evolved. Like primal therapy, feeling therapy rejected the "symbolic" qualities of pain and neuroses and sought instead to identify the direct roots of real-life experience. A troublesome thought or behavior, therefore, was viewed not as the result, say, of a "symbolic" fear of castration by an imposing (yet vague) parental figure, as in classical psycho-analysis. Rather, such problems were said to be due to an *actual experience or threat of violence* by a parent in a specific instance. Therefore, instead of sitting down with a therapist and getting one's dreams analyzed for what they said about the myths and symbols of one's past, the client in feeling therapy worked with his or her therapist to develop clear and lucid dreams, dreams that spoke directly of real encounters, present feelings, and future directions. Patients were given exercises to improve the clarity of their dreams—and their lives—by eliminating fictitious elements and concentrating on present desires and feelings.

Later, the Center's therapists, who eventually numbered a dozen or more (with a client base of over 300), abandoned dream therapy and started stressing other means of personal improvement, some of them quite abusive. People were "broken down" during their intensive introductory sessions; they were forced to strip, physically and mentally, before the "community"; they were expected to have sex with assigned partners; they were called names and beaten before the group; they were entrapped in financial schemes aimed at generating revenue; and, in some cases, they were forced to give up their children or have abortions. By the time that these practices were taking place, the Center was basically functioning as a cult organization led by zealous cult leaders. Books published by Center therapists included *Going Sane* (1975), *Dream Makers* (1977), and *Psychological Fitness* (1979)—the last one, in particular, hinting at the punishing regime.

In 1981, a group of former Center members filed a lawsuit against their onetime therapists, claiming that they had been brainwashed and abused physically and emotionally. The case came to be a scandal for clinical psychology generally, in that it called into question the limits of therapeutic practice by qualified individuals and the need for professional controls. The litigation in this case ended in a $6-million settlement, and most of the Center therapists lost their licenses while some were charged with negligence, incompetence, and other crimes. Feeling therapy never quite recovered from this scandal.

Michael Shally-Jensen

See also: Codependency Counseling; Drama Therapy; Encounter Groups; Est and Other "Human Potential" Therapies; Guided Imagery, or Visualization; Psychoanalysis; Recovered Memory Therapy, "Split Personality," and Satanism

Further Reading

Ayella, Marybeth. 1998. *Insane Therapy: Portrait of a Psychotherapy Cult.* Philadelphia: Temple University Press.

Feltham, Colin, and Ian Horton, eds. 2012. *The SAGE Handbook of Counseling and Psychotherapy.* 3rd ed. Thousand Oaks, CA: SAGE Publications.

Fox, Margalit. 2017. "Arthur Janov, 93, Dies." *New York Times,* October 2, B14.

Singer, Margaret Thaler, and Janja Lalich. 1996. *Crazy Therapies: What Are They? Do They Work?* San Francisco: Jossey-Bass.

REFLEXOLOGY

Reflexology is a therapy in which pressure, in varying amounts, is applied to specific points on the feet or hands. These pressure points are believed to match certain other parts of the body—and not just those of the musculoskeletal system, but internal organs from other systems as well. Thus, the soles (and tops) of the feet and the palms (and backsides) of the hands are taken to be maps of the body representing major organs and other bodily parts. Reflexologists examine the feet and hands to ascertain the health of the individual and to determine how best to respond by applying pressure to the areas needing attention. Massaging these reflex points on the extremities is thought to influence deep organ function and bring healing. However, the *means* by which these benefits are achieved are identified differently by different practitioners as: reducing stress, improving circulation, exciting nervous pathways, releasing energy blockages, eliminating toxic buildups, promoting balance/homeostasis, or all of the above. Few if any of these claims have been scientifically proved—although for those who practice reflexology, or find that they have benefited from it, the proof is in the pudding. It works because it works (for them).

Ancient, Modern, or Mix?

There is scant information about the existence of reflexology prior to the early 20th century. Its advocates, however, do point to an ancient wall painting in Egypt depicting a pair of figures touching the hands and feet of two other figures. (This is at the tomb of Ankhmahor, at Saqqara, which is also known as the physicians' tomb.) There is also speculation as to reflexology's relationship to early East Asian medicine, particularly acupressure and shiatsu. Both of these Asian therapies make use of pressure points that, according to the theory, allow for the movement of subtle energies elsewhere in the body when massaged or touched. Although parallels between these and reflexology are evident, any direct connection remains sketchy. Likewise, Ayurvedic medicine, as practiced in India, is sometimes alluded to as an ancient source for reflexology, but again the linkage seems tentative. Native American traditional medicine is also noted as a parallel practice, because medicine men in some tribes are believed to have manipulated or stimulated the feet as a part of their healing practice. Another remote parallel is the ancient Scythians of the Eurasian steppes, who saw connections between distant parts of the body: to treat varicose veins or lameness, for example, Scythian healers drew blood from the vein behind each ear (Kuriyama 1999, 205).

According to Harry Bressler in *Zone Therapy* (2013), one of the earliest Western works on a reflexology-like practice was published in 1582 by two European physicians, Dr. Adamus and Dr. A'tatis. A second book by a Dr. Bell was published shortly after this in Leipzig. The approach described in these books, however, differs from today's reflexology, albeit based on body areas and touching or manipulation.

It was the American doctor William H. Fitzgerald (1872–1942) who advanced the practice of reflexology in the modern era. Fitzgerald studied at the University of Vermont and graduated in 1895. For two years he practiced medicine in Boston before transferring to the Central London Ear, Nose, and Throat Hospital in England. He also practiced at a clinic in Vienna. Perhaps influenced by the ideas he encountered in Europe, Fitzgerald sought to develop a method of anesthesia for minor surgery by means of pressure points or targeted massage. In 1913 he brought his findings to the attention of the medical profession while heading the Nose and Throat Department of St. Francis Hospital in Hartford, Connecticut. Fitzgerald had discovered that pressure, when applied to certain points on the body, could relieve pain and improve the functions of certain organs of the body. In his research, Fitzgerald identified a system of ten vertical zones running from the top of the head to the tips of the toes and hands. Another researcher, the alternative medicine proponent and spiritualist Edwin F. Bowers, looked into Fitzgerald's claims, and, satisfied that they were legitimate, helped the doctor publish a book, *Zone Therapy; or, Relieving Pain at Home* (1917). Zone Therapy was considered a natural method of anesthesia and pain relief (analgesia), and in this respect differed somewhat from contemporary reflexology.

A physical therapist who worked with Fitzgerald, Eunice Ingham (1889–1974), began to promote Zone Therapy nationally, touring cities throughout North American and giving seminars and demonstrations. At the same time, she steered it in a different direction, focusing primarily on zones of the feet as access points to the body. The foot was mapped out into areas corresponding to the various glands, organs, and other systems. Ingham published illustrative charts of these zones along with two books, *Stories the Feet Can Tell* (1938) and *Stories the Feet Have Told*

(1951). Most modern practitioners of foot reflexology acquired their basic under-standing of the field from Ingham's works.

In 1961 the professional organization representing physiotherapists objected to the word *therapy* in the name Zone Therapy. Thus was the name *reflexology* born. However, the name "reflexology" too soon came under fire. In 1969, a book by Mildred Carter, *Helping Yourself with Foot Reflexology,* faced a legal challenge on the grounds that it amounted to the practice of medicine without a license. Around the same time, physicians objected to accounts that ascribed the workings of reflexology to the nervous system. It was a debate, that is, between mainstream medicine and complementary and alternative medicine (CAM). In the case of Carter's book, the publisher's attorneys successfully defended publication of the book. On the other hand, explanations about the workings of reflexology came to avoid mention of the nervous system and instead drew on metaphorical terms for how pressure and/or energy points influenced the body. Other names adopted by some for the practices of reflexology are Pressure Point Massage, Compression Massage, and Pointed Pressure Massage. (In Europe and some other parts of the world, the name Zone Therapy is still used, along with Reflex Zone Therapy and similar terms.)

There are various specializations within reflexology as well. Besides foot reflexology, which probably is the most common, there is hand reflexology, body reflexology, and even ear reflexology/acupressure, which resembles acupuncture in that 50 or more highly specific points in the ear are made use of for therapeutic purposes.

Currently, the professional practice of reflexology has been integrated into the core health-care delivery system in at least three countries—China, Denmark, and the United Kingdom. In the United States it is considered part of the CAM community and may or may not be available through CAM centers in local and regional hospitals. Nevertheless, it is widely available privately and is increasingly embraced for its provision of an enhanced sense of health and deep relaxation and pleasure coupled with its inherent simplicity and generally harmless nature (unless one is diabetic or has other issues with foot pressure and the like).

Noted Users and Uses

Diana, Princess of Wales (1961–1997), is purported to have been a regular client at a CAM clinic in England, where she underwent reflexology treatments (Health .com 2011). Likewise, the noted food tourist Anthony Bourdain (1956–2018) is said to have enjoyed reflexology (along with a variety of other exotic techniques). Additionally, the vocalist/guitarist for Metallica, James Hetfield, has stated that he and other members of that metal band have benefited from reflexology (UHR n.d.). One doesn't have to look too far to find other celebrity users.

On the other hand, experts from the (mainstream) medical community trad-itionally have not held reflexology in high esteem, saying that the system of cor-respondences it lays out between bodily organs and zones of the feet and hands is "not biologically plausible," and that no reputable scientific studies support its use as either a diagnostic tool or a therapy (Singh and Ernst 2008, 323). Recently,

ROLFING235

however, at least one study (in Britain) showed that reflexology can help people with pain relief and might therefore be used effectively to complement drug therapy in the treatment of conditions such as backache, osteoarthritis, and pain associated with other conditions like cancer (Telegraph 2013). It seems, then, that Dr. Fitzgerald and his original Zone Therapy may have come closest to the mark when it comes to identifying the best uses of reflexology.

Michael Shally-Jensen

See also: Acupuncture; Alternative Diagnostics; Ayurvedic Medicine; Chinese Traditional Medicine; Craniosacral Therapy; Naturopathic Medicine; Phrenology; Reiki and Therapeutic Touch; Shiatsu

Further Reading

Health.com. 2011. "21 Celebs Who Embraced Natural Medicine." November 15. https://www.health.com/health/gallery/0,,20543672,00.html

Kuriyama, Shigehisa. 1999. *The Expressiveness of the Body and the Divergence of Greek and Chinese Medicine.* New York: Zone Books.

Pacific Institute of Reflexology. 2017. "Reflexology History." https://www.pacificreflexology.com/reflexology-history

Singh, Simon, and Edzard Ernst. 2008. *Trick or Treatment: The Undeniable Facts about Alternative Medicine.* Uxbridge Road, Ealing, UK: Bantam Press.

The Telegraph. 2013. "Reflexology 'as effective as pain killers.'" April 9. https://www.telegraph.co.uk/news/science/9981099/Reflexology-as-effective-as-pain-killers.html

UHR—Underground Health Reporter. n.d. "Why Do Celebrities Love This Affordable Technique?" http://undergroundhealthreporter.com/reflexology-healing-technique/

ROLFING

Rolfing, formally known as Rolfing Structural Integration, is a therapy by which a practitioner attempts to improve a person's health and well-being through the manipulation of connective tissue (fascia). It is sometimes compared to a deep body massage, because both include the exertion of pressure on parts of the body in an attempt to relieve discomfort experienced by the client. However, according to the Rolf Institute of Structural Integration, when a Rolfing practitioner manipulates the fascia in the proper manner, the results go beyond those of a massage to include an "integration" of the various components of the body, allowing it to regain the desired balance. Thus, the goal of Rolfing is to help a person gain greater fascia flexibility, thereby reducing pain and discomfort by allowing muscles, and related anatomical structures, to function in a healthier manner. One's body, if properly "aligned," can perform more effectively/efficiently with less pain or discomfort.

Ida P. Rolf

The technique of Rolfing is based on the work of Ida Pauline Rolf (1896–1979). Born in New York City, she earned her bachelor's degree from Barnard College

(1916) and a PhD in biochemistry from Columbia University (1920). While working at the Rockefeller Institute of Medicine, Rolf's wide-ranging interests included studying/practicing yoga and homeopathic medicine. In part because her oldest son had medical issues, she applied herself more fully to pursuits that later became the foundation for Rolfing. In the 1950s, Rolf created the foundational Ten-Series for Rolfing. (This is the basis for the first ten sessions a client generally experiences with a practitioner.) In the early 1960s, she focused more on the effects that gravity had on the human body, publishing the foundational article "Rolfing Structural Integration." After founding the Rolf Institute of Structural Integration in 1971, she published her only book in 1977. During the last 40 years of her life, Rolf focused her work on what became known as Rolfing, both as a practitioner and in the development of the theories that underlie the approach. One quote from Ida P. Rolf, which the Rolf Institute uses to summarize her outlook is, "This is the gospel of Rolfing: when the body gets working appropriately the force of gravity can flow through. Then, spontaneously, the body heals itself." After Ida Rolf's death, the popularity of Rolfing slowly declined, until there was a revival during the second decade of the present century.

In her work, Rolf came to see the human body as a unity. Although not specifically opposed to traditional medicine or to doctors who specialized in specific areas, Rolf believed that it was important to understand that the entire body is a system, and it needs to be treated as such. Fascia is the type of tissue that, within the body, acts to unify or connect—in a sense, to hold it together. Thus, if one has problems with the fascia, this is thought to create additional problems in those parts of the body that connect with the fascia. Conversely, by manipulating the fascia to increase its flexibility and to rid it of problems that have accumulated over time, or perhaps from a specific injury, the related parts of the body can, arguably, function better, restoring the individual to a healthier state. Generally, Rolfing seeks to improve posture, relax muscle tension, and decrease pain in order to allow the body to move naturally. As stated in the Standards of Practice adopted by the Rolf Institute, "The purpose of Rolfing is to improve the organization of the person as a whole, rather than to alleviate symptoms."

Structural Integration

Although advocates of Rolfing believe that it can be used with people of all ages, including infants, the norm is for the clients to be adults who are experiencing some discomfort. Thus the introductory Ten Series visits have been structured to unify/integrate the body, from a Rolfing perspective. The first three sessions focus on loosening the connective tissue throughout the body. The fourth through seventh sessions seek to help the client develop the proper support for the body. The next two sessions attempt to focus on areas in which the individual's health issues have been overcome, while the last seeks to create "order and balance" so that the client can then live a healthy life. While Rolfing is directed only toward assisting clients to overcome physical problems, the Rolfing Institute of Structural Integration states that clients generally feel less stress and often feel other emotional and psychological benefits from the treatment. However, these types of experiences are not the reason Rolfing was created. In addition to the basic Ten Series, Rolf, toward the end of her life, created with others a therapy called Rolf Movement Integration. In this practice, the client is assisted to develop balanced movement in order to incorporate it into a healthier lifestyle.

Few medical practitioners outside the Rolfing community believe that the techniques used achieve the desired goals, with critics questioning the underlying theory. No scientifically valid study has demonstrated that Rolfing can achieve its stated results. (A rigorous scientific study must have a large number of participants and be conducted in a controlled, unbiased setting.) However, for many medical professionals, if not used to completely replace conventional medical procedures, Rolfing is deemed to have no serious harmful effects, except that it should not be used by individuals with a serious disease condition or a fresh injury. (Manipulation of tissue near a cancerous tumor can cause the cancer to spread more rapidly.) It is recognized that for many people, just as a massage helps them feel better, manipulation by a Rolfer can do the same.

The Rolfing Institute of Structural Integration, founded in Colorado by Ida Rolf in 1972, became the foundation for the expansion and continued development of Rolfing. It has created courses of study, at various levels of certification, for individuals who desire to become Rolfers. In addition, it has adopted a formal Code of Ethics and a Standards of Practice for Rolfing practitioners certified by the institute. It is the legal entity that holds the trademarks associated with Rolfing and associated groups. There are other individuals who practice a type of structural integration, with their own organizations. Some even refer to Rolf in their literature, and have a foundation in the work of Ida Rolf, but these are independent of the main movement. The Rolfing Institute has about 2,000 practitioners whom it has certified.

Donald A. Watt

See also: Aging Prevention, or "Successful Aging"; Chiropractic; Feldenkrais Method; Gestalt Therapy; Mind–Body Medicine; Osteopathy; Yoga

Further Reading
Jacobson, Eric. 2011. "Structural Integration: Origins and Development." *Journal of Alternative and Complementary Medicine.* September.
Rolf, Ida P. 1989. *Rolfing: Reestablishing the Natural Alignment and Structural Integration of the Human Body for Vitality and Well-Being.* Rev. ed. Rochester, VT: Healing Arts Press.
Rolf, Ida P. with Rosemary Feitis, ed. 1990. *Rolfing and Physical Reality.* Rochester, VT: Healing Arts Press.
Rolf Institute of Structural Integration. Rolf.org
Weil, Andrew. 2018. "Rolfing." In *Weil: Andrew Weil, M.D.* Phoenix: Healthy Lifestyle Brands LLC. www.drweil.com/health-wellness/balanced-living/wellness-therapies/rolfing/

VEGETARIANISM

While the ancient Greek mathematician Pythagoras is often called the first vegetarian, vegetarianism existed long before his time. Historians have found evidence that some ancient Egyptians followed a vegetarian diet, and there is some evidence that our Neanderthal ancestors mostly ate plant-based materials. Vegetarianism has been part of religious traditions for centuries. Early Christians were somewhat conflicted about the eating of meat, and there was a strain among them advocating for a meatless diet or the eating of fish only (a practice that carried over into modern Catholicism in modified form). Various church founders, such as John Wesley of Methodism, recommended vegetarianism. Other traditions, too, such as those tied to ancient India—Buddhism, Hinduism, and Jainism—have similarly promoted vegetarianism to one extent or another. When Americans first became fascinated by Eastern religions in the late 1800s, vegetarianism was part of that fascination. Vegetarianism saw a resurgence in the mid-1900s, as books were published that encouraged abstaining from meat for various moral and health reasons.

Varieties of Vegetarianism

There are many different kinds of vegetarians, and vegetarianism is practiced with differing levels of strictness.

- Ovo-lacto vegetarians eat dairy products and eggs, but not other meat products. An ovo vegetarian would eat eggs but not dairy, and a lacto vegetarian would do the opposite.
- Pescetarians avoid the flesh of mammals (cows, pigs, and so forth), but generally eat fish and other seafood.
- Vegans eschew all types of animal-based foods, and often avoid animal by-products as well. For example, many candies contain gelatin which may be derived from animal products, and vegans will avoid these foods.

People may call themselves vegetarians, but not follow a particular vegetarian diet very strictly. For example, they might only eat meat on rare occasions, or keep a vegetarian diet at home, but eat more freely when out socially or when having a meal at a friend's home.

Some people are unable to stay healthy on even the most carefully balanced vegetarian or vegan diets, and eventually return to eating meat for health reasons.

Becoming Vegetarian

Our oldest ancestors probably ate a mostly vegetarian diet because roots, berries, and other plant-based foods cannot, of course, run away from those seeking to harvest them. Hunting animals was both hard work and dangerous; even animals we think of as prey, like deer, can do significant damage if they charge an unprepared human.

Vegetarianism and *Diet for a New America*

While vegetarianism had already been a fad on and off in the United States for many years, 1987's *Diet for a New America* by John Robbins made a different case for being a vegetarian. Instead of focusing on religious or spiritual benefits, the book talked about the brutal treatment of animals in factory farms. Robbins did make a case for Americans eating too much dairy and meat, but his primary argument was that by eating meat of any kind, Americans were engaging in a shocking amount of animal cruelty.

The book received mixed criticism at the time of its publication. Some reviewers compared it to *Silent Spring*, the Rachel Carson book that exposed how DDT was harming bird eggs and endangering species. Others said that while Robbins's discussion of factory farm animal treatment was shocking and accurate, his discussion of the health reasons for vegetarianism were exaggerated.

Robbins's book certainly did encourage a new kind of vegetarianism in the United States and may have been a major factor in encouraging Americans to seek out "free range" meats. This can easily be connected to the trend toward "organic" produce and meats as well.

While plant-based diets are generally easy to find and consume (in fertile areas), they are not energy efficient. It takes a lot of work to gather enough berries to fuel a body for an entire day. When we were able to create tools and strategies that made regular hunting possible, meat became a more calorie-efficient food than plants. Eventually, humans set about making both plants and meat easier to gather; they developed an agricultural approach to growing food and domesticated animals to make hunting unnecessary.

Once eating meat was an option, many people began to choose to avoid it. This choice was often framed as moral or philosophical. Generally, it was based around the idea that animals had souls, and therefore killing them and eating them was wrong.

But there may be a more simplistic reason that some cultures embraced vegetarian or modified vegetarian diets. Places, such as India and Japan, that have very long growing seasons, plenty of fertile growing land, and a history of cultivating calorie-dense grains are more likely to consider vegetarianism a sensible dietary option.

In places like Europe, however, the growing season is often shorter, and growing the kind of plants that provide enough protein to maintain health is more difficult. Desert areas, like the U.S. West or much of the Middle East, make growing plants very difficult.

Those areas, however, do have vegetation that can be eaten by certain animals. Ruminants like cows, goats, and sheep thrive on virtually any kind of plant. In those situations, eating animals allows humans to convert calories that are useless to themselves—fibrous plants, for example—into usable calories through meat.

Health Benefits

Proponents of vegetarian diets claim any number of benefits to vegetarianism. They suggest that avoiding meat can prevent cancer, eliminate heart disease, prevent or reverse diabetes, and cure asthma—and plenty more. Some of these claims can be inferred from other scientific facts, but others seem less likely.

For example, saturated fat is generally considered to be unhealthy; it raises your bad cholesterol, has a large number of calories in proportion to the nutrients it provides, and can cause unhealthy rises in blood sugar. One of the most common sources of saturated fats is red meat and processed meats. Avoiding these would probably cause a decrease in bad cholesterol and more stable blood sugar.

Eating a healthy vegetarian diet (i.e., not one of pizza, candy, and bagels) also encourages more servings of fruits and vegetables. In general, whole fruits and vegetables are still one of the best foods most people can eat. The fiber and phytonutrients in them are necessary for our ongoing health.

Eliminating meats may even reduce the risk of developing certain types of cancer. Avoiding meat entirely, though, can leave someone very short on certain crucial nutrients. The biggest concerns are protein, calcium (for those who also avoid dairy), and vitamins B12 and D. It is possible to get all the necessary nutrients from a solely plant-based diet, but it is hard. Doctors generally recommend taking vitamin supplements to make sure that one is getting enough of crucial nutrients—but there are debates about how effective nutritional supplements really are for your body.

Modern Vegetarians

Roughly 5 percent of Americans consider themselves to be vegetarians, according to surveys, and for many different reasons.

- Animals have feelings, and killing and eating them is cruel.
- Factory farms are inhumane, and supporting the meat farming industry is immoral.
- Meat-based diets have a negative impact on the land, and avoiding meat is the only environmentally sound choice.
- Vegetarianism is a healthier choice that helps people lose weight and maintain weight loss.

That question of land use comes back into play when we begin to discuss the actual cost of a vegetarian diet, however. Many of the high-quality foods that make a vegetarian diet possible—quinoa, for example, or avocados—have rapidly increased in prices as demand has risen. The price doesn't just increase in the United States, however; often the countries that produce these foods see substantial increases in their prices as well. This has meant, for example, that quinoa is too expensive for the very people for whom it used to be an inexpensive staple grain.

So, is a vegetarian diet healthier than a meat-based one? Perhaps. But staying healthy while eating vegetarian takes a fair amount of nutritional research. If your reasons for becoming a vegetarian are ethically based, be prepared to do a lot of research on where your food comes from and what it takes to get it to you. You may find, in the end, that buying a whole chicken from the farm down the street and using it efficiently is more ethical and cost effective than picking up a sack of avocados.

Kay Tilden Frost

See also: Aging Prevention, or "Successful Aging"; Detox Diets; Diet and Exercise; Diet Pills and Metabolism Boosters; Juice and Juicing; Macrobiotics; Vitamins and Minerals

Further Reading

Blitz, Matt. 2017. "The History of Vegetarianism: From Plant-Eating Neanderthals to 'Diet for a Small Planet.'" *Food and Wine*, June 22. https://www.foodandwine.com/fwx/food/history-vegetarianism

Lappe, Frances Moore. 1991. *Diet for a Small Planet:* 20th anniv. ed. New York: Ballantine Books.

Peters, C. J., et al. 2016. "Carrying Capacity of U.S. Agricultural Land: Ten Diet Scenarios." *Elementa: Science of the Anthropocene* 4:000116. DOI: http://doi.org/10.12952/journal.elementa.000116

Stuart, Tristram. 2008. *The Bloodless Revolution: A Cultural History of Vegetarianism.* New York: W. W. Norton.

VOODOO AND SANTERÍA

Voodoo

Also spelled *voudou* and *vodou*, this term refers to the folk religion of Haiti, as practiced there and in Haitian and other Caribbean diaspora communities. Voodoo represents a mix of African, Roman Catholic, and local elements. It developed in Haiti among enslaved peoples formerly of the West African Fon, Yoruba, Ibo, and other ethnic groups during the period of French colonization. The word *vodun* in the Fon language means "spirit." Many of the theological and magical components of voodoo exist as well in other religious systems that share a history of Transatlantic colonialism and slavery, such as Santería in Cuba, Condomblé in Brazil, and Shango (Xangó) in other parts of Latin America.

In the United States the word *voodoo* is sometimes used to mean any type of magic, such as "voodoo economics" (a phrase that George H. W. Bush used to refer to the economic policies of President Ronald Reagan). A real-life voodoo spiritual folkway, similar to the one found in Haiti, developed in Louisiana in the 19th century and was revived in the 20th. Its practices differ from Haitian voodoo in areas such as initiation into the cult and the greater force given to magic. It was through Louisiana voodoo that such popular paraphernalia as the voodoo doll and the protective amulet (*gris-gris*) came to be widely known, along with the popular image of the zombie, or "walking dead." Voodoo's healing rituals are less well known but exist nonetheless.

Voodoo and Its Presentation in Hollywood

Like many folk religions, the presentation of voodoo in Hollywood has very little to do with how the religion is actually practiced. The tropes focus on the magical aspects of voodoo—Tarot cards and mystical readings, voodoo dolls (what's done to the doll will be done to the person), and making zombies.

Voodoo practitioners in media are almost always women; the only man or god ever mentioned is Baron Samedi. Even if the deity isn't mentioned by name, the male character almost always dresses in the fashion of Baron Samedi—a tattered tuxedo, skull makeup, and a top hat. This even carries over into media for children, such as the character of Doctor Facilier (the Shadow Man) in Disney's *Princess and the Frog*.

From *American Horror Story* to the James Bond film *Live and Let Die*, magical practitioners who are also people of color are almost exclusively shown to be voodoo practitioners. This creates intense negative stereotypes, especially for people of color from islands like Haiti and Jamaica, who are then assumed to be capable of cursing everyone they contact.

In voodoo, believers profess faith in a supreme deity (*Bon Dieu*), but it is really the lesser spirits known as *loa* that drive most of its magico-religious activities. The *loa* are variously regarded as African gods and Catholic saints. They attach themselves to individuals and to families and demand ceremonial recognition and, sometimes, specific acts on their behalf. Among the more prominent *loa* are Papa Legba (guardian of the crossroads), Erzulie Freda (spirit of love), Simbi (spirit of rain and magic), Kouzin Zaka (spirit of agriculture), and the Marasa, divine twins that embody opposites such as matter and spirit.

Voodoo ritual service consists of a gathering of devotees at a meeting place, where a priest (*houngan*) or priestess (*mambo*) leads them in activities that include singing, drumming, dancing, praying, food preparation, and animal sacrifice. Believers have obligations regarding their loa and their ancestors in the context of both the service and outside of it; sometimes the priest or priestess provides expert help in carrying out the required rites. In general, the *houngan* or *mambo* function as counselors, healers, and protectors against sorcery or witchcraft. Each group of worshipers is independent—there is no central organization, hierarchy, or official dogma. Nevertheless, groups often communicate with each other and share insights and local traditions.

The presence of the loa is solicited in the course of the ceremony, and they arrive through the idiom of spirit possession—which is to say, they enter the person of the participant and take him or her over, as it were. In a trance state, the participant assumes the gestures, facial expressions, and general behaviors of the loa. He or she might don the characteristic garb of the loa, perform stylized dances, eat and drink the loa's preferred foods, and, inspired by the loa, even give advice to others, provide medical cures, and perform magical feats. The participant may remain possessed by the loa for a short time only or perhaps for a few hours, depending on the situation. The experience of possession is said to be unremembered at its conclusion, because it was the loa, not the individual, who was present. At the same time, possession is conceived of as concrete evidence for the reality of the gods and their effectiveness in addressing human needs. Most Haitians hold that there are two categories of loas, one consisting of "cool" souls associated with Africa and called Rada loas, and the other consisting of "hot" spirits of the New World known as Petro loas. Both can be used for beneficial purposes or for the making of "black magic."

One of the more sensational aspects of voodoo is the concept of the zombie. The basic image is that of a human corpse that has been raised from the grave by magical means and can be guided to do evil or perhaps perform work. Equally prominent in voodoo, however, is the notion of a zombie as a disembodied soul that is used for magical purposes, either good or bad. In some cases in the past (and to a lesser extent today), a zombielike state could be created by a priest through the administering of poisonous substances that paralyzed the subject. Either way, the zombie is thought to have no will of its own. It has become, rather, a kind of "living dead" surrounded by mystery and creating fear and agitation wherever it roams. The zombie concept has given rise to innumerable fictional treatments in popular books and films.

The so-called voodoo doll, which is used to impart malign wishes to a person through the use of pins stuck into the doll's body, is in fact not part of traditional Haitian material culture; it is, rather, more closely associated with Africa, where wooden effigy figures and small metal spikes were used, and even with premodern Europe, where rag dolls and needles were employed. The link with Haitian voodoo seems to have come primarily from Western writers and filmmakers seeking to sensationalize their tales of pirates and zombies (Armitage 2015).

In Haitian folk medicine, the opposite of voodoo-doll pin-sticking could be said to occur when the healer, in a "possessed" state, acts to *remove* a small object from the body of the patient, thus "unblocking" the surrounding tissue and/or internal passages and allowing health to be restored. As with most such shamanic healing rites, the object—a shell fragment, for example—is typically placed in the mouth of the healer beforehand and then strategically sucked out of the victim; yet that does not necessarily lessen the overall effect of the rite. The healer may also place items such as bones, sticks, and herbs into a cauldron in order to conjure loa spirits and deploy them for magical purposes. In some cases, a chicken or goat is sacrificed in order to feed the loa and gain from their beneficial presence.

Santería

Santería is a syncretic religion that originated in Cuba during the colonial era; it is constructed of West African, Roman Catholic, and indigenous elements. It eventually spread to other Caribbean islands and is also practiced in (primarily black and mixed-race) Cuban communities in the United States. As with voodoo, it includes belief in a supreme being but primarily centers on the worship of saints or spirits known as *orichás*—indeed, *santería* is the Spanish word for "worship of saints." Each orichá represents a particular natural or worldly force as well as an individual set of human characteristics. The primary orichás are Eleguá (god of paths/ roads; associated with St. Michael), Obatalá (sky; father of orichás), Yemayá (water; mother of orichás), Changó (thunder; associated with St. Barbara or St. Jerome), and Ochún (rivers; pleasure and sexuality).

Santería ceremonies are conducted in an *ilé*, or shrine to one or more orichás, built by a priest (*Santero*) or priestess (*Santera*), who also conducts the ceremony. The ceremony is complex but involves, among other things, ritual devotions, drumming and dancing, food offerings (including a sacrificed animal), invocations using fetishes, and participants going into and out of trance states. The object is to encourage an orichá to intervene on one's behalf, aid in the resolution of problems, and cultivate a sense of spiritual wholeness.

In Santería healing practices, the person who becomes ill is thought to suffer not merely from a physical ailment but from an attack of bad spirits brought on by a disjunction between the victim and the spiritual world. Taking a holistic approach to the person's condition, and seeking to reintegrate body, mind, and spirit, the traditional healer uses botanical substances and ritual means to achieve the desired end. A key concept in this regard is *aché*, a primal life force that flows throughout the material (and spiritual) world and that must be channeled productively to keep the person on a path to health and vitality. Various orichás are summoned to assist, and, in order to harmonize the patient with the forces of nature, a number of substances, such as animal blood (from sacrifices), water (from rivers or rain), honey, tobacco, alcoholic "firewater" (*aquardiente*), or Datura (a poisonous plant) may be employed. A *pataki*, or spiritual parable, is often recited by the Santero/a and passed on to the patient for later recitation in order to stay attacks from evil spirits.

Michael Shally-Jensen

See also: Alternative Diagnostics; Cupping; Dance Therapy; Drama Therapy; Faith Healing and Prayer; Folk Medicine; Herbal Remedies; Mind–Body Medicine; Native American Traditional Medicine; Shamanism and Neo-Shamanism

Further Reading

Armitage, Natalie. 2015. "European and African Figural Ritual Magic: The Beginnings of the Voodoo Doll Myth." In *The Materiality of Magic: An Artifactual Investigation into Ritual Practices and Popular Beliefs*, edited by Ceri Houlbrook and Natalie Armitage. Philadelphia: Oxbow Books.

Brown, Karen McCarthy. 2011. *Mama Lola: A Vodou Priestess in Brooklyn.* 3rd ed. Berkeley: University of California Press.

Fernández Olmos, Margarite, and Lizabeth Paravisini-Gerbert, eds. 2001. *Healing Cultures: Art and Religion as Curative Practices in the Caribbean and Its Diaspora.* New York: Palgrave Macmillan.

Fernández Olmos, Margarite, and Lizabeth Paravisini-Gerbert. 2011. *Creole Religions of the Caribbean: An Introduction—from Vodou and Santería to Obeah and Espiritismo.* 2nd ed. New York: New York University Press.

YOGA

When Americans think of yoga, they generally think of a small studio, fragrant incense, and lots of slim women holding strange positions on padded mats. Yoga is actually a much more involved practice, both spiritually and physically. In some ways, the public practice of yoga in the West is actually opposed to the spiritual roots of the practice.

History and Development

No one actually knows how old the practice of yoga is. The original sacred texts relating to yoga, like many ancient religious texts, were passed down in an oral tradition. What was written down was written on fragile palm leaves, which were lost long ago.

What we do know is that yoga originated more 5,000 years ago on the Indian subcontinent. The word *yoga* has the Sanskrit root of *yuj*, which means "to yoke" or "to unite." The original goal of yoga was to unite the individual consciousness with the universal consciousness. It is not quite accurate to say that yoga seeks to unite the individual with god (or *a* god). An experienced yogi is someone has sought and achieved a state of oneness with the whole of existence. This state is often called nirvana in the Hindu and Buddhist traditions. But yoga is present in virtually all of the folk traditions of India, which later developed into the different religions practiced in the region. The Bhagavad Gita was composed around 500 BCE, and is generally considered one of the most important of yogic scriptures.

The document that had the greatest impact on modern yoga traditions, however, was the Yoga Sutras, written sometime before 400 CE by Maharshi Patanjali. This document laid out what is now called Classical Yoga, or the eight-limbed path.

The concept of eight limbs of yoga is a literal translation of the Sanskrit term Ashtanga Yoga. This isn't the same as the type of yoga that you would hear about in an Ashtanga class; that's a type of hatha, or physical, yoga.

The eight limbs of yoga is meant to be a complete spiritual practice to bring a person into union with the universe. The eight limbs are as follows.

- Yamas: This refers to the vows and self-discipline we use to interact in the world. There are five yamas: ahimsa (practicing nonviolence), satya (practicing truthfulness), Asteya (not stealing), bramacharaya (proper use of energy), and aparigraha (avoiding greed).

- Niyama: This refers to the way we interact with ourselves, or treat our own bodies and minds. There are also five niyamas: saucha (cleanliness), santosha (contentment), tapas (discipline or "burning of desire"), svadhyaya (self-reflection and study of spiritual texts), and isvarapranidaha (surrendering to a higher power).

- Asana: this is the part of yoga most Westerners are familiar with. Putanjali, interestingly, only uses words that mean "seat" here; he appears to be referring

Yoga: From an Indian Spiritual Practice to an American Exercise Routine

In 2016, Americans spent about $16 billion on yoga equipment, clothing, and classes. When yoga was first introduced to the United States in the mid-19th century, it was closely tied to its philosophical and spiritual roots. In the 1980s, however, hatha yoga—the physical practice of yoga—began to boom as a type of exercise, completely divorced from the practice's spiritual roots.

Now, yoga is practiced by millions of Americans, and the U.S. yoga industry tends to hold up one very specific body as the ideal: young, slim, female presenting, flexible—and white. This is complicated enough on its own, but when one recalls that during the British colonization of India, yoga itself was outlawed, the focus on white practitioners seems even more dubious.

U.S. yoga practitioners eventually tried to reintroduce spirituality to Americanized yoga, but in doing so have created a hodgepodge that most Indian Americans find hugely uncomfortable. Studios are decorated with statues of gods and goddesses that the teachers can't identify; they pronounce Sanskrit terms badly and have a limited and Americanized understanding of chakras and other yogic energy points.

One example of this disconnect is the phrase "namaste." Americans almost always use this phrase to close classes, and are told that it is a highly spiritual greeting, translating to "I bow to the divine in you." While this translation is accurate, it is simply a greeting in the Hindi areas of India, used when people arrive and leave. It's a little formal, and by liberal and urban Indians, often considered old-fashioned.

to the idea that the posture should be steady and comfortable. Hatha yoga, a later expansion of asana, uses postures and movements to help create that steady, comfortable posture.

- Pranayama: This term has to do with breathing techniques. We know that controlling breathing can affect anxiety and panic; we often tell someone who is frightened or anxious to "take a deep breath." Pranayama goes deeper than that, using different methods of breathing to help practitioners reach heightened states of consciousness.

- Pratyahara: This translates to "sense withdrawal." This could initially sound like practitioners are trying to turn off their senses; instead, the goal is to focus on internal states of being so that the outside world falls away and doesn't distract from meditation.

- Dharana: This limb of yoga refers to focused concentration. To withdraw the senses from the outside world and control the breath, the practitioners often focuses on something specific. This could be a mantra (a repeated phrase that is meant to bring quietness to the mind, somewhat similar to a Hail Mary performed on a rosary) or the physical qualities of the breath, for example.

- Dhyana: This refers to the concept of being absorbed in meditation. This is the moment when the world falls away, when the thought of "I'm meditating" is no longer present, and a practitioner simply is meditating. It's an odd concept, and makes more sense when experienced than when explained!

- Samadhi: enlightenment or bliss. This word, when broken down, means to "see equally," or simply experience the world without judgment or attachment. Putanjali is very clear in his sutras that this is not a permanent state of being for most practitioners; most people will experience moments of samadhi in their lives. The eight limbs of yoga have the goal of increasing a person's ability to exist in that place of nonjudgment.

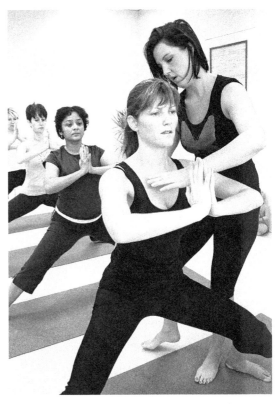

A yoga instructor adjusts a student during class. (Hongqi Zhang/Dreamstime.com)

Health Benefits of Yoga

To talk about the health benefits of yoga, one can do well by looking first at hatha yoga, or the practice of various postures and positions. In the Western world, these movements have less to do with bringing one's body into a state of spiritual readiness for samadhi (enlightenment), and more to do with increasing flexibility and improving balance and coordination. When used in this way, yoga can be very beneficial.

There are many different types of yoga that one can practice, either through group classes in a studio, through private lessons, or through videos at home. Different types of yoga bring different benefits: ashtanga yoga, for example, is focused on building strength through strong, active movements. Bikram yoga is performed in a very hot studio and aims to make your body sweat heavily while you practice the movements. Iyengar yoga combines movements with a close focus on the breath. All types of yoga will increase flexibility, but others will increase strength, improve breath control, decrease anxiety, and more.

For those suffering from significant anxiety and depression, it is possible that exploring the complete eight limbs of yoga may offer some relief from these struggles. The activity and mindfulness that are key components of yoga seem to play a useful role in this regard. As always, however, it is good to consult a doctor before starting a new exercise program or discontinuing any medications.

If you've decided that you want to start a yoga practice, the next question is usually whether you want to go to a studio or learn by practicing with a video. In some areas, there may not be any studios at all, and YouTube videos may be the only option. In other locales, there are dozens of yoga studios to choose from. Here are some thoughts to consider:

- Are you concerned about the concept of appropriation? Many Indian Americans have discussed how they feel unwelcome in yoga studios, where the trappings of their religions are used without context or consideration to give the studio the right "feel." To avoid participating in this, you might consider practicing at home, instead of in an expensive studio.

- How much money do you have to spend on a yoga practice? Technically you don't need any equipment for yoga, though comfortable clothes and a nonslip surface like a yoga mat are helpful. When you attend yoga at a studio, however, there's often a social pressure to invest in fashionable yoga attire, and classes themselves can be expensive.

- How comfortable are you with exercising around other people? Not everyone is ready to start their practice in a group. If you are new to yoga and want some time to get familiar with the terminology and the flow of movements, starting off with a few videos at home may also be more helpful.

Yoga can be a great way to improve flexibility, build strength, and increase endurance. It is important to practice yoga in a way that is mindful of its roots and respectful to those who are descended from the actual founders of the spiritual practice.

Kay Tilden Frost

See also: Breathwork; Chiropractic; Dance Therapy; Diet and Exercise; Feldenkrais Method; Meditation and Mindfulness; Mind–Body Medicine; Rolfing

Further Reading

Basavaraddi, Dr. Ishwar V. 2015. "Yoga: Its Origins, History, and Development." *Ministry of External Affairs, Government of India*, April 23, 2015.

Brown, Christina. 2003. "The Yoga Bible." *Walking Stick Press*, May 29.

McCall, Timothy M.D. 2007. "38 Health Benefits of Yoga." *Yoga Journal*. August 28. https://www.yogajournal.com/lifestyle/count-yoga-38-ways-yoga-keeps-fit

Telang, Kashinath Trimbak, trans. 2017. "Bhagavad Gita." *Digireads*, February 1.

1980s–2000

INTRODUCTION

In the 1980s the so-called New Age healing movement arrived in force, as people in growing numbers sought measures to enhance their health and wellness. For the most part, these methods—which included naturopathy, homeopathy, Ayurvedic medicine, energy healing, and others—were drawn on to boost personal health or to complement conventional medical treatments when needed; they did not necessarily replace the latter except among a population of New Age diehards who saw Western medicine as bankrupt and Eastern healing and other sources as the wave of the future. Mass-market magazines like *Self*, *Health*, *Shape*, and, later, *Fitness* marked the coming of a new consciousness about looking healthy and fit in public, and feeling like it too. These were supplemented by a few smaller-circulation magazines focusing specifically on alternative healing.

Social movements generally arise during times of unrest and change, as people become discouraged with the status quo and seek out new ideas and methods to explore. We have already seen how increased dissatisfaction with mainstream medicine in the 1960s and 1970s gave rise to the first wave of the alternative health movement. This pattern continued into the next two decades, as well, as people recognized that orthodox medicine offered no grand cure for diseases such as chronic fatigue syndrome, rheumatoid arthritis, cancer, and, the latest entry in the pantheon, AIDS, or acquired immune deficiency syndrome. Moreover, health costs continued to soar, while traditional insurance coverage shrank dramatically, leaving more of a burden for the consumer to carry. These conditions led to an ever-expanding interest in do-it-yourself health—especially in the area of prevention. New Age/alternative healers tapped into this trend toward self-improvement, common sense, and simplicity as a way of life. They advocated for equal consideration in the medical marketplace and empowered consumers to become arbiters of their own fate.

"Prevention" became a kind of watchword, used in equal measure with "holistic." Although a *Prevention* magazine had been started by the organic gardening promoter J. I. Rodale in 1950, in the 1980s sales of this publication took off, and its competition grew. Everyone was looking for "nature's cures" along with advice on weight management, health tips, popular exercises, antiaging measures, and new therapies that they might try for themselves or recommend to a friend or family member. Ideas that once were considered "on the fringe," such as magnet therapy, detox diets, or shamanic healing, were now on the table, subscribed to or at least acknowledged as possibilities by millions. A growing recognition of the important role the mind plays in healing and in fighting disease fueled the popular interest. It was now the whole person—body, mind, and spirit—that needed to be considered in making any health decisions.

This was also a time of change in the medical establishment, partly as a result of the New Age push. There were a growing number of acknowledgments by mainstream practitioners that some alternative therapies either seemed to help or "might be effective"; at a minimum, they didn't appear to pose any serious risk to those who might want to try them. (However, some qualifications were eventually added for certain populations or certain therapies.) Even as criticism of alternative techniques continued to come from leading medical organizations and journals, where they were characterized as unscientific and physically implausible, by the 1990s the tide had begun to change, and less was the overt hostility between mainstream practitioners and those from the alternative health community. Indeed, at this time, some of the first major "complementary and alternative medicine" (CAM) centers opened under the aegis of large university or public-private partnership hospitals. The rationale behind these launches had as much to do with cashing in on widespread public interest as it did with uncovering unexplored regions of pure medical science.

In 1991, the appropriations committee of the U.S. Senate decided to set aside funds for the creation, under the National Institutes of Health (NIH), of a research program in alternative medicine. The Senate committee was headed by Iowa's Tom Harkin, who had seen two family members die from cancer and was open to unorthodox remedies, and Utah's Orrin Hatch, who was an advocate of dietary supplements and had strong ties to the industry. The ensuing Office of Alternative Medicine, later known as the National Center for Complementary and Alternative Medicine, was lauded by some as a great achievement by nonconventional medicine, while others proclaimed it a waste of taxpayer dollars on bogus science. Meanwhile, in Europe CAM had always been more generally accepted, and growing number of doctors there began a process of *integrating* standard care with CAM approaches. Thus, in the United States, too, some new or existing CAM centers started to become known as centers for "integrative medicine." This did not satisfy critics like Marcia Angell, editor in chief of the prestigious *New England Journal of Medicine,* who wrote, "There cannot be two kinds of medicine—conventional and alternative. There is only medicine that has been adequately tested and medicine that has not, medicine that works and medicine that may or may not work" (Angell and Kassirer 1998.) Such cautions went largely unheeded by the general public, however, except to make them a little more certain, perhaps, to "read the fine print" when it came to utilizing CAM therapies that carried potential negative consequences or side effects (if these happened to be disclosed or appeared in a magazine article or on the new Internet).

Two of the largest growth areas in CAM during this period were energy therapies and naturopathy. The former drew on traditional methods such as Chinese Qigong and modern variants such as Japanese Reiki. For example, the Reiki-like practice of therapeutic touch, developed by a New York nursing professor in the 1970s, flourished (especially among nurses). The idea behind most energy therapies is that there is a human energy field that has polarities and that flows inside the body and can be accessed at key points and "channeled" to correct imbalances, relieve "blockages," and improve the person's overall energy profile and health. Acupuncture is perhaps the premier technique associated with such goals, although it is variously explained by its practitioners as entailing "energetics" or not. There is no definitive consensus on how it works, yet if any CAM approach has been shown to work, it is most likely acupuncture. Acupuncture, along with various other energy or "biofield" therapies, enjoyed a tremendous increase in usage during the New Age era and in many ways came to define the period.

The second major area of growth was naturopathy—primarily because, by this time, it had come to be something of an umbrella term encompassing nutrition, herbalism, homeopathy, aromatherapy, physical/manipulative therapies (especially massage), spirituality, and general lifestyle counseling. These all used to be rather distinct, even competing areas, but now they were all part of New Age "naturopathy." Each one enjoyed significant growth in its own right during the 1980s and 1990s, with massive quantities of herbal supplements, essential oils, and homeopathic remedies being marketed to consumers, who eagerly bought them up.

During this period, too, there arrived on the scene the first modern health and wellness "gurus"—physicians who had a foot in each camp and were able to present compelling stories to the public about the virtues of CAM. Andrew Weil, a Harvard-trained psychedelics researcher, published a series of best-selling books on topics such as "spontaneous healing" and "the natural mind," which catapulted him to fame. In his teaching and writing, Weil, who is still a top name in the integrative medicine field, emphasizes diet, herbal remedies, and mind–body techniques. Another major figure is Deepak Chopra, who studied medicine in India before emigrating to the United States. Chopra uses the Indian Ayurvedic system in his teaching and focuses on both the spiritual and physical aspects of healing. Chopra has written some 80 books, nearly two dozen of which have been *New York Times* bestsellers. The millions of Americans who read Weil's and Chopra's books, follow their appearances on television, visit their websites, and generally admire what they have to say, are not ill-informed innocents in matters of health and life; they are regular people who hope to "optimize" their chances of survival in a complex world filled with health hazards, impersonal institutions, and dogmatic thinking. The "integrative" form of lifestyle medicine promoted by Weil and Chopra, among others, supplies a dose of personalized care, as it were, to the individual consumer. One can choose from among dozens and dozens of different remedies and lifestyle recommendations in order to design the perfect plan for *you*. And those who have done so, say these authors, lead healthy and more satisfying lives.

Further Reading

Angell, M., and J. P. Kassirer. 1998. "Alternative Medicine—The Risks of Untested and Unregulated Remedies." *New England Journal of Medicine* 339(12): 839–41.

Baer, Hans A. 2004. *Toward an Integrative Medicine: Merging Alternative Therapies with Biomedicine.* Walnut Creek, CA: AltaMira Press.

Whorton, James C. 2002. *Nature Cures: The History of Alternative Medicine in America.* New York: Oxford University Press.

AGING PREVENTION, OR "SUCCESSFUL AGING"

As a society, our population has greatly extended the duration of human life over the decades. For the World War II generation, for example, 40 or 45 was considered the point at which more of life lay behind than ahead. Even today, teens and those in their early twenties tend to see life beyond 40 as unimaginably "old." But such age comparisons are relative. Nowadays, many Americans in their sixties still consider themselves middle-aged rather than as senior citizens. That's because people are indeed living longer and healthier today. And yet, for members of this same group, one reaches a stage where the inevitability of death is contemplated— along with the loss of independence that typically leads up to it. Some individuals deal with these thoughts better than others. In any case, both medical advances and changing cultural attitudes have pushed us toward thinking that "70 is the new 50," as the saying goes. And many older people are actively taking advantage of what the health and wellness marketplace has to offer in terms of the possible extension of life.

Collagen Creams, Hair Transplants, and the Quest to Stay Young Forever

The focus on using creams, oils, and supplements to appear youthful is nothing new. Cleopatra took baths in donkey milk (it took a stable of 700 donkeys to sustain her habit); Ponce de Leon spent his life searching for the Fountain of Youth; and modern women inject Botox, a neurotoxin, to smooth out wrinkles.

Meanwhile, Egyptian men created oils and creams that incorporated hippopotamus fat, porcupine hair, or the leg of a female greyhound to try to prevent baldness. Julius Caesar invented the comb-over; when that didn't work to hide his shining pate, he popularized laurel crowns to hide his hair loss. Wigs and toupees have been popular for centuries; some modern men opt for hair transplants to stop their hairlines from receding.

In every generation, the obsession with maintaining a youthful appearance has consumed a certain amount of the population. Modern dermatologists say that most of the oils and creams sold to "prevent aging" don't do anything but empty our wallets, but that doesn't stop us from spending more than $140 billion a year around the world to try to hold on to our youth.

Senior Living

As the percentage of persons participating in the retirement system increased in the 20th century, a new complex of retirement communities arose—replacing, for the most part, former "old-age homes" that were linked to specific localities or to labor unions, fraternal organizations, or religious societies. By the 1970s, large migrations of retirees were taking place as older citizens flocked to specially planned "adult" communities in Sun Belt states like Arizona, Nevada, and California; Florida had already cultivated a tradition of welcoming northern-state retirees. Underscoring the growing economic and cultural importance of this new population of senior citizens were a variety of targeted magazines, film and television offerings, membership organizations (such as the American Association of Retired Persons, or AARP), insurance plans, and an ever-expanding tourism industry. Growing right alongside these developments was an increasingly profitable U.S. medical sector, including a burgeoning complementary and alternative medicine (CAM) marketplace. The health and well-being of seniors quickly became a big business. Although it is difficult to find reliable statistics concerning this broad trend, consider the fact that in 2015 the nation's largest prescription drug retailer, CVS Health, purchased Omnicare, a drug delivery company that serves senior-living centers, for the sum of $12.7 billion (Lorenzetti 2015). And that is just one company among *thousands* that specialize in senior health-care services.

Among the common consequences of aging are diminished vision, loss of hearing, loss of taste and smell, declining hormonal levels, impaired immunity, increased blood pressure, atherosclerosis, decreased cardiac output, poor circulation, digestive problems, loss of muscle mass, osteoporosis, back pain, arthritis, diabetes, loss of energy, increased anxiety, cognitive decline, increased likelihood of cancers, and decreased functioning of the kidneys, liver, and lungs. Not a very pretty picture! Is it any wonder that people facing such conditions might seek to stave off their development or growth by pursuing antiaging strategies?

A first line of defense in this regard is "healthy living," which means, essentially, the complete cessation of smoking, alcohol, and any other questionable substances, along with the elimination of foods containing high levels of salt, fat, or sugar—the kinds of additives that go into fast foods and processed foods. The healthy senior should also ensure that he or she gets plenty of exercise: yoga, walking, hiking, cycling, swimming, gym workouts, and so forth. More and more, senior-living centers are designed to serve just such needs. As if that were not enough, many centers, along with most health and wellness resorts, offer such items as Rolfing, Tai Chi, detoxification, meditation, sound therapy, and many others. The basic premise of these programs is that aging is unacceptable, even a kind of disease, and that older adults must take matters into their own hands if they wish to age gracefully or to prevent or postpone the aging process until the very end.

Older persons are also advised to undergo routine medical testing for all the common conditions as well as any conditions that may "run in the family." Annual breast exams for women, annual prostate tests for men, and a host of other tests are now, or were until very recently, strongly recommended by medical authorities. Wealthier individuals can even opt for "concierge care," where, for a substantial fee, they can undergo multiple days of testing and analysis. In cases where the emperor of all maladies, cancer—or precancer—is detected, the patient is usually advised to immediately undergo major treatment, either surgery, chemotherapy, or radiation. Although this has become the norm in the medical field, some critics have countered that false positive test results and overdiagnosis are quite common, leading to unnecessary worries, costs, and treatments. Moreover, some of the standard treatments come with their own considerable risks, including mortality (Ehrenreich 2018, 36–39).

Looking for Solutions

Because of economic status or lifestyle preferences, many aging people find these kinds of healthy living regimens are not always the first choice. An easier route, for many, is to take a pill. Most products sold today to "prevent" or "combat" aging are not pharmaceutical drugs regulated by the federal Food and Drug Administration (FDA) but supplements, subject to much less stringent forms of regulation. One of the more popular antiaging remedies, for example, is any compound or solution containing antioxidants. Antioxidants have been shown to inhibit oxidation and thereby protect the body from any potentially harmful effects of free radicals (i.e., reactive atoms or groups of atoms). Although research done around the turn of the century suggested that antioxidants were always a good thing, more recently researchers have begun to ask whether maintaining some free radicals in the system might be beneficial, as they appear to perform useful functions like chemical signaling, maintenance of a consistent heartbeat, and others (Karolinska Institutet 2011).

Impressive results have also been obtained merely by restricting laboratory mice's caloric intake. Overfed, obese mice die earlier on average than those who eat very limited amounts of food—to the point of near starvation. These results have led some professionals and laypersons who follow this type of research to conclude that humans, too, could live longer by operating on a near starvation diet. While some health gurus have taken to preaching this advice, only a very small percentage of the U.S. population actually adheres to it—mainly because it makes living itself rather unsatisfactory. People, it seems, would rather eat, be merry, and die in the normal way than make do with tiny servings of celery sticks and pine nuts in the hope of living a couple of extra years.

The use of supplemental hormones represents another avenue of research. Such supplements have been touted as a remedy for everything from limping libidos to wrinkled skin. On the one hand, it is true that levels of human growth hormone (HGH) decline as one ages, but introducing synthetic versions of HGH has not been proved indisputably to slow or reverse the aging process—despite the claims of synthetic hormone makers. They may help to improve muscle strength and bone density in adults who are notably deficient in HGH, but their use, which must be prescribed by a physician, often comes with strong side effects, including pain, swelling, and increased cancer risk. A nonprescription steroidal supplement called DHEA (dehydroepiandrosterone) has been proclaimed as something that preserves youth and enhances sexual drive and performance, but there is little in the way of rigorous scientific studies to back up those claims.

Another area of research is embryonic stem cells. Research suggests that the transplantation of healthy cells into damaged organ systems can help repair ailing tissue. This indicates that one day in the near future, the use of stem cells that can differentiate into different types of tissue—cartilage, heart, liver, skin, brain, pancreatic cells—might prove key in treating many disorders and conditions, including osteoarthritis, diabetes, Parkinson's disease, and muscular dystrophy. It may also indicate that, in the more distant future, stem cell applications could be used to address "cosmetic" issues such as the appearance of the skin or the composition of the body—much as cosmetic surgery is employed today.

Michael Shally-Jensen

See also: Antioxidants; Detox Diets; Diet and Exercise; Eating Organic; Health and Wellness Gurus; Meditation and Mindfulness; Paleo Diet; Reiki and Therapeutic Touch; Rolfing; Vitamins and Minerals; Walking and Jogging; Yoga

Further Reading

Ehrenreich, Barbara. 2018. *Natural Causes: An Epidemic of Wellness, the Certainty of Dying, and Killing Ourselves to Live Longer.* New York: Twelve.

Hamblin, James. 2016. *If Our Bodies Could Talk: A Guide to Operating and Maintaining a Human Body.* New York: Doubleday.

Karolinska Institutet. 2011. "Free Radicals May Actually Be Good for You." *ScienceDaily,* March 1. https://www.sciencedaily.com/releases/2011/02/110228090404.htm

Lorenzetti, Laura. 2015. "The Ten Biggest Health Care Companies in the Fortune 500." *Fortune,* June 20. http://fortune.com/2015/06/20/fortune-500-biggest-healthcare-companies/

Mittledorf, Josh, and Dorion Sagan. 2016. *Cracking the Aging Code: The New Science of Growing Old—And What It Means for Staying Young.* New York: Flatiron Books.

ANGER AND ANGER MANAGEMENT

Anger is a normal emotional experience. Although perfectly common, in some cases it can become dysfunctional because its intensity or duration impairs people's ability to function at work or home. There has been a dramatic upsurge in the number of people referred for anger management treatment in the last few decades—in part, because it is increasingly recognized as something that can be managed. Despite the recognition that many people suffering from problems related to anger could benefit from therapy, there are no official guidelines for diagnosis or treatment of anger because it is not recognized as a disorder by the mental health field's main medical authority, the *Diagnostic and Statistical Manual of Mental Disorders* (DSM-5). Insurers generally will not cover treatment for anger because of that lack of official medical recognition. Nevertheless, for those who need anger management counseling, treatment is increasingly available out-side of standard medical/psychiatric circles.

What Is Anger?

Anger is experienced when someone or something blocks the attainment of an important goal. For example, a spouse may prevent one from feeling valued by making demeaning comments, or a computer crash may prevent one from fin-ishing a course paper. Whether a goal is still attainable with additional effort may determine whether people feel angry or sad when they fail.

Anger has a number of effects on the mind and body. It is usually accompanied by physical arousal, causing the heart to beat faster, adrenaline to release, and the body to prepare for action. Anger is also associated with changes in cognition (how people think about the world around them). When angry, people tend to focus on and remember information related to their anger. Consider a woman who hangs up her phone during a heated exchange with her partner. During their argument she likely noticed that he was not listening to what she had to say. She would remember all the other times this happened during earlier exchanges with him. As a result of these thoughts, she would become angry and shut down the conversation.

Anger is also expressed behaviorally, through aggressive facial expressions, actions, and verbalizations. These behavioral manifestations are often what observ-ers use to identify whether someone is angry, and include a glowering look, physi-cal aggression, offensive gestures, yelling, and cursing. Men and women are equally likely to experience intense anger, but men are more likely to aggress directly against people or objects, while women are more likely to aggress indirectly (e.g., gossiping, excluding people from groups).

Anger and Aggression

Overt aggression does not inevitably follow from the experience of anger, but it is one of the possible behaviors that is commonly associated with it. Aggression refers to emotionally laden actions that are elicited by intense frustration and can involve hostile, destructive behavior. Aggressive activity may be directed toward another person, toward the individual's surroundings, or even toward the subject him- or herself. Aggression may also be displaced—that is, directed toward outlets that are in no way related to the frustrations originally provoking them. Thus, senseless acts of vandalism, physical injury to other persons, wanton destruction, self-injury, and crimes readily witnessed by others or easily detectible by police officers are conceived of as aggressive behaviors carried out by frustrated individuals moti-vated by rage.

Often, young children respond to frustrating circumstances by having a "tem-per tantrum." A key part of socializing the young is teaching them how to inhibit expressions of extreme anger or rage. As they become adults, they will be expected to master their childish emotions by developing psychological resources to handle frustration. In dealing with aggressive tendencies, the person is faced with intersecting problems. If those tendencies remain pent up, serious personality difficulties may ensue. If, on the other hand, they are expressed, social problems can occur: rejection by a lover, a career derailed, family relations upturned.

Dysfunctional Anger

Anger per se is often adaptive and undeserving of its bad reputation, but it can precipitate violence and aggression. Anger can cause people to remember things that made them angry in the past, and prime them to respond aggressively. It can also reduce normal restraints and make aggressive responses feel more justified. In addition, anger may strain the cognitive resources required to control behavior. Consider a man who becomes angry over an insult. He is cognitively distracted by his anger and thus is less likely to suppress his urge to shove or punch the person who maligned him. In addition, anger causes physiological arousal, which can facilitate physical aggression.

Anger can be considered dysfunctional when it is out of proportion to the situation, experienced frequently, or elevated to the point where it impairs the person. Whether anger impairs a person often depends on his or her response to an angry episode. Consider a man who wants to spend time with his girlfriend, but she wants to have a night out with her friends. His goal of spending time with her has been blocked, and he becomes angry. He could discuss the matter with her and reach a compromise that allows both people to attain their goals. Or he could attempt to make her feel guilty every time she wants to spend time with anyone else, resulting in arguments and an end of the relationship, putting him even further from his original goal. In the first case, anger was functional in that it motivated a resolution; in the latter case, anger was chronic and dysfunctional because it resulted in goal failure and harm to a social relationship.

Another approach for identifying dysfunctional anger includes looking at whether or not expressions of anger are inappropriate. The uncontrolled expression of anger is generally considered inappropriate and conflicts with societal norms, although these norms vary by gender and culture. For example, acts of physical aggression are perceived to be less appropriate when committed by women. In the same vein, acts of physical and verbal aggression are viewed more negatively in some cultures than others. Some anger and aggression is valued in Western cultures in order to preserve independence and "stick up" for oneself; other cultures view anger as destructive, and people who express anger are ostracized from social groups (Briggs 1998).

A final approach to determine if anger is dysfunctional is to look at its effect on the health of the individual. Feelings of anger toward the self and others are associated with higher rates of mental and physical ailments. Anger has consistently been linked to hypertension and coronary problems, along with increased release of adrenaline and other hormones. People with chronic anger also tend to be slower to recover from blood pressure increases while feeling angry, which may put undue stress on the body. Anger may also influence health indirectly, through an increase in unhealthy habits associated with attempts to cope with intense emotion, such as smoking.

What Causes Dysfunctional Anger?

There is a tendency, by both clinicians and the general public, to dismiss anger as a problem. The assumption often is that there is some other, deeper issue (such as depression) that causes problematic anger. In contrast, no one would ever ask what was "really" causing someone's depression instead, they accept that intense and chronic sadness is a problem that results from biological predispositions and negative experiences. This may lead individuals with anger disorders to feel misunderstood and decrease the likelihood that they will seek and adhere to treatment regimens.

As anger is not currently recognized as a psychiatric condition (except in rare cases involving *intermittent explosive disorder*), its potential causes have not been systematically studied. The experience of problematic anger and referrals to anger management are associated with poor social and coping skills, which are generally necessary to deal with anger in an effective and socially acceptable way. Individuals lacking in social skills have difficulty accurately processing social events and the intentions of others. For example, they may interpret an ambiguous situation as being overly hostile, and react with anger out of proportion to the situation (Lochman et al. 2010). A lack of effective coping skills may also increase problematic anger as people repeatedly fail to resolve a problem. Over time, they are likely to experience even more frequent and intense anger as they struggle to find a way to overcome obstacles to their goals. Further, ineffective attempts at coping may affect their social and professional relationships as they may react in negative or inappropriate ways to stress.

When faced with stress, people with effective coping skills take steps to change the situation or how they perceive the situation in ways that result in positive emotions. Examples of effective coping strategies include problem solving, looking for positive results ("seeing the silver lining"), and finding positive meaning from events (Lench 2004). In contrast, people with ineffective coping skills tend to make a problem worse because the situation remains unresolved. Examples of ineffective coping strategies include less of a focus on problem solving and the use of more aggressive and antisocial actions, such as retaliation (ibid). People with problematic anger also report that they have fewer positive ways to express their anger. They use less reciprocal communication and are less likely to take time to calm down, and generally report an inability to control their reactions in situations that trigger anger (Denson et al. 2011). This lack of control over impulsive behavior may explain many of the problems experienced by people with problematic anger, including physical assault on other people or objects, verbal assault, and nonverbal actions such as glaring or "giving the finger" (Lench 2004). Interventions targeting increased control over impulses might therefore prove beneficial.

Treatments for Anger and Aggression

What is anger management therapy? Unfortunately, because anger is not currently recognized as a mental disorder, it can mean many things and there are no firm guidelines for what kind of therapy should be given for different anger problems, to whom it should be given, or who should administer the therapy. Despite the lack of guidelines, anger management therapy can effectively lower angry persons' blood pressure and improve their behavioral control. Reviews of the potential therapies to treat anger suggest that multiple types of therapy may be effective, especially those that target a variety of components of anger at one time. One such multi component treatment that has shown success is stress inoculation therapy. This therapy focuses on addressing the cognitive, emotional, and behavioral aspects of anger through cognitive preparation, skill acquisition, and practice of these skills in mildly stressful situations (Tafrate and Kassinove 2009). Other promising therapeutic approaches include techniques to increase the ability to tolerate physical and emotional distress and family therapy approaches. Complementary and alternative therapies may also have a role to play in getting the client to learn how to recognize his or her dysfunctional reactions and to work to remain calm, or calmer, in stressful situations.

In addition to these therapies, there is some evidence that dysfunctional anger may be reduced by medication. Individuals suffering from "anger attacks"—brief episodes of intense anger, similar to the anxiety during panic attacks—may experience fewer attacks while taking low doses of antidepressant drugs that target the neurotransmitter serotonin. Other studies have found that medications, including mood stabilizers and antipsychotics, are helpful in treating dysfunctional anger.

Dysfunctional anger is a growing problem in today's society. The news is filled with examples of violence and aggression committed by people who are angry at some insult or stressful situation. Unfortunately, anger problems often go unrecognized and untreated. Anger is a normal emotional experience that can become problematic and disrupt the lives of many individuals. Hopefully, there will one day be ways to identify and treat such anger before it results in harm to the self or others.

Kathleen E. Darbor,
Heather C. Lench, and Michael Shally-Jensen

See also: Behavioral Theories and Therapies; Biofeedback; Meditation and Mindfulness; Primal Therapy and Feeling Therapy ; Self-Help

Further Reading

Briggs, Jean L. 1998. "Never in Anger: Portrait of an Eskimo Family." In *Human Emotions: A Reader*, edited by Jennifer M. Jenkins et al., 45–54. Malden, MA: Blackwell.

Denson, Thomas F., et al. 2011. "Self-Control Training Decreases Aggression in Response to Provocation in Aggressive Individuals." *Journal of Research in Personality* 45:252–56.

Lench, Heather C. 2004. "Anger Management: Diagnostic Differences and Treatment Implications." *Journal of Social and Clinical Psychology* 23:512–31.

Lochman, John E., et al., 2010. "Anger and Aggression." In *Practitioner's Guide to Empirically Based Measures of Social Skills,* edited by Douglas W. Nangle et al., 155–66. New York: Springer.

Tafrate, Raymond C., and Howard Kassinove. 2009. *Anger Management for Everyone: Seven Proven Ways to Control Anger and Live a Happier Life.* Atascandero, CA: Impact.

ANTIOXIDANTS

The human body continuously produces energy by building up and breaking down, at the cellular level, substances introduced to it in the form of food and drink. In the course of this process, called oxidation, certain molecules are produced that can be missing an electron. These "electronless" molecules are called *free radicals*. Because of their structure (or lack thereof), free radicals are unstable and seek to "borrow" electrons from surrounding matter, working to restore themselves to a balanced state. When such borrowing occurs, the chemical structure of the cell from which the free radical has taken an electron itself becomes altered.

Free radicals are strange beasts because, on the one hand, they break down toxins and help to fight disease, and on the other hand, when present in excess they can create a condition known as oxidative stress. To maintain a healthy level of free radicals, the body produces *antioxidants,* or makes use of antioxidants present in certain foods. Antioxidants are able to give up one of their electrons to a free radical molecule and still remain in balance themselves. In doing so, they may help prevent the damaging effects of free radicals.

Some people may have a "shortage" of antioxidants in their system as a result of genetics or illness or exposure to harmful substances or a host of other situations that are not completely understood. In these cases, cellular damage can occur. In the most extreme cases, it can lead to degenerative diseases like nervous system disorders or damage to the eyes, as well as cancers, atherosclerosis, or diabetes. Again, these are far more the exception than the rule, but they illustrate the problem.

Boosting Antioxidant Intake

Many claims have been made about the health benefits of antioxidants. As noted, these are substances that counteract the harmful free radicals created by oxidation. Oxidation, for example, can rust cars. Some oxidation in the body is good because it produces energy and kills bacterial invaders. But, in excess, it can damage tissues. Antioxidants are found naturally in many foods, primarily fruits and vegetables. They are also available as supplements, but whether or not they are helpful is still a matter of debate. There are claims that antioxidants in large quantities can help prevent or reduce the effects of a variety of diseases, including cardiovascular disease, diabetes, Alzheimer's, and various forms of cancer. Vitamins with antioxidant properties include vitamins E, C, and A as beta-carotene. Some minerals such as selenium, lutein, and lycopene are also considered to have antioxidant properties.

Research on the effect of antioxidants is continuing. In 2014, for example, two studies found that the carotenoid lycopene, found in tomatoes, pink grapefruit, and watermelon, may decrease the risk of prostate cancer. On April 10, 2000, a panel at the Institute of Medicine of the National Academies of Science reported that megadoses of antioxidants haven't yet been proven to be helpful and might in fact be dangerous. According to the press release announcing the findings, "A direct connection between the intake of antioxidants and the prevention of chronic disease has yet to be adequately established," said Norman I. Krinsky, chair of the study's Panel on Dietary Antioxidants and Related Compounds, and a professor of biochemistry at Tufts University School of Medicine, Boston. "We do know, however, that dietary antioxidants can in some cases prevent or counteract cell damage that stems from exposure to oxidants, which are agents that affect a cell's molecular composition. But much more research is needed to determine whether dietary antioxidants can actually stave off chronic disease" (Bijlefeld and Zoumbaris 2014, 8).

As such, the panel established the following recommendations for dietary supplementation of antioxidants. It increased recommended intake levels of vitamin C to 75 milligrams per day for women and 90 milligrams per day for men. Smokers, who are more likely to be impacted from the cell-damaging biological processes and deplete more vitamin C, need an additional 35 milligrams per day. The report set the upper intake level for vitamin C, from both food and supplements, at 2,000 milligrams per day for adults, saying intakes above this amount may cause diarrhea. Food sources for vitamin C include citrus fruit, potatoes, strawberries, broccoli, and leafy green vegetables.

Vitamin E recommendations were also increased, and men and women are now advised to consume 15 milligrams of vitamin E from food. Food sources for this vitamin are vegetable oils, nuts, seeds, liver, and leafy green vegetables. Synthetic vitamin E from vitamin supplements should not exceed 1,000 milligrams of alpha-tocopherol per day for adults. Alpha-tocopherol is the only type of vitamin E that human blood can maintain and transfer to cells when needed. People who consume more than this amount place themselves at greater risk of hemorrhagic damage because the nutrient can act as an anticoagulant, according to the report.

The report also recommended that men and women need 55 micrograms of selenium per day. Food sources include seafood, liver, meat, and grains. The upper level of selenium, including natural and supplement sources, should be less than 400 micrograms per day. More could result in selenosis, a toxic reaction that can cause hair loss and nail sloughing.

The report did not set a recommended daily intake or upper intake level for beta-carotene and other carotenoids, which are found naturally in dark-green and deep-yellow vegetables. However, it cautioned against high doses, recommending supplementation only for the prevention and control of vitamin A deficiency.

The report stressed that a balanced and varied diet will provide adequate amounts of these vitamins and minerals without requiring supplements. The American Heart Association concurs in a February 1999 Science Advisory, "Antioxidant Consumption and Risk of Coronary Heart Disease: Emphasis on Vitamin C, Vitamin E, and Beta-Carotene," which concluded, "The most prudent and scientifically supportable recommendation for the general population is to consume a balanced diet with emphasis on antioxidant-rich fruits and vegetables and whole grains. This advice, which is consistent with the current dietary guidelines of the American Heart Association, considers the role of the total diet in influencing disease risk. Although diet alone may not provide the levels of vitamin E intake that have been associated with the lowest risk in a few observational studies, the absence of efficacy and safety data from randomized trials precludes the establishment of population-wide recommendations regarding vitamin E supplementation" (Bijlefeld and Zoumbaris 2014, 9).

Marjolijn Bijlefeld,
Sharon K. Zoumbaris, and
Michael Shally-Jensen

See also: Bottled Water; Detox Diets; Diet and Exercise; Eating Organic; Herbal Remedies; Juice and Juicing; Naturopathic Medicine; Vegetarianism; Vitamins and Minerals

Further Reading

"Antioxidants: Beyond the Hype." The Nutrition Source. Harvard School of Public Health. http://www.hsph.harvard.edu/nutritionsource/antioxidants/.

Bijlefeld, Marjolijn, and Sharon K. Zoumbaris. 2014. "Antioxidants." In *Encyclopedia of Fad Diets: Understanding Science and Society. Second Edition*, by Marjolijn Bijlefeld and Sharon K. Zoumbaris. Santa Barbara, CA: Greenwood.

Charnow, Jody. 2014. "Lycopene May Decrease Prostate Cancer Risk." *Renal and Urology News*, February 28. http://www.renalandurologynews.com/lycopene-may-decrease-prostate-cancer-risk/article/335907/.

"DRI: Dietary Reference Intakes for Vitamin C, Vitamin E, Selenium, and Carotenoids." 2000. Institute of Medicine of the National Academies, August 3. http://www.iom.edu/Reports/2000/Dietary-Reference-Intakes-for-Vitamin-C-Vitamin-E-Selenium-and-Carotenoids.aspx

CODEPENDENCY COUNSELING

We often think of "seeing a therapist" as just one type of treatment; in fact, there are many different kinds of therapists, and many different kinds of therapy treatments. A therapist trained in cognitive behavioral therapy (CBT) will work differently than a therapist trained in psychodynamic therapy; a therapist who specializes in couples work will have a different perspective from someone who works primarily with children. Therapists who specialize in codependency recovery, similarly, do a specific kind of work.

What Is Codependency?

Put simply, codependency refers to a relationship in which one person puts the other person's needs above his or her own, even if the situation tends to be harmful. If someone is codependent, that is, they might focus on providing for the needs of a spouse, a parent, or a particular friend—while the other person relies on his or her to do so. Codependency can be a general trend in one's life, but therapists most often talk about two people being in a codependent relationship: one person provides for the needs of the other without necessarily seeing the act reciprocated—except in the form of more demands and expectations. And, somehow, together, the two people manage to go on like this, the relationship growing ever more routine and predictable.

Codependency often comes up when therapists are treating people who have addictions. Their partners have often hurt themselves emotionally or financially trying to support or "save" someone with an addiction, all the while merely enabling them to carry on as before, addiction and all. Abused children can also be codependent on their abusers, trying to prevent the behaviors they see as leading to their abuse—that is, keeping quiet about it and not making a fuss. These cycles can be painful and violative for everyone involved.

Technically, codependency is not a mental health diagnosis—meaning that it is not listed in the official *Diagnostic and Statistical Manual* (DSM), the book that therapists and psychiatrists use as a guideline for their diagnoses and treatment choices. Still, these sorts of relationships can cause anxiety, behavioral outbursts, and severe depression, so managing them is important. (It has been proposed that codependency be included in the DSM as a personality disorder, but, to date, the authorities have not accepted it, preferring to see it merely as a normal trait taken to excess, or, possibly, as an "attachment" issue.)

There are many stories that show examples of codependency, breaking down the difference between supporting someone and trying to save them from themselves.

- *Sid and Nancy* (1986) is a biopic about the real-life relationship between the Sex Pistols' star punk rocker, Sid Vicious, and his girlfriend, Nancy Spurgen. Both Sid and Nancy are heroin addicts, and their relationship quickly causes them to spiral out of control.

- The movie *When a Man Loves a Woman* (1994) looks at the aftereffects of someone trying to fix her role in a codependent relationship. Alice is an alcoholic. When she and her husband, Michael, agree that she should enter rehab, Alice works toward sobriety and Michael manages the household. But when Alice returns home, healthier and stronger as a sober woman than she ever was as an alcoholic, Michael is lost; he doesn't know what to do without taking care of Alice in a drunken stupor. The couple breaks up for a time, and the movie ends without a real declaration of whether their relationship can work without Alice's alcoholism. In real life, many people find that when they begin to assert themselves to move out of a codependent relationship, the other person has extreme reactions that are often negative.

- Harley Quinn is a great example of a codependent character (1992) in the *Batman* series. She partners up with The Joker (Mr. J) even though she knows that he's bad for her, and she regularly saves him when Batman knocks him around. In fact, many superheroes are often described as somewhat codependent; they need villains in order to be superheroes, which is why they never kill their villains and instead push for their redemption. Saving villains from themselves, sometimes as a symbol of redeeming a corrupt or lost society, is where the average superhero is at.

- The movie *Benny and Joon* (1993) included Johnny Depp in one of the roles that originally made him famous. Joon is living with schizophrenia and resides with her brother, Benny. Benny is so accustomed to taking care of her that when Joon does try to find ways to be more independent, he immediately pulls her back, trying to force her into the same relationship they've always had. Joon's story eventually ends with Benny at least considering his own needs, and supporting Joon in moving into her own apartment.

- *Heavy* (1995) is about an obese, unhappy man who works as a cook and is in a codependent relationship with his mother. A new waitress shows up at work and the man begins to see how he might approach his life differently, even if the prospect is frightening.

Other movies to watch for their theme of codependency include *In the Bedroom* (2001), *The Deep End* (2001), and *Dreamland* (2006).

Codependency Counseling

In some ways, counseling for codependency is very similar to other kinds of talk therapy. The individual discusses problems and concerns with a trained counselor/therapist, who offers feedback, suggestions, and strategies that will help the client handle situations differently, to better his or her emotional health.

With codependency, it is important that a therapist help identify what in the past has created the need to care for other people. Codependent people often feel lost without someone to take care of, and they can end up seeking out others to "save." A counselor who specializes in this area can help identify such behavior and look for ways to create relationships with healthy, stable people who won't feed the client's need for a codependent relationship.

Therapists can help people ease the urge toward "perfectionism" that they tend to experience, and help them improve their self-esteem. Counselors can help them establish healthy social boundaries and learn the difference between caring about, supporting, and saving people. Group therapy can also be helpful in many cases; there is a 12-step program for codependent people called Co-Dependents Anonymous, or CoDA. There are also, as always with mental health conditions, self-help guides available. Some assertiveness training is often part of the solution, as the person learns to stand on his or her own. Role-playing can also help in this regard, allowing the person to try out a new identity, as it were.

Codependency can make it difficult to maintain healthy relationships with other people. Seeing a therapist is a positive way to make the kinds of changes necessary to create a healthier life all around.

Kay Tilden Frost

See also: Behavioral Theories and Therapies; Client-Centered Therapy; Depression and Its Treatment; Drama Therapy; Recovery Movement; 12-Step Programs

Further Reading

Beatty, Melody. 2009. *The New Codependency*. New York: Simon and Schuster.
Esposito, Nancy. 2016 "6 Signs of a Codependent Relationship." *Psychology Today.* September 19. https://www.psychologytoday.com/us/blog/anxiety-zen/201609/6 -signs-codependent-relationship
"Recovery from Codependency." *Good Therapy.* November 21, 2018. https://www .goodtherapy.org/learn-about-therapy/issues/codependency/recovery

CRYSTALS

Crystals have long fascinated laypersons and experts alike. Why is that so? What is it about crystals that makes them so special? Do they have some unique qualities? Do they have certain "powers" that make them beneficial to humans?

Crystal Basics

Crystalline materials vary from gemstones to salts to snowflakes. While the shape and characteristics of a naturally formed crystal are determined by the substance of which it is composed, all crystalline materials are marked by an ordered, repetitive arrangement of the atoms making them up. That is, they exhibit a so-called crystal lattice, or regular array of their constituent parts. The basic geometry of the crystal lattice is different in each material—for example, diamond, topaz, quartz, mica, ice, table salt—and that geometry determines the outward form of the crystal, or how it appears to the eye.

Most all crystals display *symmetry,* because the matter composing them is homogeneous (the same throughout) and the atomic arrangement is repeated over and over. Besides affecting the external shape and markings of the crystal, that symmetry affects other characteristics, such as the crystal's optical properties—how it refracts light—and its electrical conductivity. It is generally this combination of symmetry, optical qualities, physical beauty, and, conductivity that has long attracted observers to crystals and crystallography (the study of crystals). The same combination has led many people to conclude that crystals have unique "powers" that can be utilized for the benefit of human beings, including in the maintenance of human health and wellness.

Different cultures around the world, including Celtic, Native American, and Chinese, have traditionally valued crystals and used them for spiritual and healing

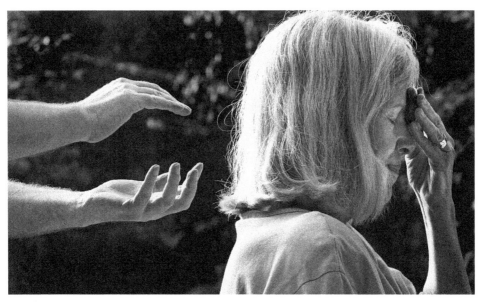

Energy healer Ken Klee works with a client during a healing session. The woman holds a "pulsor" over her forehead (and heart). Pulsors contain microcrystals that, Klee says, remove energy blockages and restore integrity to the body. (Gina Ferazzi/Los Angeles Times via Getty Images)

purposes. The purple gem amethyst is mentioned in the Book of Exodus as part of a bejeweled breastplate worn by Moses's brother (and fellow prophet) Aaron, echoes of which are still seen in the formal garb of Catholic bishops. Plato cites the use of crystals among the inhabitants of Atlantis, and the legendary Arthurian magician Merlin is said to have lived in an enchanted cave featuring crystals. The U.S. clairvoyant and healer Edgar Cayce (1877–1945) was known to have favored crystals; Cayce even held that a giant crystal charged by the sun had been used by the Atlanteans to power their world.

The earliest scientific observations of crystals were made by the German physician and alchemist Andreas Libavius in 1597, when he noticed that crystals of different substances often have characteristic shapes. Nearly a century later, two Danish naturalists, Nicolas Steno and Rasmus Bartholin, studied, respectively, the angular faces of crystals and their ability to refract light. In the 18th century two French crystallographers, Jean-Baptise de Romé de l'isle and Abbé René Jüst Hauy, examined the angles and shapes of crystals in order to identify their underlying structures; and another Frenchman, François Arago, explored the polarization of light by crystals. In 1880 the brothers Pierre and Jacques Curie of France demonstrated the piezoelectric effect in crystals—that is, the creation of an electrical charge under mechanical pressure, a phenomenon that causes a small spark to jump across a gap, as in a modern cigarette lighter. All of these scientific discoveries, to the extent that they became widely known, only added to the mystery and allure of crystals in the popular consciousness.

In the modern era crystals are used in a variety of technologies. Early telegraph and radio equipment used a crystal called galena as a crude means to detect wireless signals. Phonographic record players used crystal pickups and a sapphire stylus ("needle") to capture vibrations from the vinyl record groove as a step in the process of producing sound. Electric guitars, too, in addition to magnetic pickups, often used a piezoelectric "sandwich" of quartz crystals at specific points beneath the strings to pick up vibrations. A quartz watch is a timepiece that makes use of the piezoelectric qualities of quartz to keep accurate and reliable time. Display screens on clocks and calculators typically consist of liquid crystal diodes. Semiconductors, fiber optics, and lasers also make varying use of crystal physics in performing their functions.

Crystal Healing

One of the key qualities of crystals commonly mentioned in connection with their use in healing and wellness is the "energy" that crystals contain and/or the "vibrations" they give off. As noted, some crystals do have conductive (or semiconductive) properties, but they do not actually store or "contain" that energy; it passes through them or otherwise dissipates. Crystals do have some internal energy associated with molecular vibrations, but so too do many noncrystalline solids. In addition to molecular vibrations, crystals can exhibit mechanical vibration—like a tuning fork does when it is struck. Here too, however, other substances, including metals, display this type of vibration. In short, the energetic or vibratory qualities of crystals are notable, but they don't necessarily have a magical or metaphysical aspect to them, as popular healers suggest. Still, combined with the other characteristics noted above, the electroenergetic qualities of crystals add to the aura of these objects as something to behold and from which to draw inspiration or, perhaps. even a feeling of strength or power.

Crystal healers say that the "energy fields" surrounding crystals can be manipulated to help restore balance in the body.

> All life, in order to exist and be meaningful, must be in a state of balance. When life becomes polarized in one direction or the other, there is an imbalance and interference with the natural pattern of living. Quartz crystals, blood, and water all have an affinity for each other because they all share common elemental properties. Crystals [can] store energy, . . . color, and memories, as well as sound, fragrance, light, emotions, dreams, and specific experiences. (Knight 2009, 472)

The idea, then, is that crystals can serve to connect one with the wider universe through their energy fields and the specific vibrational frequencies attributed to individual crystals, or types of crystals. Each crystal has a particular application, though some applications are quite broad. Red garnet, for example, is recommended to arouse or invigorate a patient; it can also be placed on the lower back to help alleviate menstrual cramps or lower back pain. Black obsidian, in contrast, is used to "ground" the individual who feels emotionally scattered or unstable.

Clear quartz is suggested for achieving insight, clarity, or higher consciousness. Jasper is used for endurance, fortitude, protection. Lapis lazuli is employed for divination, wisdom, creativity. Onyx is advised for building structure in one's life, for accessing memories, stimulating the telling of stories, and enhancing communication. Turquoise helps to put one in touch with spirits and ancestors and to build knowledge, wholeness, and self-realization. Most crystals also have applications for various physical ailments, from headaches and muscular pain to respiratory or digestive issues.

In addition to "aligning" one's energies in a health-producing way, crystals are said to aid in the removal of energy "blockages" that may be causing an unhealthful attitude or condition. Many crystal healers refer to the classical chakra points of Eastern healing traditions when devising a plan of action for their clients: crystals are to be set on or about the body according to a layout suggested by these points. The layout optimizes energy flows and facilitates the coming together of mind, body, environment, past, present, and the spiritual and material worlds. Thus, crystal healing is both New Age medicine and traditional medicine combined. Although it grew very popular in the last part of the 20th century, it draws on older principles and methods and continues today to be a popular touchstone of emotional well-being and, to a lesser extent, of physiological health and healing. While skeptics point to the likely operation of the placebo principle in any application of crystal healing, practitioners and consumers point to their own personal experiences with crystals, experience that suggests crystals are everything they are thought to be. Indeed, one of the highlights of crystal usage is the discovery of one's personal stone

> All crystals and stones are naturally tuned to particular frequencies, vibrations, and harmonies of energy. When you are in attunement with a stone, you will experience sensations of balance, harmony, clarity, and wholeness. Choosing [a personal stone] is an intuitive act. Take a deep breath and notice which stones feel good to you. If a stone feels right, it's probably the right one for you. If it doesn't feel right, try another one. (Knight 2009, 479)

Michael Shally-Jensen

See also: Alternative Diagnostics; Aromatherapy and Essential Oils; Ayurvedic Medicine; Chinese Traditional Medicine; Magnet Therapy; Mind–Body Medicine; Naturopathic Medicine; Yoga

Further Reading

Frazier, Karen. 2015. *Crystals for Healing: The Complete Reference Guide.* Berkeley, CA: Althea Press.

Knight, Sirona. 2009. "Healing with Crystals and Gemstones." In *Natural Healing Wisdom and Know-How: Useful Practices, Recipes, and Formulas for a Lifetime of Health,* edited by Amy Rost, 470–89. New York: Black Dog and Leventhal Publishers.

Walker, Barbara G. 1989. *The Book of Sacred Stones: Fact and Fallacy in the Crystal World.* San Francisco: Harper and Row.

DETOX DIETS

While many modern Americans think of detox diets as the latest craze, the concept of detoxification is an ancient practice that has been present in almost every culture throughout history.

The basic concept of detoxification is this: the body carries toxins that affect it in ways that traditional Western medicine either can't identify or can't treat. Some religious cultures have looked to detoxify spiritual impurities; other cultures looked to balance humors or elements in the body. In the modern world, the focus of detoxification is usually removing toxic chemicals from the body.

Why Detox?

Proponents of detox diets and other detoxification methods believe that we live in a world that has more potentially dangerous chemicals in it than ever before. They believe that the food we ingest, the air we breathe, and the water we drink are polluted with toxic chemicals that must be removed from our bodies in order for us to live our healthiest lives. Although many detox diets are vague about what toxins they will be removing, or "flushing," from the user's system, some of the most common targets are heavy metals (like mercury), synthetic chemicals, and environmental pollutants.

It is definitely true that too much of any chemical can cause health problems. Western medicine has ways of testing for most of these chemicals, such as mercury or lead. But those who favor detox diets say either that the Western methods of treating these problems is even more harmful than the initial exposure, or that doctors will allow someone to have too much of any given chemical before treatment begins.

Detox diets are said by their advocates to improve:

- obesity
- inflammation
- digestion issues
- allergies
- autoimmune diseases
- bloating
- other chronic illnesses

What Does a Detox Diet Involve?

While there are many different detox diets in the news and on the Internet, they share some similarities. A detox, or cleanse, usually begins with a period of fasting. This means that you avoid all foods and generally drink only water for a period of time. When you're allowed to eat again, you focus on specific "clean" juices, fruits and vegetables, and water. This continues for a certain amount of time; eventually you're allowed to return to a normal diet, though you're often encouraged to "eat clean" to maintain your newly healthy body.

How Gwyneth Paltrow Convinced America to Detox

If you first noticed Gwyneth Paltrow in her films from the late 1990s—*Seven, Emma,* and *Shakespeare in Love,* or even her more recent role as Pepper Potts in the Marvel cinematic universe—learning about her lifestyle company, Goop, can be a jarring experience. Goop offers its fans a "clean" beauty, fashion, and health experience.

Founded in 2008, Goop has promoted a wide variety of practices that don't have backing from the scientific community, such as "vaginal steaming" and coffee enemas. By that measure, popularizing a Goop-branded detox experience is one of the more mainstream practices she has promoted.

Paltrow says that natural beauty comes from within; in this case, natural beauty refers to great skin, and within refers to the diet. In 2016, Paltrow said "a diet rich in nutrients and poor in processed foods is optimal for getting that lovely glow." At first, Paltrow was recommending a few extrahealthy recipes. Some of the ingredients were expensive or esoteric—bee pollen, acai, and buckwheat groats—but foods like grilled salmon and an avocado salad are healthy and tasty.

But then things got intense. The past few years, Goop has encouraged its followers to engage in a 30-day (at least) cleanse that forbids gluten, corn, soy, caffeine, added sugar, red meat, white rice, and more. Paltrow also recommends expensive supplements and workout routines, and she states that the diet plan is endorsed by her doctor.

While most people scorn older detox plans like the Master Cleanse, Paltrow's celebrity has expanded to encompass Goop and its "clean living" brand. Whether detox diets are helpful or not, Paltrow has clearly increased the number of people who are interested in following them.

Many diets also encourage you to use various supplements, teas, herbs, and colon cleanses to make your detox more effective. The same company advocating for the detox will usually sell these products. Many companies make significant amounts of money selling these items that are marketed as doing basically the same thing that your liver does naturally.

Some detox diets argue that some chemicals built up in the liver can't be cleansed naturally; others claim that toxins build up in your body because your liver is overwhelmed by the amount of toxins it needs to process, and that it can get sluggish. This is not dissimilar from Hippocrates and his theory that sluggish humors needed to be stimulated so that the body could function properly. Most likely if someone had such a high level of chemical exposure, their symptoms would be evident and they would be smart to seek medical help.

Do Detox Diets Work?

There are many celebrities and regular people who absolutely swear by cleanses and detox diets to keep their bodies in excellent health. Jennifer Aniston, Gwyneth

Paltrow, and Jennifer Lawrence have all talked to celebrity magazines about the various ways they give their bodies an early start on staying healthy. And there certainly is something to be said for waking up to light, healthy, nutritious foods instead of the heavier, fattier breakfast foods that many Americans have become accustomed to.

But do detox diets really eliminate chemicals that would otherwise not be eliminated? The science is slim.

For most people, the liver does the hard work of eliminating toxic chemicals from the body. This is, in fact, the bulk of its role in the body. It makes various chemicals harmless, and then excretes them from the body in feces, urine, and sweat. If the liver is overworked—for example, when someone drinks too much alcohol—it becomes larger in order to handle the additional workload, and can actually become scarred and stop functioning (cirrhosis of the liver). If the toxic overload is removed, the liver can actually heal, to a certain degree.

But the amount of work the liver can perform, and the length of time it can continue to do so, before it ever reaches this critical state is impressive. It takes years of heavy drinking, in most cases, to damage the liver. People who work with dangerous chemicals for many years can also sustain liver damage. Hepatitis B, a blood-borne disease that primarily affects the liver, can also cause long-term damage, and can eventually require a transplant. Outside of problems such as these, the liver generally does its job amazingly well.

There are a few chemicals that the liver either cannot, or has a difficult time, removing from the body. These include substances like phthalates (all that BPA that we stopped putting in plastics after 2010), or heavy metals like mercury and cadmium in big amounts. But these chemicals are generally stored in the body's fat, rather than in the bloodstream. The typical detox diet will not do anything to remove them; they can take years to be gradually cycled out of the body. If they are causing other health problems, doctors can use a process called chelation to help remove them from the body.

Can Detox Diets Be Harmful?

It depends on how they're handled. In general, focusing on reducing or removing foods with heavy, saturated fats, increasing servings of fruits and vegetables, and minimizing foods with added sugar is going to help improve anyone's health. Some people advise shopping at the "edges" of the grocery store: most stores have the produce, the dairy, and the meat and fish areas around the edges, while snack foods, prepared frozen foods, and cookies and desserts tend to be in the inner areas. Most detox diets also encourage you to reduce or remove alcohol from your diet; this is one goal that can absolutely help a person's liver stay healthy.

But spending days eating nothing but fruits and vegetables can starve your body of essential nutrients that it needs to function. The supplements and teas that are sold—usually at a considerable price—to support your cleanse are unregulated by the Food and Drug Administration, and can potentially contain even more harmful ingredients than the chemicals a detox diet is meant to remove. And spending days drinking only water can absolutely be dangerous, causing low blood sugar, low energy, and more. If a person really does have heavy-metal exposure, lowering calorie intake can actually make things worse; remember that heavy metals are stored in fat, and when you starve your body, it burns fat for energy. This can dump huge amounts of heavy metals into the bloodstream, causing serious illness. If you believe that you've been exposed to heavy metals, you should see a doctor.

So, if detox dieting seems right for you, make sure to proceed with caution.

It is important to note, however, that when doctors are trying to diagnose a food allergy, they may try something called an elimination diet. This means that the person eliminates all suspected allergens from their diet, then slowly adds them back in to see what is causing the allergic reaction. This is done carefully, and under medical supervision; this makes it very different from a detox.

Other Types of Detox

Some cultures have incorporated methods of detoxification that are not diet-based and are generally safer. Ritual sweating, for example, is commonly associated with Native American tribes, such as the Chumash tribe of California. Many cultures across northern and eastern Europe, however, have created saunas and similar experiences. The Chumash sweat lodge rituals were part of incredibly intensive religious and spiritual ceremonies, and white people who try to copy them are being somewhat "appropriative." That said, the average health club will often have a sauna room where one can sit and encourage the body to sweat out the toxins. As long as it's not dangerous to be in the heat and humidity, the experience can be very relaxing—and less dangerous than a detox diet.

Kay Tilden Frost

See also: Aging Prevention, or "Successful Aging"; Antioxidants; Bottled Water; Eating Organic; Juice and Juicing; Macrobiotics; Paleo Diet; Sweat Lodges and Saunas; Vegetarianism

Further Reading

Cosgrove, Ben. 2018. "The Truth about Detox Diets," *University of California, Berkeley, Wellness.* March 19. http://www.berkeleywellness.com/healthy-eating/diet-weight-loss /nutrition/article/truth-about-detox-diets

Foroutan, Robin. 2017. "What's the Deal with Detox Diets?" *Eat Right: Academy of Nutrition and Dietetics.* April 26. https://www.eatright.org/health/weight-loss/fad-diets/whats-the -deal-with-detox-diets

Zeratsky, Katherine. 2018. "Do Detox Diets Offer Any Health Benefits?" *Mayo Clinic.* April 27. https://www.mayoclinic.org/healthy-lifestyle/nutrition-and-healthy-eating/expert -answers/detox-diets/faq-20058040

DIET PILLS AND METABOLISM BOOSTERS

It is only recently (in historical terms) that the word *diet* has become synonymous with a weight-loss regimen of restricted eating and drinking. The ancient Greeks employed the word *diaita*, but for them it referred not simply to the foods a person consumed but to an entire way of life—what the person ate and drank as well as the type of exercise he or she did and his or her lifestyle as a whole.

Modern Americans have taken dieting, in the modern sense, to the extremes. The physical ideal for women tends to be extremely slim, and for men it tends to be very muscular. Both genders are thus idealized as having very little body fat. Most people cannot achieve this ideal appearance on their own. Many of them turn to weight-control medications and commercially sold metabolism boosters in addition to watching their food intake and doing a little exercise.

The Body and Dieting in History

If one studies ancient Greek art, it is clear that the idealized male form was strong, muscular, and slim. Athletic youths were idealized. Early Christians also contributed to this social ideal; gluttony was and is considered one of the cardinal sins, after all, and many Bible passages warn against succumbing to such a temptation. Then as now, it seems, being slim was socially approved; being fat was not.

There have also been times when plumper, more rounded figures in women were considered desirable. The painter Peter Paul Rubens (1577–1640) famously painted women who had fleshy rolls, full breasts, and large thighs. The word *Rubenesque*, to refer to a woman with a heavier, rounded figure, comes from his paintings.

Although men have certainly been pressured to have a certain physical appearance, much of the societal pressure to remain thin has been directed toward women. Modern science is gathering more and more evidence that what we eat and how much we exercise have only limited effect on our weight, given the power of genes and individual development. This, however, has yet to turn around social attitudes regarding the ideal-typical body and how to achieve it. Dieting remains a multibillion-dollar industry.

Here are just a few of the fad diets that have existed throughout history.

- The Immortality Diet: Luigi Cornano, an Italian man living in 1558, allowed himself to eat only 12 ounces of food and 14 ounces of wine a day. He lived to be 102 years old.

- The Apple Cider Vinegar Diet: a modern variation on Lord Byron's explanation for his pale, thin look, participants in this diet drink three tablespoons of apple cider vinegar before each meal to, supposedly, curb hunger and burn fat.

- The Master Cleanse or Lemonade Diet: Created in 1941 by Stanley Burroughs, one drinks only a particular liquid, like lemonade, for at least 10 days. There are many modern variations on this diet—which actually can be quite dangerous because of its lack of nutrients.

- Miracle Food Diets: These come in endless varieties. Eating one magical food—half a grapefruit, cabbage soup, or peanut butter—is supposed to "melt away" the fat.

Diet pills and metabolism boosters are recent additions to this history.

Medications and Supplements

One major difference between diet medications and metabolism boosters is that diet medications are regulated by the FDA and prescribed by doctors, while metabolism boosters are often marketed as dietary supplements—and such supplements do not fall under the jurisdiction of the FDA; they can be manufactured and sold by anyone.

Diet medications work in various ways. Most of them, however, either block the body's ability to absorb fats or suppress the appetite so that one will not want to eat. There are a number of commonly prescribed, brand-name pharmaceutical products that serve these purposes. There are also a variety of over-the-counter products that make some of the same claims, but these are generally poor substitutes. In some cases, as with the drug Fen-Phen in the 1990s, regulators have had to call for the removal of a product from the market because of its negative side effects. Sometimes, too, doctors will prescribe certain antidepressants and diabetic medications to help patients lose weight, if their situation warrants it.

For diet medications to work, patients are generally advised to eat healthily and perform exercise on a regular basis while taking the medication. When used according to proper medical protocols, most patients can lose between 5 and 10 pounds. Most patients, however, will immediately regain the weight once they stop taking the medication or revert to old eating and exercise habits. Nonetheless, because these medications are regulated and require a doctor's prescription (and, presumably, a doctor's oversight), they are generally safe to use as prescribed and probably more effective than metabolism boosters.

Metabolism refers to the physiological process of converting the nutrients we eat and drink into usable energy. The rate at which this process occurs tells us something about an individual. One's basal metabolic rate (BMR) is a gauge of how much energy (how many calories) one's body needs to function. Specifically, it indicates the energy that your body would need if you remained at rest, and it is generally linked to genetic makeup and developmental history.

Metabolism boosters—also called "fat burners"—are commercial products that claim to change the body's metabolic rate so that one burns more energy, either at rest or during workouts. Some of the marketing slogans used for these products are "Kick your metabolism into high gear" and "Supercharge your metabolism." These dietary supplements often contain ingredients like caffeine, L-carnitine (an ammonium compound), or green tea, perhaps along with sugars (especially in the case of "energy drinks") and other ingredients. Theoretically, they work by increasing the level of internal activity in the body, which in turn causes the body to burn more calories.

TV Advertising and Diet Pills

As one of just two countries that allow TV advertisements for prescription drugs and other medications, Americans are bombarded with ads for the newest pills on the market. From heart disease to antidepressants to diabetes complications, new and expensive medications are regularly advertised to TV viewers with the goal of getting their viewers to ask their doctors for new, brand-name medications.

But another segment of TV advertising revolves around "metabolism boosters," the more recent name given to diet pills. Just like diet pills, these supplements are paired with claims that they will get your body working more efficiently, burn fat, increase muscle strength, and drop weight—all without your even getting off the couch.

While some viewers might, in seeing such ads, roll their eyes and use the opportunity to switch to another channel or get a glass of water, and while studies show that many of these supplements are either useless or dangerous (or both!), the ads can have a powerful psychological effect, especially on preteen and teen girls. A great deal of pressure is put on girls to maintain a certain physical appearance. In studies, girls at this age are less likely to understand the emotional manipulation of advertising and are more likely to believe the claims of weight loss and other benefits as true.

The FDA has little to no power over the industry of supplements, and so they are rarely if ever able to charge companies with false claims or make sure that what is listed on the bottle is what's actually in the supplement itself. The truth is that these supplements rarely work and are often dangerous. You just would never know it from the ads.

The problem with these supplements is essentially the same as that with diet medications: they work, arguably, only during the time that you are taking them. As soon as you stop, the body reverts to the status quo in terms of its normal metabolic rate. Moreover, there is no strong evidence that they work all that well in raising metabolism to begin with—unless they happen to include or are supplemented by carbohydrates and sugars to temporarily push the body in that direction. There is even some evidence suggesting that when you stop taking them, your metabolism will become *slower* than it was before you started. Thus, the experience can be like a sugar rush gone cold.

Risks and Benefits

The potential for abuse in the case of both diet medications and metabolism boosters is significant. Doctors generally recommend them only for patients who are both significantly overweight and prepared to follow through on the exercise and lifestyle changes needed to support the weight loss and weight maintenance goals they have set for themselves. Cheating by relying solely on pills is unhelpful at best and potentially dangerous at worst. Nevertheless, abuse does occur: people with eating disorders, for example, often use medications and supplements to suppress their appetite and keep weight off, even as they risk any number of serious medical consequences in doing so.

For very heavy patients who are showing other signs of illness, such as poor cardiovascular health, high blood sugar, or increased pain in their hips and knees, diet medications may be helpful when prescribed by a doctor. Sometimes doctors will use them to help a patient prepare for weight loss surgery, or other surgical procedures, since doing surgery on heavier patients carries a comparatively higher risk than does performing the same procedure on those who are of average size.

Yet diet medications can cause rapid heart rates and high blood pressure and can increase the risk of a stroke. Since metabolism boosters are unregulated supplements, those using these pills cannot be sure what is in them, whether the amount of the ingredient is consistent across batches or bottles, or whether any of the claims made by the manufacturer really hold water.

Ultimately, if people are concerned about their weight or health, the best thing for them to do is to make lifestyle changes. Instead of snack foods, unhealthy desserts, and lots of red meat they should eat plenty of fruits and vegetables, moderate levels of carbohydrates, and lighter/whiter meat, among other strategies. And they should get and stay active: taking walks at lunch, say, and participating in a sport of some kind or purchasing a gym membership (and using it).

Overall, diet pills are useful only for a limited number of cases and for a very short period of time. They might help people see the kind of early weight loss that can help them jump-start the healthy lifestyle changes that may help them keep the weight off and stay more fit overall. But in the long term, there are other, better solutions involving making healthier choices and sticking with them. In addition, social attitudes could stand to adjust to the reality of the body as we see and experience it in most people every day versus the idealized forms that we encounter in the media.

Kay Tilden Frost

See also: Antioxidants; Bottled Water; Detox Diets; Diet and Exercise; Eating Organic; Fat and Obesity Surgery—and Other Weight-Loss Methods; Juice and Juicing; Macrobiotics; Paleo Diet; Self-Help; Vegetarianism; Walking and Jogging

Further Reading

Foxcroft, Louise. 2012. *Calories and Corsets: A History of Dieting over 2,000 Years.* London: Profile Books.

Morris, Susan York. 2016. "Diet Pills: Do They Actually Work?" *Healthline.* July 29. https://www.healthline.com/health/healthy-eating/diet-pills

Popper, Pamela. 2013. *Food over Medicine: The Conversation that Could Save Your Life.* Dallas, TX: BenBella Books.

Wdowik, Melissa. 2017. "The Long Strange History of Diet Fads," *The Conversation.* November 6. https://theconversation.com/the-long-strange-history-of-dieting-fads-82294

GUIDED IMAGERY, OR VISUALIZATION

Guided imagery is a form of therapy that makes use of mental images to produce positive outcomes in patients/consumers. The images are created in the "mind's eye" of the person, but they may also involve all the major senses (sight, hearing, touch, smell, taste, and movement/kinesthesia). Guided imagery, also called visualization, relies on human imagination, memories, dreams, and fantasies to sharpen the connection between the mind and the body. It is a technique that encourages relaxation and the use of thought processes and the senses to promote physical healing and a change in attitude or behavior.

Guided imagery is based on the idea that the mind can affect the body. In fact, research has shown that stimulating the brain through visualization can have significant impacts on human physiological processes and biochemistry (especially endocrine and nervous systems) and might well produce positive changes in immune responses and other functions (Ernst et al. 2008, 76). "Seeing is believing" when it comes to images in the brain: imagining oneself in a particular setting or activity activates the same areas of the brain as does actually being there or doing that. A person who imagines a scenic vista, say, activates optic centers in the cerebral cortex, which in turn send signals to parts of the lower brain controlling emotional responses; this region likewise relays the message to the endocrine and autonomic nervous systems, which govern a broad range of bodily functions like heart rate, respiration, and blood pressure (Bauer 2010, 100). A positive, welcome image can have a beneficial effect—just as a *frightening* image can have the opposite effect. (A famous example of the latter is a scene in the Stanley Kubrick film *A Clockwork Orange,* in which the protagonist is forcefully exposed to violent images for an extended period of time.)

Practitioners of guided imagery use this knowledge to guide their clients toward beneficial outcomes. Alternatively, individuals may employ visualization on their own, once they have done a little training and become adept at practicing it. Guided imagery has been used to treat many conditions ranging from phantom-limb syndrome, the effects of stroke, posttraumatic stress disorder, anxiety/depression, pain (including fibromyalgia), tension and/or migraine headaches, diabetes, burn trauma, arthritis, and even cancer—as well as recovery from cancer treatments. It is often used in conjunction with other forms of medicine, including other applications of complementary and alternative medicine (CAM).

Imagery in Time

The idea that mental imagery has a role to play in thinking and feeling, in sickness and in health, goes back a long way. Before the rise of Western culture, shamanic healers around the globe practiced elaborate rites consisting of images, sounds, and smells to encourage patients to venture beyond ordinary experience and imagine themselves as healthy and satisfied. Modern-day neo-shamans use the same techniques.

In Greek thought, Plato famously held that the things we perceive in the world are but instances of ideal forms. A triangle that we construct, for example, is not the same as the triangle that a geometer knows, which has no particular size or thickness of line and no place of existence. If a person wants to understand the world, therefore, he must fix the eye of his mind on these ideal forms and grasp how they connect with one another and the world. In learning about our perceptions, we each become philosophers, as it were—and become the better for it.

The Greek physician Hippocrates had a *very* different approach. He believed that images inside the head released spirits within the body, thus animating the heart, the brain, the muscles, and other parts. Moreover, he believed that a strong image of disease could be enough to cause illness, for the same spirits were released. Hippocrates was, in a way, far ahead of his time, anticipating by centuries the view that we now have from PET scans and fMRI data proving that parts of the body and mind are activated upon envisioning an object or scene, as they are activated upon directly perceiving them.

The 17th-century English philosopher John Locke said that the mind at birth is a blank slate. As we grow and learn, we fill in the blank with ideas based on our sense perceptions. To be conscious as a functioning person is to be conscious *of* something—a table, the blue of the sky, et cetera. Thus, to see something in the world is to lay down the idea of it in the mind. Knowledge, therefore, similar to Plato's conception of it, is a relation between and of ideas. Unlike Plato, however, Locke also examined the relevance of consciousness and perception to personal identity, or an individual's sense of self.

In the early 20th century, Sigmund Freud explored people's ability to use the imagination in making sense of the world and constructing their place within it. Pain and pleasure also played and important part in the Freudian worldview, as did the images and symbols that often represent these sensations in the individual. Freud's one-time protégé, Carl Jung, gave images and symbols even more weight, claiming that they represent archetypes drawn from the "collective unconscious" of humankind. In order to assist a patient in the healing process, said Jung, the psychiatrist must guide him or her toward understanding these archetypes and the patient's relation to them.

Two literary movements also contributed to the modern appreciation of images and symbols. In the late 19th century, members of the symbolist movement sought to convey individual emotional experience through the use of suggestive and highly metaphorical language. Symbolist poets used subtle, indirect expression to communicate meaning; symbolist painters eschewed realistic portrayals in favor of fantasy and imagination; and symbolist dramatists made use of myth and mood to uncover truths of human existence. Then, a few decades later, another movement, imagism, took to avoiding mystical and romantic themes to focus instead on concrete, precise imagery in order to provoke thought and feeling. The imagists drew on Chinese poetry and the Japanese haiku. Ezra Pound, for example, once wrote a 30-line poem about seeing faces in a Paris Metro station, which was later reduced to 15 lines—and finally to 2:

The apparition of these faces in a crowd;
Petals on a wet, black bough.

Of course, images later became the stock-in-trade of Hollywood as well as of the video game and virtual reality industries. We pursue them incessantly, it seems, as a natural part of the human makeup. It should not be surprising, therefore, that they can play a role in illness and health. We can and do manipulate images to change people's attitudes, alter their moods, and produce physical changes in the body.

A couple of best-selling books helped put medical visualization on the map for both popular health enthusiasts and those facing serious illness: O. Carl Simonton and Stephanie Matthew-Simonton's *Getting Well Again: A Step-by-Step Self-Help Guide* (1978), and Bernie Siegel's *Love, Medicine, and Miracles: Lessons Learned about Self-Healing* (1988). Since then, the field has exploded.

Types of Visual Healing

There are different types of visualization techniques for different situations (and different preferences). The basics of applied imagery are often taught in small classes. Such classes usually begin with a demonstration of relaxation exercises and move on from there to more specialized methods. Participants may be guided toward the building up of highly specific images. If a particular medical condition is at issue, subjects may be asked to imagine the body free of that condition. Alternatively, they may be asked to focus closely on the organ or tissue or physiological processes involved, and imagine harmful cells dying, healthy tissue emerging, and proper functioning being restored. Dancers or athletes, for example, may be asked to see themselves as moving well and competing once again. People from other walks of life likewise will be urged to view themselves as returning to a normal existence. Some mental health conditions—anxiety, depression, and the like—can also be treated in this way.

Other techniques involve the use of symbols. A person with cancer, for example, might be advised to regard radiation therapy as involving targeted "bullets" or "lightning bolts" that do away with the cancerous growth. Similarly, those suffering from pain might be asked to see their pain as a "dark cloud" or "heavy weight" of some kind, which then must be pushed out by the patient's force of will. A combination of imagery, symbolism, and story, or narrative, can also be used. One example is an exercise called the "magic carpet ride," in which the person is encouraged to imagine a sensational trip involving this classic symbol of fantastic travel (Mason 2016, 577). Music can be an essential component of the visualization experience. Such an exercise can help relieve stress or "reset" the person's mental attitude. Although it is not widely practiced, in recent years some advocates have pushed for the use of psychotropic drugs as health aids in visualization. These substances can make something like a magic carpet ride seem almost second nature to the user. (Obviously, one is advised to be careful with this procedure.)

In addition, over-the-counter guided imagery "packages," with music or ambient sound, are now widely available. Consumers can try such themes as "The Awakening Forest," "Ocean Escape," or "Stars in Real Time," among many others.

These media are mostly for relaxation and stress-relief as opposed to making real images inside one's own head for therapeutic purposes. Self-help books, with video accompaniments, are also increasingly popular. Today, imagery and visualization have become a key part of the overall mix of alternative and complementary medicine.

Michael Shally-Jensen

See also: Anxiety and Its Treatment; Aromatherapy and Essential Oils; Art and Music Therapy; Biofeedback; Dream Interpretation; Jung and Jungian Analysis; Psychedelic Drugs; Self-Help; Shamanism and Neo-Shamanism

Further Reading

Bauer, Brent A., ed. 2010. *Mayo Clinic Book of Alternative Medicine.* 2nd ed. New York: Time Inc.

Ernst, Edzard, et al. 2008. *Oxford Handbook of Complementary Medicine.* New York: Oxford University Press.

Hall, Eric, et al. 2006. *Guided Imagery: Creative Interventions in Counselling and Psychotherapy.* Thousand Oaks, CA: SAGE.

Mason, L. John. 2016. "Mind–Body Healing Techniques." In *Natural Healing: Wisdom and Know-How,* edited by Amy Rost, 557–607. New York: Black Dog and Leventhal.

HEALTH AND WELLNESS GURUS

For as long as humans have tried to make sure that their bodies are healthy and well, they have looked for those in the know—experts—who might show them the way. After all, if we knew how to be healthy, wealthy, and wise on our own, we would just do it, no? From Aristotle to Andrew Weil, health and wellness "gurus" have made their knowledge and guidance available to the public, and people have followed it. The problem, of course, is that some advice is better than others. The rule of thumb in this crowded field is "buyer beware."

What Is a Guru?

The word *guru* comes from Eastern religions; in Buddhism and Hinduism, a guru is a spiritual teacher; in the Sikh religion, gurus are the 10 spiritual leaders of the religion. The term became popular in the United States in the 1960s and 1970s as Americans became fascinated with Eastern culture and philosophy. Over time, Americans have started to use the term to describe any teacher whose teachings they want to follow, and the word has become largely divorced from its religious meanings (except in the case of religious cults and the like).

Thus, in the United States, we tend to say that someone is a health and wellness guru whenever he or she has a significant following among those who are seeking such advice. In many cases, the people giving this advice have few, if any, medical or professional credentials; in fact, often they are celebrities from the world of popular entertainment who have turned themselves into a spokesperson for health topics. The evident good looks and fame of such celebrities usually play a large role in their success in the health and wellness field.

Real public health researchers and experts are fascinated by our enchantment with celebrities and their wellness advice. They have thoughts on why we are more likely, at times, to listen to, say, the Kardashians than to our own doctors. There is a phenomenon called *self-conception* that is at work here: if we see someone as the best potential version of ourselves, we will try and replicate what that person does in the hope of achieving that best version. If someone wants to be muscular like Dwayne "The Rock" Johnson, he can try following Johnson's training regime; if someone thinks that Chrissy Teigen's relaxed approach to health and living matches her own self-image, she can try and model herself after Teigen.

When celebrities are serving up good basic advice, such as building up your own self-confidence or finding time to relax after a busy day, the results are often good. When public health experts can get celebrities to encourage habits they would like us to follow—like former First Lady Michelle Obama encouraging kids to eat well and move around, or Angelina Jolie talking about her risks for breast and ovarian cancer—an important service is performed. But when celebrities with no expert knowledge about a subject espouse dubious or even potentially dangerous practices, doctors and public health professionals become concerned.

Celebrity Extravaganza

Although some health and wellness gurus have medical backgrounds—Andrew Weil and Deepak Chopra, for example—or training in other areas, like nutrition, psychology, or physical fitness, many others have neither. We can look at a few examples of both types here.

Gwyneth Paltrow. Actress-turned-health "expert" Gwyneth Paltrow runs the website Goop. The site is frequently in the popular health news, but rarely for good reasons. Paltrow and Goop have advocated intense cleanses, sold pricey rings related to spirit animals (appropriating Native spirituality), and suggested that total body yeast infections and undetectable parasites could be causing your health problems. Goop has also suggested doing various things to the vagina, such as inserting a small "jade egg" to make one feel "grounded," that are simply unnecessary and even risky.

While many people have mocked Paltrow's postfilm career as a health guru, the Goop website continues to be visited by legions of consumers and her products and her advice are in wide circulation.

Jillian Michaels. Jillian Michaels got her start on TV's *The Biggest Loser*, a reality show (2004–2016) that encouraged people who are obese to lose weight through diet and exercise as part of the show. Michaels is a fitness trainer who offers a variety of exercise videos and programs, books on metabolism and diet, and more. Many people have found her approach to fitness encouraging, and have found

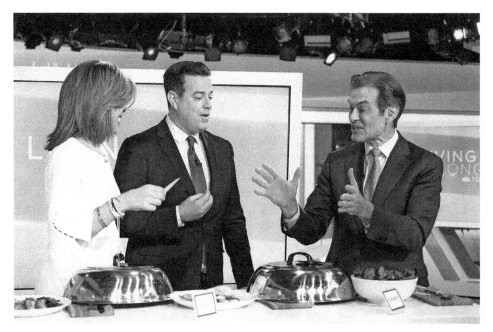

Dr. Mehmet Oz, host of *The Dr. Oz Show*, speaks with Hoda Kotb and Carson Daly of the *Today* show about how to match diet to circadian rhythms in order to live longer, lose weight, and achieve greater overall health. (Nathan Congleton/NBC/NBCU Photo Bank via Getty Images)

better exercise routines and improved strength and cardiovascular health through her training.

Michaels has occasionally come under fire: a lawsuit alleged that some supplements she was selling were either dangerous or useless, although the case was dismissed. It was alleged, too, that she had practiced as a personal trainer when her license had expired, yet in this case again the media outlet was forced to publish a retraction. Michaels has also appeared in TV ads for other products, such as the SodaStream sparkling water system.

Dr. Oz. Dr. Mehmet Oz got his original boost from the Oprah Winfrey show, where he was a frequent guest in the early 2000s. Eventually, he won his own program, called *The Dr. Oz Show*. Trained as a heart surgeon, Oz also espouses the benefits of complementary medicine, holistic healing, and alternative treatments. He has invited guests onto his show who are passionately opposed to vaccines, for example, or who believe that baking soda can cure cancer. Oz himself has said that science is just another religion. Many doctors and scientists have expressed horror at how a man they describe as a brilliant surgeon (with many peer-reviewed articles in medical journals to his name) could have morphed into the celebrity they now see striving for ratings on daytime television.

Jenny McCarthy. Prior to 2007, Jenny McCarthy's main claims to fame were her history as a *Playboy* model, her stints on MTV shows, and a couple of small acting jobs. In 2007, however, she announced that her son, Evan, had been diagnosed with autism, and that he had been cured by chelation therapy (a procedure for removing heavy metals from the body). She stated that Evan had begun showing signs of autism after receiving a standard childhood vaccination, and she launched virtually a whole movement around the idea that autism is caused by vaccines. (It unequivocally is not.)

Several professionals have suggested that McCarthy's son was misdiagnosed to start with. He began to have seizures at a young age, and when the seizures were treated, his development caught up and expressed the autistic symptoms. Such a turn of events is arguably more consistent with other disorders than autism, but it cannot be entirely ruled out that that's what happened. McCarthy, nevertheless, has insisted that Evan's original diagnosis was correct and that he only later "contracted" autism. The antivaccination movement, bolstered by other leaders as well as McCarthy, has had an effect and vaccination rates have fallen slightly in recent years.

Dr. Phil. Another wellness guru who got his start with Oprah Winfrey is Dr. Phil McGraw, a trained psychologist whose show has to do with mental health and wellness. Dr. Phil offers advice to those who are struggling with addiction, relationship issues, and other mental health issues. He has come under fire, however, for shady business practices, derogatory statements about people with mental health issues, and for setting his guests up to be part of a spectacle on his show. Nevertheless, his daytime program remains very popular and has consistently been nominated for an Emmy Award.

Outlook

At first, Americans had to journey to East or South Asia to find their gurus. Later, they found their experts in the self-help section of the bookstore or on daytime TV. Nowadays, social media has changed the way people access health and wellness information. Anyone who can take a picture of their special food preparation or shoot a video of their fitness routine can create a wellness program that can generate followers. Even so, the other media continue to perform in the popular health marketplace, as people continue to subscribe to magazines, buy books, and watch television to learn the latest techniques and find out about the latest products.

Many wellness accounts focus on body appearance and health, on healthily prepared and tasty meals, and on emotional positivity to approach the day. The modern-day gurus and programs that fall into this category can be a beneficial addition to people's lives. Those people, on the other hand, who promote questionable dietary supplements, suggest that their diet will cure cancer, or claim that modern medicine has nothing to offer over their own system, do not serve the public interest and can cause serious damage to the field of health and wellness generally.

Kay Tilden Frost

See also: Aging Prevention, or "Successful Aging"; Anthroposophic Medicine; Dianetics; Diet and Exercise; Est and Other "Human Potential" Therapies; Faith Healing and Prayer; Infomercials and Wellness Promotion; Macrobiotics; Meditation and Mindfulness; Reiki and Therapeutic Touch

Further Reading

Offit, Paul. 2018. *Bad Advice: Or Why Celebrities, Politicians, and Activists Aren't Your Best Source of Health Information.* New York: Columbia University Press.

Stieg, Cory. 2018. "Why We Trust Celebrity Health Advice—Even When It's Wrong." *Refinery29.* July 26. https://www.refinery29.com/en-us/2018/07/205460/goop-gwenyth -paltrow-health-wellness-advice-celebrities

INFOMERCIALS AND WELLNESS PROMOTION

If commercials and infomercials are both trying to sell something to you, what's the difference?

In the 1990s and early 2000s, the difference between the two was fairly obvious. A commercial ran for about thirty seconds during television ad breaks. It promoted a few main features of a product, but it was pretty clearly a product that the audience was expected to already understand. We all know what a vacuum is, for example, so the ad for it would briefly summarize how this vacuum was different from the competition.

Infomercials, in contrast, introduced a new concept or product to the audience. They ran longer than typical commercials—sometimes for a full half-hour—and they often featured the different ways a product could function, and the concept behind it, instead of just highlighting a few important details. They often aired during daytime TV, when homemakers were expected to be watching, or during late-night television, when people were tired and more likely to react to something they saw since their inhibitions were lowered.

Another major difference was that infomercials were a kind of *direct* selling, meaning that viewers were given a phone number or website to use to purchase the product directly, rather than having to find it at a retail outlet. The prices of the items often differed as well, with infomercials featuring products that sometimes cost hundreds or even thousands of dollars, instead of, say, $19.99. Informercials, then, are essentially a type of paid programming, usually preceded by disclaimers saying that "the following is a paid advertisement for X brand," even as the ad might present the information as newsworthy or some kind of "breakthrough" human development. The key change occurred in 1984, when the Federal Communications Commission (FCC) removed rules limiting the length of advertisements.

Yet, with the modern Internet being what it is, the infomercial, too, has gotten an update. Today they are rarely a full half-hour long; most fit into a five-minute YouTube ad. They also appear in ads for crowdfunded products, where having videos to explain how a product is used and what benefits it has means that the project is much more likely to be fully funded by third parties. In early morning or late night, however, one can still find classic infomercials for health products on television.

Of course, all of this ultimately goes back to the era of patent medicines and professional hawkers at medicine shows, which were all the rage in the later 19th and early 20th centuries. The field of health and medicine has long been on the cutting edge of advertising to consumers. Where once various "cure-all" tonics were promoted face-to-face, nowadays an amazing variety of dietary supplements and other health aids are widely advertised on all media. Even hospitals and cancer centers have gotten into the act, presenting high-quality promotions intended to attract paying (or well insured) customers. The medicine show has moved to the media.

From Information to Health and Wellness

Wellness programs can be a variety of things. A lot of employers now have wellness programs attached to their health insurance policies. If someone takes actions that are likely to keep them healthy—maintain a certain body-mass index (BMI) and weight, avoid or stop smoking, have a good cholesterol level and other indicators of heart health—they usually pay less for their health insurance. They may also get certain other benefits in the workplace (like free bottled water) for participating in wellness programs.

But there is a lot more to wellness programs than those designed to just keep your premiums low at work. There are many different products, supplements, and exercise programs being promoted that are designed to get and keep you well—often without you doing any work at all. As most people know, that doesn't always work, yet it didn't stop people from spending $171 million in 2017 on health and wellness products.

Some wellness programs are actually quite effective if they are followed properly. Eating more fruits and vegetables and fewer sweets and starches, getting into a regular exercise program, and avoiding smoking and excessive alcohol use are all good general rules to maintain health. But these are not necessarily the stuff of infomercials, which frequently feature quirky "quick fixes" as they did in the days of the medicine show.

Here are some notable examples of health improvement tools that caught on in the popular consciousness through media promotions.

- The Ionic Breeze Air Purifier. Marketed by the Sharper Image, which prided itself on bringing cutting-edge consumer items to the market, this air purifier was part of a big campaign that saw the item entering into millions of homes in the 1990s. It actually did effectively remove excess airborne dust, allergens, and pet dander, in limited spaces, but most people today manage to live with these things on a daily basis without any serious health effect.

- The Thigh Master. This was an exercise product for the thighs promoted by Suzanne Somers, of TV's *Three's Company* fame (1977–1984). It was claimed to be a "shaping" as well as a strengthening device. Moreover, like many fitness products marketed to homes, the ads presented the Thigh Master as something that could be used while the consumer was doing something else, such as watching television. It was created by a marketer (Josh Reynolds) who had made a fortune previously by selling mood rings. Somers herself went on to become an icon of the popular health industry, creating and selling a number of branded items linked, apparently, to her own recognizable health and beauty.

- The Squatty Potty. According to people who favor bathroom items like the Squatty Potty, we as humans are not meant to defecate in modern toilets. Being in a squatting position (knees higher than the hips) is said to be an ideal position to properly clean the colon and poop more easily. But the people who made Squatty Potty realized that most people in the West find it difficult to squat over a hole in the ground, as was traditionally done worldwide. Their device therefore is a stool that sits in front of the toilet and raises the knees to the ideal defecating position. All of this basically seems sound—but the product was advertised with a unicorn ejecting what looked to be a rainbow-colored ooze of soft-serve ice cream!

- Bow-Flex, Tae-Bo, and other fitness videos. From Jane Fonda to Billy Blanks to Jillian Michaels, fitness videos have a strong appeal to audiences hoping to avoid couch-potato status. They are usually competitive with the cost of enrolling at a gym, and they have the added advantage that you don't have to worry about how you *look* as you would if you were going to the gym. Modern fitness programs like Tae-Bo often also offer customized workouts that can be used depending on how one is feeling, what parts of the body feel weak or need toning, and more. Some programs also come with a consultation with the fitness leader.

- P90X. While Jane Fonda encouraged women in the 1980s to "feel the burn!" P90X was (and remains) an "extreme" fitness program that took things to a whole new level. It combined a home exercise regimen based on cross-training and "periodization" (cycles of intensity) with a nutrition and dietary supplement program. Endorsed by the likes of Sheryl Crow, Michele Obama, and Paul Ryan, this fitness craze (which peaked in 2010) really did provide impressive results, as long the user could manage to keep up with its stringent workout and dietary demands—and, of course, could afford the whole package.

Advertising has changed a lot since the old style of 30-second ads during commercial breaks. Companies have more freedom and flexibility, not just with ad breaks on platforms like Hulu and YouTube but with the ability to post video on one's own website. Companies use social media platforms constantly to get and keep our attention. The job of the consumer, then, is to sort the wheat from the chaff, especially in the area of fitness and diet programs.

Kay Tilden Frost and
Michael Shally-Jensen

See also: Aging Prevention, or "Successful Aging"; Detox Diets; Diet and Exercise; Fat and Obesity Surgery—and Other Weight-Loss Methods; Health and Wellness Gurus; Juice and Juicing; Medicine Shows; Patent Medicines; Self-Help

Further Reading

Cook, Karla. 2017. "Are Infomercials Cool Now?" January 9. https://blog.hubspot.com /marketing/infomercials-examples

Miller, Stephen. 2018. "Does A New Study Underestimate Wellness Programs?" February 5. https://www.shrm.org/resourcesandtools/hr-topics/benefits/pages/does -study-underestimate-wellness-programs.aspx

Sugget, Paul. 2017. "What Exactly Is an Infomercial?" November 13. https://www .thebalancecareers.com/what-exactly-is-an-informercial-38542

JUICE AND JUICING

When we think of juice, a simple glass with breakfast probably comes to mind—orange, apple, grape, or maybe cranberry. Juices that incorporate vegetables aren't really new: V-8, a spiced tomato juice, has been popular for decades, and there are plenty of other such "cocktails" made with tomato and celery juice. But the idea that consuming juice and juiced vegetables gives you health benefits beyond that of simply eating the fruits or vegetables themselves has become popular in the past century, and really popular in the last few decades. Fans of juicing say that it can keep you slim, stave off cancer, and generally make your skin dewy and perfect. Juices are also closely tied to different types of cleanses and so-called colon health.

What's in Your Juice?

Juice has been bottled and sold in the United States since the original Welch's company (founded 1869) realized that by selling "unfermented sacramental wine" (grape juice), he could give Christians obsessed with temperance a way to take communion without drinking a drop of wine. After some bumps in the road, Welch's Grape Juice became something that everyone wanted at home.

Oranges got their day as well. Every home had an orange juice squeezer. You could buy your own oranges, lemons, or limes, half them, and then twist them down and get a disappointingly small amount of juice out of the fruit—or go commercial and buy bottled juice from a company like Minute Maid or Tropicana.

Modern juices, however, tend to go farther out on a limb. They include all sorts of vegetables—carrots, kale, cucumber, and celery are popular—and are often thick enough to count as smoothies. Prune juice is still around too, repackaged from an aid for constipation to a fiber- and vitamin-and-mineral bearing fruit treat. You can also get a number of different juicy-fruity flavors in gummy form, replete with added sugars and thickeners.

We eat fruits and vegetables for the micronutrients and phytonutrients they provide, many of which are not found in meat or dairy. Eating fruits and vegetables is important; but *eating* is the key here: fruits and vegetables have a lot of carbohydrates, which means that they have a lot of (natural) sugar. When you eat them, you get fiber along with that sugar, which makes your body absorb the sugar more slowly. When you drink the juice alone, then, you lose out on that crucial fiber. Your body absorbs the sugar quickly, giving you a big energy rush—generally followed by a big crash. Your blood sugar spikes; over time, those spikes and falls can contribute to Type 2 diabetes.

One of the claims about juicing is that by drinking just the juice, your body can absorb all those micronutrients more efficiently. Science, however, says otherwise; studies have consistently shown that both eating fruits and vegetables and drinking their juice give you the same amount of nutrients—but still without that crucial fiber in the case of juice alone—unless it is added back in by the manufacturer.

Popular Drinks?

If you really dislike eating vegetables, it is better to juice them than to skip them altogether; but one way to get all the nutrient benefits without cutting out the fiber is to make a smoothie with your veggies. Since smoothies pulverize the fruit rather than just squeezing out the juice, the fiber is still present. You don't even have to use only veggies, either; you can add a handful of spinach to your apple-blueberry-yogurt smoothie and you won't even taste the greenery—although the color may look a little strange.

But if you are dedicated to juicing, then know that you are in good company. Numerous celebrities shout about the benefits of these drinks.

- Drew Barrymore, who posted about her love of green juice on her Instagram, talking about how drinking green juice made her feel like an adult.
- Zac Efron says that he drops a fizzy tablet into his water every day that turns it into an amazing green juice extravaganza.
- Michelle Williams has said that she is obsessed with any and all green juices, that they're easy to use and make her feel great.
- Blake Lively favors juice that includes kale, beets, and half a lemon. She says it's better than any po'boy you'll ever eat.
- Debra Messing starts her day with a juice that includes kale, celery, beet, and cucumber. She says this is great for her, since she "isn't a green vegetable person."

Of course, these are celebrities doing and saying things that celebrities do and say; it doesn't mean that they know what they're talking about, nutritionally, or that you should necessarily follow them.

The Juice-Cleanse Tie

It is hard to talk about juicing without talking about how it links to the fad of juice cleanses. Several different cleanse options start with nothing but water for a day or two, then gradually add in fruit and vegetable juices to help "flush toxins" out of the body. The Master Cleanse may be the most famous juice-related cleanse on the market, but now there are dozens of others specifically designed to help you cleanse your system.

Doctors say that all of these cleanses are basically a bad idea, and can backfire in a big way. First of all, cleanses for weight loss do not work. Any weight loss based on juicing tends to be temporary, with an immediate weight gain once one starts eating again.

Second, your body naturally cleanses itself through your liver. Eating healthier is usually a good idea, but you shouldn't need any special juices to accomplish it.

Juice diets can actually put significant strain on your kidneys. If you're prone to kidney stones, for example, heavy juicing can cause them to become much worse.

Juice: Yea or Nay?

The occasional glass of fruit juice is certainly not going to hurt you. Know, however, that it is high in natural sugars. Vegetable juice is often a better option than fruit juice, if only because the ingredients have lower sugar overall and typically they contain added fiber as well. And, yes, drinking your fruits and vegetables is a good way to make sure you are getting them into your body period, if you would not be likely to do so otherwise.

But if you are looking for the healthiest way to support your system, a green smoothie may be better for you than any glass of juice. Toss some spinach, a chopped apple, and a little water if necessary into a blender, and you'll have a delicious veggie-fruit smoothie that is also healthy. And, obviously, you can experiment with other combinations until you find just the one for you.

Kay Tilden Frost

See also: Antioxidants; Bottled Water; Detox Diets; Diet and Exercise; Eating Organic; Herbal Remedies; Macrobiotics; Paleo Diet; Vegetarianism; Vitamins and Minerals

Further Reading

Arnold, Amanda. 2016. "License to Kale." *Broadly.* May 23. https://broadly.vice.com/en_us/article/qkg777/history-of-juice

Jennings, Karry Ann. "Health Benefits of Juicing." *Food Network.* November 21.https://www.foodnetwork.com/healthy/articles/health-benefits-of-juicing

Nall, Rachel. 2018. "What Are the Pros and Cons of a Juice Cleanse?" *Medical News Today.* September 21. https://www.medicalnewstoday.com/articles/323136.php

MIND–BODY MEDICINE

Mind–body medicine is generally conceived of, in the West, as a subdivision of the broad field of complementary and alternative medicine (CAM)—or those approaches that, to one degree or another, fall outside conventional medicine.

According to the National Center for Complementary and Alternative Medicine (NCCAM website 2016), a branch of the National Institutes of Health (NIH), CAM consists of a variety of holistic health and natural approaches, including herbal products, dietary supplements, mind–body medicine, manipulative and body-based practices, energy medicine, exercise and movement therapies, expressive art therapies, and a broad array of other practices that do not fit neatly into one category. Complementary practices "complement" mainstream practices (e.g., exercise and movement therapies) while alternative practices are "alternatives" to mainstream practices because they are based on different premises (e.g., homeopathic theory). Some practices fall under both categories—for example, Chinese traditional medicine.

According to NCCAM, the main premise behind mind–body medicine is that a focus on the interactions between the mind and body (i.e., brain, and behavior) will impact physical and mental well-being and promote health. The historical roots of integrating the mind and body as an important element in the treatment of illness dates back over 2,000 years to traditional Chinese medicine, ancient Greek medicine, Ayurvedic medicine, and similar holistic approaches. In the past few decades, CAM has gained increasing popularity in Western cultures, as indicated in the 2012 National Health Interview Survey (NHIS), which revealed that over one-third of Americans used some type of CAM (NCCAM website 2016).

The approaches, or modalities, that fall under the domain of mind–body medicine include yoga, meditation, acupuncture, guided imagery, hypnotically facilitated psychotherapy, progressive muscle relaxation, Qigong, Tai Chi, and biofeedback, to name a few. However, it could be argued that all healing modalities fall under the mind–body domain to some extent, since at a deeper level there is no justifiable way to delineate mind from body. However, CAM approaches are geared toward integrating what a culture considers "body" and what that culture considers "mind" (including "emotions" and "spirit") to improve health; whereas more conventional medical approaches segment these into separate domains. For example, Reiki—which also falls under the "energy medicine" domain—is geared toward the movement of the hypothetical construct of some sort of "energy" to remove mind and body blockages in order to promote health. While this technique does not use physical touch, its clients are typically passive recipients of its treatment. Clients do not have to meditate, visualize, or relax. The hoped-for result is that the effects of this treatment will impact the mind and the body by at least inducing relaxation and perhaps by more deeply affecting other mechanisms that remain unknown.

Although the full range of mind–body approaches is fairly diverse, some are more popular in the United States than others. For example, the 2012 NHIS survey found that nearly 11 percent of adults practiced some sort of deep breathing; 10.1 percent practiced yoga, Tai Chi, or Qigong; 8 percent practiced meditation; 6.9 percent practiced massage; 2.2 percent had used homeopathy; and 1.7 percent made use of guided imagery (NCCAM website 2016). Smaller percentages reported employing other practices such as acupuncture, biofeedback, healing touch, Reiki, movement therapies, and more. The 2012 NHIS survey showed that utilization of mind–body approaches had substantially increased as compared with previous NHIS survey results.

Because many of the major mind–body approaches are discussed separately in the present volume, here we just provide some background information and describe a few general principles.

Background

Until about 300 years ago in the West, virtually all medicine and philosophy treated mind and body as an integral whole. With the Enlightenment of the 18th century, however, new paradigms emerged that considered the body and mind as separate and each as functioning according to mechanistic principles. Those mechanistic models, and the scientific reductionism on which they were based, worked well enough in dealing with the many infectious diseases—smallpox, tuberculosis, cholera—that devastated populations in earlier periods. In the contemporary era, however, the diseases that kill most people in developed nations are not infectious diseases but chronic, degenerative diseases like heart disease, hypertension, cancer, and diabetes along with substance abuse and addition. These conditions are tightly linked to psychological, lifestyle, social, and environmental factors. They are conditions whose treatment with mind–body medicine and a holistic health approach can generally be useful.

Interest in mind–body medicine has been advanced by the introduction, and increasing acceptance, of Asian healing systems into mainstream U.S. culture. In the last half of the 20th century, for example, researchers discovered that people who practice yoga proficiently are able to regulate bodily functions that once were thought to lie outside the control of conscious thought, including electrical activity in the brain, body temperature, heart rate, and blood pressure. In examining some of these Asian healing systems, researchers found them to be beneficial in helping to prevent or even heal conditions that, earlier, had been accepted as a natural part of the adult aging process or of life in the contemporary era.

Medical research on aging has shown that those who live longer often display psychological, social, and lifestyle characteristics that contribute positively to their longevity or "successful aging." Those characteristics include staying socially connected with others, maintaining a sense of purpose, sustaining a positive attitude, remaining physically and mentally active, and making optimal use of conventional medicine as well as appropriate CAM therapies (Pelletier 2000, 60). Discovering the overall health benefits of mind–body connections such as these has helped propel mind–body medicine to the forefront of popular awareness and within the complementary and alternative medicine field generally.

Eastern Principles

In contrast to the West's fascination with distinguishing between body and mind, matter and energy, Eastern healing methods, particularly those of China, traditionally concentrate on pattern and process. Instead of asking what things are made of and how they work, the Chinese philosophers wondered why, if everything in the universe is in a state of flux, the forms we see maintain a constant, though evolving, presence. Western scientists focused on identifying chains of cause and effect, whereas Eastern naturalists observed correspondences between things and events at two different scales—microcosm and macrocosm. Europeans examined things and their parts through systematic study; Chinese thinkers and practitioners, on the other hand, examined relationships, patterns, and processes from a holistic perspective. As the historian of science and sinologist Joseph Needham has written,

> The key-word in Chinese thought is *Order* and above all *Pattern*. . . . The symbolic correlations or correspondences [they saw] all formed part of one colossal pattern. Things behaved in particular ways not necessarily because prior actions or impulsions of other things, but because their position in the ever-moving cyclical universe was such that they were endowed with intrinsic natures which made that behavior inevitable for them. If they did not behave in those particular ways they would lose their relational positions in the whole (which made them what they were), and turn into something other than themselves. They were thus parts in existential dependence upon the whole world-organism. And they reacted upon one another not so much by mechanical impulsion or causation as by a kind of mysterious resonance. (quoted in Milburn 2016, 257)

Thus, in Chinese medicine, and in Eastern medicine generally, practitioners think differently about the occurrence of a disease. Rather than look solely for material causes, they seek to identifying the underlying patterns of imbalance, taking mind–body to represent a single, complete system in which a given illness is set. Both mental and physical signs and symptoms are included in understanding any pattern of disharmony. For example, a patient seeking help for a digestive problem may be asked about any emotional disturbances or family problems—if these are not already evident to the physician. Similarly, a patient referred for excessive irritability or anger will likely have his or her liver considered during the examination, as that is considered the seat of such feelings and could also produce accompanying digestive troubles. And no matter what the final "diagnosis" is, the treatment will center on adjusting the qi (energy), which serves as the bridge between the body and the mind.

Likewise, in the Ayurvedic healing tradition of India, two fundamental principles, matter (*prakruti*) and spirit (*purusha*), are said to be present in everything. These principles operate through the five elements (space, air, fire, water, earth) and, according to the three basic human constitutions (*vata, pitta,* and *kapa*), to bring health or illness to the individual. The Ayurvedic system of healing is designed to restore harmony to the mind, body, and spirit by rebalancing the primary life forces. As one noted researcher and practitioner, David Frawley, has written,

> Ayurveda is the medicine of nature, the medicine of life. It does not give us a set of theoretical principles to impose upon our biological functioning. Rather, it seeks to

present to the human mind the principles and powers of Nature herself. It teaches us to put into practice Nature's great principles of health and natural living. For this reason it employs the language of nature—an energetic system of the elements and biological humors, a simple yet profound system of correspondences, not a complex, scientific, materialistic or biochemical terminology. (quoted in Cantin 2016, 316)

For these reasons and more, mind–body medicine has become enormously popular in Western countries among those seeking complementary or alternative strategies in treating their own medical conditions or in helping others to heal. After all, even in the West we say, "Your health is not a debt you just cancel. The body collects" (both mental and physical damage; *Sharp Objects* 2018).

Michael Shally-Jensen

See also: Acupuncture; Aging Prevention, or "Successful Aging"; Anger and Anger Management; Ayurvedic Medicine; Chinese Traditional Medicine; Guided Imagery or Visualization; Health and Wellness Gurus; Herbal Remedies; Meditation and Mindfulness; Naturopathic Medicine; Reflexology; Reiki and Therapeutic Touch; Shiatsu; Tai Chi and Qigong; Yoga

Further Reading

Cantin, Candis. 2016. "Ayurvedic Healing." In *Natural Healing: Wisdom and Know-How*, edited by Amy Rost, 316–55. New York: Black Dog and Leventhal.

Harrington, Anne. 2008. *The Cure Within: A History of Mind–Body Medicine.* New York: W. W. Norton.

Milburn, Michael P. 2016. "The Foundations of Chinese Medicine." In *Natural Healing: Wisdom and Know-How*, edited by Amy Rost, 250–71. New York: Black Dog and Leventhal..

Pelletier, Kenneth R. 2000. *The Best Alternative Medicine.* New York: Simon and Schuster/ Fireside.

Sharp Objects. 2018. "Falling," season 1, episode 7. HBO.

NATUROPATHIC MEDICINE

Drawing on the resources available from the earth, naturopathic medicine relies for its healing methods on natural products and a repertoire of tried-and-true techniques. In fact, naturopathic medicine—or naturopathy—is not a single type of therapy but rather an umbrella term for a wide array of complementary and alternative health-care strategies. What these strategies have in common within the naturopathic paradigm is the use of interventions based on natural substances and a focus on the particular needs of individual patients—as opposed to the treatment of disease in a "generic" fashion à la conventional medicine.

Some naturopaths prefer to think of naturopathic medicine as a system of "classical" or "traditional" medicine rather than as a complementary or alternative medicine, because of its historical roots and the fact that it served as *the* form of medicine before there was (modern) medicine. Naturopathy goes back to a time when trained healers or physicians studied aspects of health, in the broadest sense, as well as the formation of disease. They drew on the healing power of plants and the elements that surrounded them along with the body's ability to heal itself under the proper conditions. The combination of natural products and the innate healing power of the body was, and is, viewed as a reliable way to help patients "rebalance" physiological systems and produce health and well-being.

Naturopathic medicine stands on the idea that one should treat diseases by treating individuals. A series of patients complaining of cold or flu symptoms may visit a naturopath's office during a seasonal outbreak, yet each one may leave with a different treatment plan. In truth, there is often some overlap among treatment options, but the intent is to address the individual and his or her physiological circumstances. The philosophy of naturopathic medicine allows for the use of an array of substances and a diverse group of practices.

During a visit, the naturopathic doctor, or ND, will likely take a medical history, perform an exam, possibly order lab tests, and make a diagnosis. Once the nature of the illness has been determined, the treatment plan may include nutritional counseling, for example, along with a homeopathic prescription and a discussion of how a particular exercise or movement regimen might be beneficial to the patient's health. The discussion could touch on overlying factors such as job pressures or family issues and how they impact the patient's life.

As students, those pursuing careers in naturopathy study most of the major medical sciences—anatomy and physiology, biochemistry, pathology, clinical and physical diagnosis, pharmacology, and the like—in courses like those taught in medical schools. Additionally, they spend months and years studying courses that have largely vanished from the medical school curriculum, including nutrition, exercise therapeutics, homeopathy, herbal/botanical medicine, hydrotherapy, physical therapy, counseling, and more.

It is especially in the area of illness prevention and the promotion of health that naturopathic medicine has left its mark in U.S. consumer culture. Both of these have become big business as more and more people seek natural, over-the-counter supplements and methods and the knowledge with which to use them. Naturopathy helped spur the growth in this market and has benefited from it, in turn. At the same time, people living with chronic conditions have sought naturopathic solutions too. Those who experience migraine, eczema, osteoarthritis, back pain, atherosclerosis, irritable bowel syndrome, recurring infections, and other conditions have often turned to naturopathic remedies, either out of preference or in order to complement treatments they receive through conventional medicine.

Naturopathic medicine, then, is very much a "lifestyle" medicine. It rejects the idea that some "magic bullet" in pill form from a pharmacy is going to cure all of one's ills; instead it embraces the idea of working to support the body and mind to bring out the healing powers intrinsic to all living matter. Clients who assume that they can eat processed food, avoid exercise, live mostly indoors, smoke, drink in excess, keep an irregular schedule of sleep and work, and spend much of their time using screens, and then be spared illness through the wonders of modern drugs are fooling themselves, in the eyes of naturopathic practitioners. Naturopathy's preferred medicines are plant and mineral preparations combined with healthy lifestyle choices.

A naturopath's recommended treatments tend to reflect his or her specialty, such as herbal/botanical treatments, homeopathic remedies, or nutritional solutions. Most naturopaths will focus initially on understanding the biological and physiological factors that might be causing an illness and then use herbal medicines or other interventions. They may also seek to enhance one's general health, thereby encouraging prevention. A healthy body is understood to make for a less severe, less lasting illness and to prevent recurrence. Naturopathic medicine, in short, is holistic medicine.

One of the naturopathic doctor's primary duties is to educate people about their conditions, thus encouraging them to monitor and improve their own health. Part of the time in a naturopath's office is spent in consultation, as naturopaths provide information about their suggested approach. Following the traditional physician's creed, the naturopath seeks, above all, to "do no harm." The ideal is to use the least invasive treatment possible, hoping thereby to avoid the side effects associated with pharmaceutical drugs or similar strong measures common to a clinical setting.

Ultimately, therefore, naturopathic medicine is a philosophy and a way of life. Consider this passage, written by a noted naturopathic physician:

> True preventative medicine requires making daily investments in our health: eating foods that nourish our bodies, exercising, developing loving relationships and supportive communities, contributing to the health of the Earth. Healthy people live in healthy environments. Preventative medicine means working for clean air, land, and water. Human health is inseparable from the health of the planet. (Boice 2016, 15)

Historical Background

The chief early proponent of naturopathy was the German-American businessman Benedict Lust (1872–1945). Lust had come to America at the age of 20 to launch his business career but immediately contracted tuberculosis and nearly died. On returning to Germany, he underwent hydrotherapy (water treatment) at a "bath" (*bad*) in Wörishofen run by a popular practitioner, Sebastian Kneipp. Lust then resumed his pursuits in New York, only now his main interest was in promoting hydropathy and Kneipp's herbal bath products. By 1900 he had expanded his vision to include a wide variety of natural components and certain activities to promote one's health. Lust's naturopathic system consisted of baths, herbs, and other "drugless" cures as well as programs in diet, exercise, massage, and sunbathing. One practice he borrowed from Kneipp was that of walking barefoot in snow or wet grass to harden the constitution. One that he added himself was mud baths, which he saw as a means to absorb the magnetic properties of the Earth. The overall idea was to cultivate a natural robustness in order to ward off disease and function optimally. Lust opened the first school of naturopathy in midtown Manhattan in 1901, from which he also sold health foods and other wares. An advertisement for the school noted that "within every human" was the potential for "Massive Muscle, Surging Blood, Tingling Nerve, Zestful Digestion, Superb Sex, Beautiful

Body, Sublime Thought, Pulsating Power," and more (quoted in Whorton 2002, 196). With his wife, Louisa, Lust also opened a resort for paying clients, Yungborn, in the Ramapo Mountains of New Jersey.

By the 1920s Lust's enterprises were booming and naturopathy was competing with chiropractic, osteopathy, and other burgeoning alternative medicines on the scene. There were now more than a dozen schools of naturopathy, a professional society (the American Naturopathic Association), and several naturopathic journals. One devotee of naturopathy who went on to popularize his own version of physical robustness, Bernarr Macfadden, published the widely circulated *Physical Culture* magazine. All the while, Lust and other naturopaths were forced to fend off criticisms from medical professionals about the unproven claims they made and the lack of control over licensing—almost anyone could claim to be a naturopath or to hold the title ND.

During the Depression naturopathy, like most everything else, suffered a decline. When Lust died in 1945, from complications related to smoke inhalation during a fire at Yungborn, the founding era of naturopathy died with him—and what was left of the field was in trouble. The rise of modern biomedicine and drug therapy saw most patients going to regular doctors for their ailments, not complementary clinicians. Through the 1950s and most of the 1960s, naturopathy remained a small player. It reemerged in the 1970s, however, as "naturopathic medicine" during the rise of the holistic health movement, and it took off in the 1980s as a broad *category* which now included things like herbalism, traditional/tribal medicine, homeopathy, aromatherapy, massage, energy medicine, and even acupuncture and various other nonpharmaceutical approaches.

With a new generation at the helm, and vastly changed circumstances in the medical marketplace, naturopathic doctors came to embrace research and more rigorous training in their field. Medical doctors, in turn, came to appreciate naturopathy's emphasis on health maintenance and "knowing one's body." Today, NDs and MDs are not inevitably in sharp opposition, though a clear gap remains to be bridged. Meanwhile, patients often make use of both systems to serve their own purposes.

Michael Shally-Jensen

See also: Ayurvedic Medicine; Bottled Water; Eating Organic; Folk Medicine; Health and Wellness Gurus; Herbal Remedies; Homeopathy; Hydrotherapy; Magnet Therapy; Mind–Body Medicine; Paleo Diet; Spas and Mineral Waters; Vegetarianism; Vitamins and Minerals; Walking and Jogging

Further Reading

Boice, Judith. 2016. "Naturopathy." In *Natural Healing: Wisdom and Know-How,* edited by Amy Rost, 13–46. New York: Black Dog and Leventhal.

Cayleff, Susan E. 2016. *Nature's Path: A History of Naturopathic Healing in America.* Baltimore: Johns Hopkins University Press.

Whorton, James C. 2002. *Nature Cures: The History of Alternative Medicine in America.* New York: Oxford University Press.

PAST LIFE REGRESSION THERAPY

Consider this scene from a medieval Japanese classic:

> The Emperor had turned eight that year, but seemed very grown up for his age. His face was radiantly beautiful, and his abundant black hair reached below his waist. "Where are you taking me, Grandmother?" he asked, with a puzzled look.
>
> She turned her face to the young sovereign, holding back her tears. "Don't you understand? You became an Emperor because you obeyed the Ten Good Precepts in your last life, but now an evil karma holds you fast in its toils. Your good fortune has come to an end. Turn to the east and say goodbye to the Grand Shrine of Ise, then turn to the west and repeat the sacred name of Amida Buddha, so that he and his host may come to escort you to the Pure Land. This country is a land of sorrow; I am taking you to a happy realm called Paradise." (McCullough 1990)

Reincarnation, or the rebirth of the soul in successive bodies, is a widely held belief. For example, the Orphics of ancient Greece believed that the soul was reborn several times and that it became purified each time by one's living a good life (or, alternatively, fouled by one's living a bad life). Similarly, Hindu religion holds that rebirth in a higher form depends on the moral rectitude and positive acts one shows in the present life. This is the doctrine of karma, or the impact of an individual's past actions on future lives. Likewise, in Buddhism in order to escape the endless cycle of birth, death, and rebirth and achieve nirvana—release from existence and realization of the ultimate state of bliss—one must first attain enlightenment by progressively learning about spiritual devotion and exhibiting righteous behavior. Among various Native American peoples, too, there has long been a belief in one's ability to return to life in another form. The Caribou Inuit, for example, believe that the dead are brought back to Earth, with the help of the moon, to live again not as human beings but as animals, birds, and fishes. In Pueblo Indian religion, the kachinas, or supernatural beings, are thought when killed to become deer. The Venda of southern Africa believe that when a person dies, the soul stays near the grave for a period of time and then seeks a new body—human or animal. For that matter, although Christianity does not have an explicit doctrine of reincarnation, some early Gnostics believed in it, and the Christian doctrine of salvation does allow for the migration of the individual's soul to another, "higher" existence (in heaven) after death.

Toward the end of the 19th century, the Russian spiritualist and author Helena Petrovna Blavatsky, otherwise known as Madame Blavatsky (1831–1891), explored Hinduism in India and came to establish the Theosophical Society there. She later lived in and traveled extensively in the United States, Europe, and elsewhere in Asia, spreading the message of theosophy. Theosophy draws on Eastern religions and Western mystic traditions in laying out a vision of "divine wisdom." It argues that a deeper spiritual reality exists and offers extensive discussions of the ways and means to access that reality. Although initially denying the existence of reincarnation, Blavatsky later became convinced that it was real, and that knowledge of karma helped to ensure that people lived according to moral principles. She brought international notice to the young Jiddu Krishnamurti (1895–1986), who himself later became a popular writer and lecturer, advancing the cause of theosophy in the United States and Europe. In short, the theosophists, together with another cross-cultural phenomenon, Annie Besant (1847–1933), helped pave the way for later movements like the International Society for Krishna Consciousness (or Hare Krishnas), transcendental meditation, Zen Buddhism, and yoga—all of which contain or are sympathetic toward the idea of reincarnation.

It might be added that the Church of Scientology also has a doctrine of reincarnation, according to which the *thetan*, or the spiritual being living in the body, can live hundreds or even millions of times over the centuries and millennia before leaving the world permanently as an elevated being. The therapeutic part of Scientology, called auditing, in part gauges the status of the thetan and how close it is to achieving immortality.

Past Life Therapy

In light of this history, it is not all that surprising that forms of *treatment* arose that explicitly address the problem of past lives and how they might affect one's current life. It is based on the idea that the soul is eternal and incarnates again and again, retaining knowledge and awareness of events that occurred in each successive lifetime. The person's past actions in any one lifetime condition the situations, behaviors, reactions, and outcomes of the next life. Thus, if in a previous lifetime one was murdered, say, or died in a terrible accident, then in one's current life the person may have to deal with more than the usual amount of grief and violence, for example, or with dark moods and attempts to escape or run away.

While the notion of past lives began as an Eastern religious doctrine, since the dawn of the New Age movement in the late 1960s and 1970s it has been a part of the alternative therapeutic community in the United States and Europe. Today, therapists use hypnosis, guided imagery, or other means to bring to light the past lives of individual clients in order to resolve situations and disturbances affecting their current lives and bring healing. The focus is on helping people to "reframe" their understanding of the present by uncovering the nature and meaning of their past(s), thus serving to "unblock" their minds and their bodies and allow them to live according to a deeper "harmony" cutting across generations (Talbot 1987).

Needless to say, this whole approach is frowned upon by the mainstream medical community, whose members see it as unscientific and mystical, at best, and delusionary and regrettable, at worst. The use of hypnosis, in particular, to direct clients to "remember" their pasts has come under fire. Critics claim that it encourages the fabrication of false memories and fantasized experiences. In this respect, past life regression shares something with the recovered memory movement, which likewise claims to be able to help people remember long-buried memories (in this life)—usually of a horrific nature. Both have been the subject of critical scrutiny and public controversy.

Popular Portrayals

Although there do not seem to be, as yet, any blockbuster works for general audiences treating the subject of past life regression therapy specifically, there are a number of published accounts by those who have gone through the process and found it helpful, as well as books by those who conduct therapy sessions using the technique and sing its praises.

One such advocate, who has achieved a degree of renown, is Brian Weiss (1944–). Weiss followed a traditional trajectory in medicine, attending Yale University School of Medicine and doing a two-year residency at the Yale Psychiatric Institute. He went on to become head of psychiatry at the Mount Sinai Medical Center, Miami—a prestigious position. In the early 1980s Weiss began researching past life regression after one of his patients, under hypnosis, began speaking about the past lives she had led. Weiss became convinced that the phenomenon was real and that patients could benefit from having them explore their past existences. He wrote a popular book on the subject, *Many Lives, Many Masters* (1988), in which, besides declaring the existence of an eternal soul and reincarnation, he claimed to have found evidence of certain "super-evolved, nonphysical souls," or "Masters," who communicate with the living about transgenerational life and other matters. Despite criticism from his medical colleagues, Weiss continued practicing past life therapy, lecturing, and publishing books, including one about the notion that each of us has a "soulmate" from a past incarnation waiting to reunite with us in the present. He founded the Weiss Institute in Miami to promote his message and has been interviewed on television by Oprah Winfrey, among other activities.

Moving beyond the subject of therapy per se, one can find a number of notable novels and/or major motion pictures that have dealt with the topic of reincarnation and past lives. These include *A Dog's Purpose* (2017; Lasse Hallström, dir.; based on 2010 novel by W. Bruce Cameron), starring Josh Gad (voice), Britt Robertson, and others; *I Origins* (2014; Mike Cahill, dir.), starring Michael Pitt and Brit Marling; *Cloud Atlas* (2012; The Wachowskis, dirs.; based on 2004 novel by David Mitchell), starring Tom Hanks, Halle Berry, and other top actors; *The Lovely Bones* (2009; Peter Jackson, dir.; based on 2002 novel by Alice Sebold), starring Saoirse Ronan (voice), Mark Wahlberg, Rachel Weisz, and others; *The Fountain* (2006; Darren Aronofsky, dir.), starring Hugh Jackman and, again, Rachel Weisz; and *Birth* (2004; Jonathan Glazer, dir.), starring Nicole Kidman, Cameron Bright, and others.

It seems that as long as there is life, death, and a struggle in between, the concept of reincarnation is going to be with us, and people are going to examine that concept for its potential benefits in therapeutic situations.

Michael Shally-Jensen

See also: Astrology; Dianetics; Existential Psychotherapy; Faith Healing and Prayer; Jung and Jungian Analysis; Recovered Memory Therapy, "Split Personality," and Satanism; Spiritualism; Voodoo and Santería

Further Reading

Barham, Ann C. 2016. *The Past Life Perspective: Discovering Your True Nature across Multiple Lifetimes.* New York: Simon and Schuster, Atria/Enliven Books.

McCullough, Helen Craig, trans. 1990. *The Tale of the Heike.* Stanford, CA: Stanford University Press.

Talbot, Michael. 1987. *Your Past Lives: A Reincarnation Handbook.* New York: Harmony Books.

Weiss, Brian L. 1988. *Many Lives, Many Masters.* New York: Simon and Schuster/Fireside.

RECOVERED MEMORY THERAPY, "SPLIT PERSONALITY," AND SATANISM

How are a type of memory-centered psychotherapy, the phenomenon of "split personality" (or "multiple personality"), and the scourge known as Satanism related? The story of their connectedness is one of the more strange and fascinating tales in the history of U.S. popular culture and mental health care.

Deep Memory

Recovered memory therapy (RMT) is, or has been in the past, one of the most controversial mental health treatments. Indeed, RMT is not a specific method or approach but rather a mixed bag of investigatory and therapeutic techniques that include hypnosis, guided imagery, psychoanalytic-like inquiry, and even drug-assisted interviewing involving the use of "truth serums" such as sodium amytal. The phenomenon of "recovered memories"—or the retrieval of images, thoughts, and feelings linked to supposedly long-hidden, long-forgotten experiences from childhood—lies at the heart of RMT and has been the subject of major disputes in and out of psychology, psychiatry, and counseling. Both recovered memories and recovered memory therapy are, and forever will be, associated with events that took place in California in the mid- to late 1980s and that entailed accusations of sex abuse and "Satanic ritual abuse" at a children's daycare facility called the McMartin Preschool. RMT is *not* to be confused with the recovery movement (q.v.), which has an entirely separate origin and trajectory. However, it does share some superficial similarities with the technique known as past-life regression (q.v.).

RMT is also associated, historically, with another sensational human mental condition, that formerly known as "split personality" or "multiple personality disorder" (MPD) but more recently, owing to evolving understandings within the mental health community, referred to as dissociative identity disorder (DID). A couple of decades ago, after MPD had already been long established, psychologists and psychiatrists began to recognize something about their MPD patients: the person so diagnosed did not inevitably have "multiple personalities" but rather had a personality structure that was fractured or compartmentalized. Thus, instead of thinking in terms of separate and distinct individuals or "alters," each with his or her own personality, the new perspective encouraged clinicians to see each fragment or compartment of a personality structure as being tied to a situation or experience in which the person responded in a particular way. The human self was there, more or less, but was unable to integrate, or remain constant, across different scenarios. Dissociative states were more a matter of failing to hold together as oneself, as it were, than of "split" personalities operating totally outside of each other. With DID, two or more conscious personas, or alters, control behavior, but usually only one of them dominates at any given moment and both operate essentially from the same underlying "self structure." It is a puzzling and disturbing phenomenon.

In order to understand how MPD/DID is related to recovered memory therapy, and to Satanism, we need to go back in time and look at some old movies.

Multiple Personality Goes to the Movies

Originally identified in the medical literature as a rarity, "multiple personality" was known at least since the late 19th century when *The Strange Case of Dr. Jekyll and Mr. Hyde* made its debut. In that famous story, Dr. Henry Jekyll is portrayed as a fine fellow who nevertheless is besieged by evil thoughts and, indeed, an evil character hiding within. The disorder from which Jekyll suffered remained relatively obscure, however, until it gained notoriety once again with the release, in 1957, of the film *The Three Faces of Eve*. Starring Joanne Woodward in the role of a woman with three personalities—Eve White, Eve Black, and Jane—the film was based on a popular case study by two psychiatrists concerning one of their patients. One of the book's coauthors, Hervey Cleckley, earlier had researched the nature of psychopaths (or sociopaths), and both authors, in collaboration, had practiced coma shock therapy, electroshock therapy, and lobotomy—all rather heavy-handed measures to treat those suffering from serious mental illness. In *The Three Faces of Eve*, however, both the book and the film, the patient is depicted as being "cured" by remembering, through counseling, a traumatic event in her childhood and coming to terms with it. It is said that she had "split" away from herself as a defense mechanism against the threatening memory. That outcome stands at odds with the recollections of the actual patient in the case study, Chris Costner Sizemore, who later reported that she was never really cured but only managed to function better following therapy. Costner Sizemore also steadfastly maintained that, contrary to the most recent theories, "my former alters were not [just] fragments of my birth personality. They were entities, whole in their own rights, who coexisted with my birth personality before I was born. They were not me, but they remain intrinsically related to what it means to be me" (Costner 1989, 211). Quite well said, and quite frightening if true.

Another milestone in the popularization of MPD was the best-selling nonfiction book *Sybil* (1973), also made into a hugely popular movie (1976) starring Sally Field. Sibyls, of course, were, in ancient Greece, oracular women thought to possess prophetic powers. In this case, Sybil Dorsett was a Columbia University grad student who in the mid-1950s visited the office of a psychoanalyst named

Cornelia Wilbur and ended up staying in her care for eleven years. The case was written about in a mass-market paperback—*Sybil*—by the journalist Flora Rheta Schreiber. Oddly enough, the film based on the book saw the return of Joanne Woodward to the screen in the role, this time, of Sybil's/Field's therapist, Dr. Wilbur. More momentous than that, however, is the recognition, ex post facto, that some or most of the real Sybil's supposed 16 personalities probably were generated by the very therapy that was meant to cure her. Dr. Wilbur, that is, did not "discover" those personalities simply by exploring matters with her patient; she seems, instead, to have helped create them. Audiotapes of the therapeutic sessions with Sybil reveal that various "truth serums" were administered, leading questions were asked, hypnotic states were induced and manipulated, and so on. All of this amounted to a clear case of psychological "suggestion," at best, or coercion, at worst. The numerous Sybil alters, in other words, were formed in the crucible of the therapeutic situation itself.

A similar observation could be made with regard to the mass media and its treatment of MPD. As the popularity of the *Sybil* movie and book expanded, the incidence of reported cases of MPD among young women (and, to a lesser extent, young men) began to increase. The media, in other words, helped bring about the illness it had meant merely to portray. This was because a suggestible or fragile personality, when exposed to an apparently fitting diagnosis—not to mention an increasingly famous one—is likely to take on symptoms of that diagnosis or condition. Books, movies, and pop psychology stories in magazines can have real effects in this regard. The psychology of human deception and self-deception is powerful in that way. In the era of *Sybil*, professional therapists helped too, by regularly coaching patients toward the conclusion that they must be suffering from MPD. By the 1980s, a raft of new

"Sybils" had emerged on the scene and MPD was practically normalized. Some patients were found to have 100 or more alters. As one scholar noted about the mainly female pool of victims, "literary and social history suggest . . . that for over a century, multiplicity has offered women a way to express forbidden aspects of the self" (Showalter 1997, 164). Thus, perhaps the proliferating alters were a means to get to new places—both in the mind and in society. Maybe MPD should be construed (in the manner of Eve) as a psychic solution to a troubled existence—an existence often involving sexual abuse. Dissociation, after all, basically means to "get away" via mental means.

Looking at the condition more closely, MPD can be said to have one prominent characteristic: the young child, in order to make sense of what is happening to her, begins to form "parts" of herself (or himself). Such "compartmentalizing" can start at a very early age, often as young as two or three years. It invariably starts with abuse—verbal, sexual, physical, or some combination of the three. And it is often familial abuse (i.e., taking place within a dysfunctional family). Because of such abuse, the child has to get away, so she does so through her imagination. She escapes mentally to "somewhere else." The child "leaves" or dissociates in order to feel safe. She can be somewhere safe, psychically speaking, somewhere where she can regain a sense of personal control. The situation is such that the abuse or trauma seems to be happening to "that girl over there" rather than to oneself (Hunter 2013).

From MPD to "Satanic Ritual Abuse"

Now, also happening in the 1980s was the rise of a new breed of "tabloid" television talk show in which hosts invited ordinary people—as opposed to celebrities—onstage to tell their personal stories and get reactions from audiences. These were shows like *Phil Donahue, Oprah Winfrey, Geraldo, Morton Downey Jr.,* and, later, *Jerry Springer, Maury Povitch,* and *Ricki Lake.* Typically, the more surprising, unbelievable, or outrageous the story, the better the viewer ratings for a show; thus, show hosts worked hard to outdo one another in bringing ever more incredible stories to their viewers. Tales of tragedy and suffering might be complemented by stories of amazing rescues or uncommon compassion. Portraits of murder and mayhem by gangs or skinheads could be contrasted with enlightened tales of perseverance in the face of adversity. Occasionally, too, there were guests who claimed to have multiple personalities or similarly rare psychological maladies. And there were even weirder stories still, stories about satanic rituals involving babies, stories about UFO abductions, and so on. Before the advent of "reality television," these tabloid talk shows presented a heady brew of fact-based and fact-free commentary and conversation to their media-hungry audiences.

It was at this time that MPD, with its roots in childhood trauma, became linked to satanic ritual abuse (SRA) and the controversial new technique of recovered memories. As more victims came forward, or therapists/spokespersons came forward for them, a popular narrative emerged in which victims were said to have endured not just "ordinary" sexual abuse but "ritualized" sexual abuse as part of one satanic cult or another. It seems that both satanism and MPD were far more widespread than one might have imagined. Recovered memory specialists advanced the notion that victims held memories of unthinkable acts committed against them as young children or babies; the therapist had only to methodically "release" those memories to discover the details of the crimes. Feeding the fantasy was an ever-growing crop of relatively untrained recovered memory therapists and book authors who sought to popularize—or cash in on—the phenomenon.

In the context of these "satanic ritual abuse" cases, one of them looms especially large. The McMartin Preschool, a southern California daycare center, faced accusations from a disturbed parent that quickly exploded into multiple accusations regarding terrible events alleged to have taken place there—ritual murders, cannibalism, pedophilia, and so on. As unprepared investigators and unqualified therapists began looking into the matter, they unwittingly led young children to give testimony that reflected the then-prominent belief in the scourge of satanism and the prevalence of buried memories. The McMartin case, not unlike the case of Sybil in that it involved clear examples of leading the witness or interviewee, also became a modern-day example of how a witch-hunt mentality can arise among otherwise sane individuals. In this instance, the same mentality came to animate not only media coverage of the story but also law enforcement agencies, state educational authorities, and ordinary families living in an average U.S. town. Ultimately, the court case arising from the McMartin accusations would become one of the most expensive and longest-running (1983–1990) criminal trials in U.S. history. At its peak, thousands of satanic sacrifices were alleged to have taken place, but none of them were proved. Seven years after it started, the McMartin trial ended without any convictions. By that time, satanic panic in the United States was beginning to wane—although it did spill into the 1990s. Some scholars (e.g., Beck 2015) have suggested that the panic likely was fueled or caused by a fear of women working outside the home and leaving their children in the hands of others (strangers)—this being a powerful new trend in the 1980s. It is difficult to say for sure whether that insight is correct or whether something else lay behind the satanic eruption. Somewhere in the mix, however, lay the effects of the fluidity of memory and the power of self-deception.

Most of the time memory serves us well. Yet, because memory is a constructive process prone to enhancement, omission, and general distortion, it can be quite faulty at times. While we usually remember the gist of past experience, we often forget the details. Sometimes, we incorrectly recall aspects of an experience, and at other times we may "remember" an event that never occurred—or certainly did not occur in the way we remember it. False memories arise when an individual "remembers" details or events from the past that did not actually occur. Further, such false or corrupted memories are especially common when misinformation is put before the person who is remembering. Biased or leading questions, for example, can readily distort people's recollections—all the more so when the one recalling is a young child. Research shows that an interviewer can alter a true memory in an adult or a child, just as an interviewer can also plant complex false events in memory and make them seem true. With repetition and corroboration, false memories begin to harden into "true" memories. In the case of children, the malleability of memory is all the greater.

Eventually, the MPD and SRA epidemics subsided, the court cases stopped coming, and the mental health profession took stock of what had happened. In 1994 the American Psychiatric Association officially dropped MPD from its *Diagnostic and Statistical Manual of Mental Disorders* (DSM), replacing it with dissociative identity disorder (DID) and rethinking the condition as a whole. Recovered memory therapy was (and is) not mentioned in the DSM, being frowned upon by the mainstream medical community. It does, however, survive as an alternative therapy, and it has built up around it a set of more rigorous guidelines to prevent the kind of abuses that occurred in the McMartin case. Meanwhile, popular interest in "split personality" and other dissociative disorders remains high, with strings of movies, television series, and mass-market books about the subject continuing to come out on a regular basis.

Michael Shally-Jensen

See also: Dianetics; Past Life Regression Therapy; Primal Therapy and Feeling Therapy; Psychoanalysis; Shamanism and Neo-Shamanism; Voodoo and Santería; Witch Trials and Exorcisms

Further Reading

Beck, Richard. 2015. *We Believe the Children: A Moral Panic in the 1980s.* New York: Public Affairs.

Costner, Chris. 1989. *A Mind of My Own: The Woman Who Was Known as "Eve."* New York: William Morrow and Co.

Hunter, Marlene E. 2013. "Dissociative Disorders." In *Mental Health Care Issues in America: An Encyclopedia,* edited by Michael Shally-Jensen, 202–208. Santa Barbara, CA: ABC-CLIO.

Loftus, Elizabeth F. 1997. "Creating False Memories." *Scientific American.* September, 70–76.

Showalter, Elaine. 1997. *Hystories: Hysterical Epidemics and Modern Media.* New York: Columbia University Press.

RECOVERY MOVEMENT

The popular term *recovery* in contemporary mental health has been at times ambiguous and a focus of ongoing debate. Broadly speaking, the recovery approach to mental illness involves people feeling better about their illness, taking the lead in managing their symptoms, living a satisfying life even in the context of their illness, engaging in a holistic approach to treating illness (one that often includes but is not limited to psychiatric medications), reengaging in their communities, finding meaning in and even positive aspects to their illness, and directing their own psychiatric treatment in conjunction with medical professionals—who are viewed more as "expert consultants" than as dictatorial providers of care.

Traditionally, the term *recovery* is thought to mean that a person would return to a previous, more "pristine" state; but it can refer to the movement, a philosophy, a model, and a method of healing or getting better. Recovery, for the individual, often has a turning point or low point and is felt to be a process or a "journey."

The recovery model for treatment strongly contrasts with the medical model of psychiatric treatment, which has dominated the field since its inception. The medical model focuses largely if not solely on the patient's illness and not on the patient's life outside of the illness. It is based on the presumption that the clinician's responsibility is to reduce symptoms and, ideally, remove or cure the illness. The means reducing symptoms, in modern psychiatry, has strongly, and increasingly, been based on psychiatric medications. The Recovery Movement can largely be viewed as a reaction again the medical model, and among its greatest champions are consumers (or patients) and former consumers who feel they were ill-served by the narrowness and rigidity of the biomedical approach.

History and Philosophy

In the 1950s, the height of the inpatient era of psychiatry, state-run institutions became increasingly regarded in negative terms, for by then abuses, such as the rampant use of lobotomy procedures, were better understood by the public at large. By the 1960s, the public became more suspicious of long-term institutional care. This sentiment, coupled with the various civil rights and liberation movements of the 1970s, created a sociocultural shift. The goals of the ex-patient movement included empowerment and liberation. The highly charged and politicized environment of the 1970s gave an epistemological privilege to individual subjectivity, and accordingly, the new methods and practices in mental health emphasized the rights and preferences of the individual consumer.

The Recovery Movement itself was so named around that time but grew markedly in the 1980s and particularly the 1990s, with additional support from physical disability activists and the increasingly outspoken role of ex-patients. The movement has continued to thrive since then. One of the most visible indicators of the adoption of the recovery approach, for example, has been the hiring of former consumers of psychiatric services to provide support to current patients and work alongside trained professionals.

As noted, the Recovery Movement is diverse and continually evolving, but there are six consistent tenets of the movement across its many constituents.

- The Recovery Movement utilizes a positive, strengths-based approach that focuses on the strengths of individuals rather than pathologizing people and focusing on their "illnesses."
- The movement seeks to empower individuals by allowing them greater involvement and choice in their treatment.
- Recovery is best thought of as a nonlinear process whereby the consumer may not ever become completely asymptomatic.
- The movement is a grassroots one that is often led and championed by consumers/survivors of the mental health system.
- The Recovery Movement promotes mental health advocacy to end the stigmatizing and discrimination of mental health consumers through education and coalition building.
- The subjectivity of the recovery movement replaces the objectivity of the medical model. Instead of a subject-object relationship, consumers are part of an I-You relationship with medical professionals.

Outcomes

Recovery has been called a lot of things, including nonscientific, impractical, not evidence based, and a "fad." However, Fred Frese (Frese et al. 2001, 2009), a psychologist who himself was recovering from schizophrenia, and others sought to counter the claim that there is a lack of evidence-based practices by creating and looking at longitudinal studies concerning the positive as well as the potentially negative results of the recovery method in the lives of consumers. Since the goal of the recovery method is not necessarily to rid the consumer of all symptoms pertaining to his or her mental health diagnosis, the outcomes largely focus on management versus remission.

One of the more contentious illnesses, for example, is schizophrenia. People with a diagnosis of schizophrenia are often stigmatized by society and told they will never recover by mental health professionals. The *Diagnostic and Statistical Manual* of the American Psychiatric Association (2013) states that schizophrenia leads to deteriorated functioning over time and notes that a cure is rare. However, some studies have suggested that many people diagnosed with schizophrenia recover, or at least experience a reduction in psychotic systems, an increase in life satisfaction, and better awareness and knowledge of the illness (Harding and Zahniser 1994; Resnick, Rosenheck, and Lehman 2004). In other words, there is a link between the individual's sense of empowerment, agency, and overall well-being even in cases of serious mental illness.

Other evidence of the strength of the recovery approach comes from the testimonials of consumer-professionals who have "come out" of the mental health closet to show that even serious mental illnesses can be overcome. Individuals sometimes hide their mental health diagnosis due to the stigmatizing effect of labels, the negative depictions in the media of people with serious mental illness (including reports of violent behavior), and the very real consequences of housing and employment discrimination. Fred Frese's (1940–2018) life and work provides a concrete example of someone who shattered people's assumptions about the prognosis of schizophrenia. Frese was diagnosed with schizophrenia at age 25 while serving as a U.S. Marine. He founded the Community and State Hospital Section of the American Psychological Association and has faculty appointments at both Case Western Reserve University and the Northeastern Ohio Universities College of Medicine. He spent his career studying schizophrenia and advocating for evidence-based practice within the Recovery Movement. Other high-profile contributions to the Recovery Movement have come in the form of revelations by various celebrities who have shared their personal experiences with mental illness. Among them are Adele (depression), Miley Cyrus (depression), Lena Dunham (anxiety, OCD), Amanda Seyfried (depression), Carrie Fisher (bipolar disorder), Lady Gaga (anxiety, depression), and J. K. Rowling (depression).

There is a five-stage model to recovery that has generally proved useful for consumers and clinicians in trying to assess outcomes of the recovery method. The stages commonly accepted are (1) moratorium, (2) awareness, (3) preparation, (4) rebuilding, and (5) growth. The moratorium stage is when a consumer is in denial about his or her mental illness or is confused about what to do about it or how to assist in his or her own treatment. This is a familiar stage for anyone trapped inside the mental health "closet"—like Frese before he made his own illness public.

Awareness is characterized by self-reflection and hope, including hope in a possible recovery or in better management of symptoms. This stage is critical for someone needing to know and trust that recovery is possible. Preparation, the third stage, involves a commitment on the part of the consumer to begin working on his or her recovery process, to go to group meetings, to undertake skill building, and to learn about his or her personal strengths and weaknesses. Rebuilding is the stage that involves working toward set goals; it involves the consumer taking responsibility for the costs and benefits (in all senses) of the recovery process. In this fourth stage comes the inevitable rebuilding of one's identity. (Frese, for example, had to transition from viewing himself as an indestructible marine, to a man with an "incurable" mental illness, to a PhD with enormous capacity for growth and self-sufficiency.) The final, growth stage is the outcome of recovery according to Andresen and colleagues. In this stage an individual can manage his or her symptoms even in the face of setbacks and can lead a meaningful and positive life. By then the person has made many overall improvements, including a greater sense of generativity, or looking toward and planning for the future.

Conclusion

The Recovery Movement is no longer regarded as a fad. In no other time in history have consumers played such an important role in their own recovery. The recovery method has given birth to innovation within mental health care by allowing experiential evidence and consumer feedback to become valid forms of treatment review and measures of progress. Many states are developing recovery curriculums, conducting trainings, and holding state, regional, and national conferences on recovery. Along with recovery-oriented education and training, agencies are adopting consumer-run services, relapse and prevention management, and crisis planning.

More studies could still be done to broaden the body of knowledge and evidence of the efficacy of the Recovery Movement. But it appears that the widespread adoption of a recovery-oriented paradigm is enduring and will offer consumers increasingly broad-based and diverse services. There is a growing recognition in the mainstream of psychiatry, too, that medical professionals need to move away from stigmatizing labels and to respect and empower consumers by treating them as people who live a life well beyond the confines of their illnesses.

Charles Barber,
Dave Sells, and Sarah Raven

See also: Client-Centered Therapy; Encounter Groups; Gestalt Therapy; Mental Hospitals; Milieu Therapy and Therapeutic Community; Moral Treatment; Narrative Therapy and Writing Therapy; Neurodiversity; Self-Help

Further Reading

Amering, M., and M. Schmolke. 2009. *The Recovery Movement in Mental Health: Reshaping Scientific and Clinical Responsibilities.* Hoboken, NJ: Wiley-Blackwell.

Davidson, L., J. Rakefeld, and J. Strauss. 2010. *The Roots of the Recovery Movement in Psychiatry: Lessons Learned.* Hoboken, NJ: Wiley-Blackwell.

Frese, F., E. Knight, and E. Saks. 2009. "Recovery from Schizophrenia: With Views of Psychiatrists, Psychologists, and Others Diagnosed with This Illness." *Schizophrenia Bulletin* 35(2):370–80.

Frese, F., J. Stanley, K. Kress, and S. Vogel-Scibilia. 2001. "Integrating Evidence Based Practices and the Recovery Model." *Psychiatric Services* 52:1462–68.

Harding, C., and J. H. Zahniser. 1994. "Empirical Correction of Seven Myths about Schizophrenia with Implications for Treatment." *ACTA Psyciatrica Scandinava* 90 (suppl. 384):140–46.

Resnick, S., R. Rosenheck, and A. Lehman. 2004. "An Exploratory Analysis of Correlates of Recovery." *Psychiatric Services* 55:540–47.

Travis, T. 2009. *The Language of the Heart: A Cultural History of the Recovery Movement.* Chapel Hill: University of North Carolina Press.

REIKI AND THERAPEUTIC TOUCH

The term *Reiki* is derived from two Japanese characters, *rei* (universal) and *ki* (energy), that when combined refer to what is usually translated as "life energy." Reiki is a form of therapy in which practitioners place their hands above a client's vital energy fields—similar to the chakras of Ayurvedic medicine or the centers of *qi* (*chi*) in traditional Chinese medicine—to help "unblock" any restricted energy flows and stimulate the client's own healing mechanisms.

Today Reiki is popular far beyond Japan, where it was developed in the late 1910s and early 1920s by Mikao Usui (1865–1926) after he experienced a period of fasting and meditation at the top of Mount Kurama. In the United States Reiki is found mainly in complementary and alternative medicine (CAM) settings, which includes CAM units in some mainstream clinics and hospitals. Its proponents say that it can be used to treat a variety of diseases and disorders, among them anxiety, stress, headaches, asthma, bodily pain, circulatory problems, recovery from surgery, and nausea from chemotherapy. It can also be used simply to enhance well-being.

A treatment session consists of a fully clothed patient lying down on a massage table. The healer holds his or her hands above different areas of the body to optimize energy circulation and bring relaxation and healing. In some cases the fingertips are brought into contact with the patient's body while the palms remain suspended. Each area is addressed in this way for from three to five minutes, the patient typically being asked to turn over midway through the session. A full session can last up to 90 minutes, but more often it lasts an hour or less.

There are two main types of Reiki, referred to as traditional Japanese Reiki and Western Reiki, both of which consist of three levels of knowledge. Level 1 practitioners are able to heal both themselves and others; level 2 practitioners can perform healing from a distance (often using standard symbols); and level 3 practitioners (the so-called master's level) are able to teach others. Depending on the type of Reiki practiced, there are between 12 and 20 different hand positions. The idea is that the healer feels the energy emanating from the patient's body, particularly at key locations, and uses the energy flowing through his or her own hands to bring the patient's energy field into balance.

Please Like Me Looks at Reiki

The popular Australia-based comedy series *Please Like Me* has a fun moment with Reiki in Season 2, Episode 4 ("Gang Keow Wan"). The episode opens where the main character, Josh (played by Josh Thomas, the show's creator) is on a date with a long-haired vegetarian mate named Cosmo (Josh Schmidt).

Josh: So what did you do today?
Cosmo: Well, my dance class was canceled, so I got a Reiki massage—and I just feel incredible, man.
J: Reiki. That's the massage where they *don't* touch you?
C: Yeah, it's about energy. They put energy into your body.
J: Yeah, well, why would you pay someone to *not* touch you?
C: Okay, well, like I said, they align your energy . . .
J: (expressing disbelief): Would you go to a restaurant and pay them to *not* feed you?

Reiki practitioners must go through a series of "attunements" with Reiki masters in order to learn the basics of energy healing and begin their advancement in the field. The masters teach the students how to activate the vital life force in themselves and how, using the correct technique, to work with it in order to bring healing to others. Certification is traditionally a nonformal affair, with the master simply approving the student's qualifications when the expected level of achievement has been reached. In recent years, however, certification has become somewhat more formal and standardized.

Recipients of Reiki treatment generally describe a sense of deep relaxation at the end of a session, accompanied by a feeling of well-being. They also report sensations of warmth, tingling, sleepiness, and/or a sense of refreshment or renewal. Occasional unwanted responses, such as anxiety or sadness, are typically said by masters to represent the release of negative energies that had been bottled up inside the patient. A number of Hollywood celebrities, including Gwyneth Paltrow, Cameron Diaz, and Angelina Jolie, are known to enjoy Reiki treatments. The novelist Eric Van Lustbader, who continued the Jason Bourne series after the death of its creator, Robert Ludlam, is a Reiki practitioner.

Although Reiki practice has not been well researched using modern scientific methods, many of the benefits that come from it may be due to its ability to promote relaxation, which in turn stands to reduce blood pressure and improve heart and respiration rates. Because the concepts of Reiki fall outside mainstream understandings of the laws of nature and the nature of medicine, it is often thought that positive outcomes could also be due to the placebo effect and to the individualized attention that the patient receives during a session. Obviously, its supporters discount such thoughts.

Different strains of Reiki claim different lineages from the founding master, Usui. In Kyoto, before his death, Usui passed on his concepts and methods, based partly on ancient techniques, to a disciple, Chujiro Hayashi, who in turn passed them on to a former patient and associate living in Hawaii, Hawayo Takata. Takata in due course initiated her granddaughter Phyllis Furumoto into the practice, and the two of them, Takata and Furumoto, trained a number of other masters, who founded, in 1983, the Reiki Alliance. The Alliance's vision is stated as follows:

> We nourish and empower our members with opportunities for personal and spiritual growth. Guided by the precepts, members deepen their mastery and connection with the Spiritual Lineage through worldwide gatherings, accessible communications, educational development and mutual support. (Reiki Alliance 2018)

Another Takata student, Barbara Weber Ray, founded a separate organization called the American Reiki Association, which later came to call itself Radiance Technique International Association (RTIA). In a statement, RTIA says that Reiki

> is the science and art of accessing, directing and applying Radiant, universal life energy to promote energy balancing and wholeness. . . . Reiki is a powerful tool for positive wellness and balance in all aspects of life and can be used safely and effectively in conjunction with any medical techniques. (RTIA 2012)

Other professional organizations for practitioners arose as well, each having a slightly different philosophy, purpose, and membership. In most cases, however, lineage and technique are important identifiers for members of the Reiki community.

Therapeutic Touch

Also called Healing Touch, this is another "energy field" technique first developed in the 1970s by Dolores Krieger, a professor of nursing at New York University. Having experienced in her nursing career the healing power of touch, Krieger began experimenting with methods for relieving patients' pain using the hands. She discovered that in many cases it was just as beneficial, if not more so, to keep the hands a couple of inches away from the surface of the patient's body rather than to make contact. It was also essential to communicate to the patient a sincere desire to assist in the healing process, and to demonstrate a commitment to doing so.

Krieger linked her method to similar techniques found in Ayurvedic medicine from India. Thus, illness is considered by practitioners of Therapeutic Touch to be the result of an imbalance of energies, and moving the hands around the patient's body is a way of redistributing those energies. As in Reiki, the practitioner channels his or her own energy field to targeted areas of the patient's body. In this way, such conditions as pain, inflammation, nausea, premenstrual syndrome, thyroid conditions, and a variety of others can be addressed.

Over a period of some 15 years, Krieger passed on her techniques to thousands of nursing students, and nursing became a center of enthusiasm for this and other CAM methodologies. By the 1990s, the North American Nursing Diagnostic Association (NANDA) had entered the diagnosis of "energy field disturbance" into its lexicon (Whorton 2002, 278). Many more thousands of nurses trained in Therapeutic Touch. Eventually, however, there was some pushback by physicians and others in the medical community—including insurers. In the 2000s, NANDA, now known as the International Nursing Knowledge Association, along with some nursing schools, began to take a more skeptical approach to energy field concepts even while still recognizing the undoubted value of human touch in the healing process and the utility of CAM approaches generally. Therapeutic Touch continues in its "traditional" form today but it is not as widespread a technique as it once was.

Michael Shally-Jensen

See also: Acupuncture; Alternative Diagnostics; Ayurvedic Medicine; Chinese Traditional Medicine; Crystals; Magnet Therapy; Tai Chi and Qigong

Further Reading

Lindquist, Ruth, Mariah Snyder, and Mary Fran Tracy, eds. 2013. *Complementary and Alternative Therapies in Nursing.* New York: Springer.

Radiance Technique International Association. 2012. "Clarification about Things Called 'Reiki.'" http://www.trtia.org/CRCorrection.htm

Reiki Alliance. 2018. http://www.reikialliance.com/en

Stein, Diane. 1995. *Essential Reiki: A Complete Guide to an Ancient Healing Art.* New York: Crossing Press/Crown.

Whorton, James C. 2002. *Nature Cures: The History of Alternative Medicine in America.* New York: Oxford University Press.

SELF-HELP

While self-help can mean many things, it is generally defined as the act of helping or improving oneself, typically without the formal assistance of a trained professional. Reasons for pursuing self-help treatment typically stem from the person's quest to change in an effort to reach his or her personal goals. Self-help in relation to health and wellness, although having some links to traditional and folk medicine in an earlier era, is a fairly recent phenomenon. One of the main applications of self-help, emerging in the last half of the 20th century, has been dietary supplements, herbal remedies, and alternative therapies generally (e.g., aromatherapy, meditation, nutritional therapy); these topics are discussed elsewhere in this volume. Self-help interventions in the mental health field, the focus of the present entry, tend to be based on professionally developed resources, often drawing on cognitive-behavioral therapy (CBT) techniques; they are typically self-administered or delivered with limited therapeutic contact.

The self-help movement has exploded in recent decades and is now a large and profitable industry. As indicated by best-seller lists, past and present, many of those seeking self-improvement (not limited to mental health recovery) have turned to works by such self-help gurus as Dale Carnegie (1888–1955), Norman Vincent Peale (1898–1993), Stephen Covey (1932–2012), and Eckhart Tolle (1948–). Others, including those seeking help with relationships, personal health,

Self-Help and the Star Power of Ram Dass

In the 1970s and 1980s, a man known as Ram Dass rose to incredible prominence in certain counterculture circles. Ram Dass was famous for his ties to psychedelic experimentation and Timothy Leary, for his travels to India and relationship with his guru Neem Karoli Baba, and for his book *Be Here Now*.

Ram Dass was born Richard Alpert. He grew up in a Jewish family living in Massachusetts but stated later in his life that he didn't have any belief in God at all until he began experimenting with psychedelics. It was *Be Here Now*, an accounting of his spiritual journey and a manual for how others could follow in his footsteps, that made him into a household name.

Be Here Now is the most well known of Ram Dass's 11 books, having been originally published in 1971 and selling more than 2 million copies. Ram Dass opened the door for other self-help books that approached self-improvement through spirituality, such as those by Stephen Levine, Deepak Chopra, Thich Nhat Hanh, and Pema Chodron.

While both Americans and Europeans have been fascinated by both Eastern and South Asian spirituality for centuries, Ram Dass was the most recent "guru" to bring a version of these spiritual concepts into the U.S. public eye. Although his writings may be considered a very diluted version of the actual spirituality from which they originate, the basic concepts have helped many Americans find a better balance in their lives.

and mental health, follow the lectures of such popular speakers as Dr. Phil (Phil McGraw; 1950–), Dr. Laura (Laura Schlessinger; 1947–), and John Gray (1951–). Still others utilize social media or online support groups to read posted comments, post topics themselves, and privately communicate with others regarding similar areas of interest and/or need.

According to Ian Dowbiggin, author of *The Quest for Mental Health* (2011), the time when self-help became a big business dates back to the late 1970s and early 1980s. There had been earlier works, of course (Carnegie, Peale), including the founding text of Scientology, *Dianetics* (1950), which began as a mental health self-help book before it became the basis of a religion. (The overlap between spiritual development and self-help has long been part of this field's history.) Things really began to take off, though, with the publication in 1976 of Thomas A. Harris's *I'm Okay—You're Okay*, complemented in the same year by Wayne Dyer's *Your Erroneous Zones*. Henceforth, authors of self-help books could become media celebrities, or, as they are more commonly known, health and wellness "gurus." People like Dr. Phil, Tony Robbins, Deepak Chopra, and Robert Fulghum have sold millions of books and appeared on daytime television shows like *Oprah* and *Donahue*. The book publishing industry, the television industry, the magazine industry, and the public/motivational speaking industry each received a large boost as a result. And interest continues to remain extraordinarily high today, with gurus like Chopra,

Andrew Weil, and Dr. Oz having raised the profile of personal health and medi-cine/alternative medicine through a variety of means.

There is a strong culture, too, of *spiritual* self-help, or spiritual development, in the United States. Besides Peale, authors such as M. Scott Peck and Marianne Williamson, among many others, have contributed to this genre. In an earlier period, the stories of Horatio Alger (1832–1899) offered narratives about virtu-ous youths rising from rags to riches on the merits of their personal integrity. One of the more extreme, yet hugely popular, contemporary versions of this genre is known variously as the "health and wealth gospel," the "prosperity gospel," or the "gospel of success." Largely an Evangelical phenomenon, prosperity doc-trine preaches self-realization through consumerism as a sign of God's blessing. It suggests a productive relationship between God's will and capitalist enterprise, especially individual entrepreneurship and personal investment in the church and the "success" movement as a whole. Purchases of lectures and course materials are sometimes, but not always, part of the program; philanthropy is encouraged as well. Those who prove themselves adept at attaining financial and spiritual "success," it is believed, stand to be rewarded here on Earth and in the afterworld. Again, the connection between self-help and spiritual growth is demonstrated by this uniquely U.S. movement.

Self-help was not a widely studied topic and did not receive significant atten-tion from social scientists until the early 1970s. Since then, however, systematic research on self-help has been more abundant. with much of it suggesting that self-help methods can indeed be helpful. Self-help is recognized by many in the health profession as an integral aspect of successful, sustained health and mental health treatment.

Self-Help Methods

There are a number of different self-help philosophies and corresponding types of activities. Sometimes, mental health professionals may assign or suggest clients' use of self-help materials. Research into how psychologists in clinical practice per-ceive and use self-help materials (with clients who have anxiety and depression) shows that a large majority (73%) recommend self-help interventions primarily as a supplement to individual or group therapy (Nordgreen and Havik 2011). Furthermore, 16.6 percent recommended self-help approaches to prevent relapse, 6.8 percent recommended self-help as an alternative to therapist contact, and 1.2 percent recommended it help for clients on a waiting list. Written materials in the form of brochures or books were recommended most frequently (79.1%), with CBT-based self-help books being the most common (14.2%). Internet resources were recommended by 41.9 percent, and recorded materials (e.g., videos, CDs, and audiotapes) were recommended by between 6 percent and 10 percent in the sample. Reportedly, the primary aim of such self-help materials was to provide clients with general information about mental health disorders and how to cope with them.

Peer support groups are one type of self-help method that gained increasing popularity over the years. Peer support provides an opportunity for those seeking self-improvement to draw on the collective wisdom of peers to learn coping skills that can assist in recovery. Peer support involves one person supporting another person who has a similar need for change or recovery. Some believe that people who have similar experiences and needs are, in these situations, better able to provide authentic empathy and validation. There is a growing body of evidence indicating that peer support provides a solid context for recovery and healing.

Alcoholics Anonymous (AA), established in 1935, is likely the most prominent peer support group in the world and has been successful in helping millions of people overcome severe alcohol abuse. Narcotics Anonymous is another influential self-help group that has as its focus helping people to eliminate their use of addictive drugs. Owing to the perceived benefits of these self-help groups, a myriad of different peer support groups have been developed along similar lines—for example, Overeaters Anonymous, Online Gamers Anonymous, and Sex Addicts Anonymous.

In the United States, three basic types of self-help peer support groups have emerged over time. These include (1) individuals with similar problems, motives, and goals (e.g., AA); (2) groups that are interested in a similar cause and volunteer their services; and (3) groups that include a paid professional and may be more of a mixed population seeking both collaboration and guidance in the self-improvement process (e.g., Weight Watchers, Regional Tobacco Treatment Center programs).

Self-Help Benefits, Drawbacks, and Points to Consider

There are a number of practical benefits to self-help. First, self-help options are both readily available and relatively inexpensive. They also can provide ways to privately explore issues without meeting others face to face. Finally, self-help approaches allow individuals to customize and take responsibility for their own therapeutic plan, which may lead to a sense of ownership and empowerment.

Despite the apparent advantages, when incorporating self-help strategies into a treatment plan, individuals may lack the perspective needed to properly understand the nature of key issues, including the choice of the best self-help strategy for their situation. Laypersons may also misunderstand, and consequently incorrectly implement, treatment plans. Furthermore, individuals may lack the motivation to stick with a self-help plan without assistance, especially if they are misled by exaggerated claims about treatment effectiveness. And, to be sure, there is no shortage of such exaggerated or false claims.

Naturally, the exclusive usage of self-help approaches, without consultation with a qualified professional, can increase the possibility of misdiagnosis (self-diagnosis). Furthermore, because so many self-help resources are available, it is difficult for those who are untrained and inexperienced in the field to correctly identify and individualize treatment. Finally, unsupervised self-help approaches provide no objective method to detect worsening of clinical symptoms. Thus, for those with more severe symptoms and complicated issues, clinical monitoring by a trained professional is generally recommended as a complement to self-help.

Victoria E. Kress, Melinda Wolford,
Richard Van Voorhis, and Michael Shally-Jensen

See also: Dianetics; Faith Healing and Prayer; Folk Medicine; Health and Wellness Gurus; Homeopathy; Medicine Shows; Spas and Mineral Waters; 12-Step Programs; Yoga

Further Reading

Dowbiggin, Ian. 2011. *The Quest for Mental Health.* New York: Cambridge University Press.
Lamb-Shapiro, Jessica. 2014. *Promise Land: My Journey through America's Self-Help Culture.* New York: Simon and Schuster.
McGee, Micki. 2005. *Self-Help, Inc.: Makeover Culture in American Life.* New York: Oxford University Press.
Nordgreen, T., and O. Havik. 2011. "Use of Self-Help Materials for Anxiety and Depression in Mental Health Services: A National Survey of Psychologists in Norway." *Professional Psychology: Research and Practice* 42(2): 185–91.
Salerno, Steve. 2005. *SHAM: How the Self-Help Movement Made America Helpless.* New York: Crown.

SHAMANISM AND NEO-SHAMANISM

Traditional shamanism is a supernatural art in which the healer, or shaman, goes into a trance state and is believed to be possessed by a spirit that speaks and acts through him or her. Among the Evenki of Siberia, from whose Tungus language the word *shaman* comes, a shaman was responsible for the health and wellness of family members and others belonging to the wider kin group. Though the position was often inherited, the selection was ultimately made by the spirits, who informed a novice of their interest in his or her candidacy during his or her first trance experience. At that point a lengthy training process began, usually under the guidance of an established shaman. During healing rites, specific actions had to be carried out with exactness to produce the expected outcomes. Siberian shamans, like those of other regions, were called in to diagnose and cure illness, control forces or events, and foretell the future. In many cases trance was induced by accelerating rhythms of song, dance, and drum or other instruments. Such was the case among American Indians, for example. Fire, smoke, and incense of some kind were also often employed, as well. In ancient Babylonian myth, the sweet aroma of a burnt offering made to the gods by a hero figure attracts the spirits so that they hover over the scene like moths and can be interacted with.

In parts of Africa, the shaman generally works while possessed by ancestor spirits. (Christianity has changed some traditional practices, however.) The ancestral connection helps to add weight to any determination that is made during the course of a shamanistic rite, supplying a sense of deep truth to what is said regarding a client's situation. Among the Dayak of Borneo, hereditary female shamans officiated (or officiate, to the extent that the practice still occurs) at the reinterment ceremonies for the dead held every few years. At such religious events, where the bones of the deceased are gathered together for permanent storage, the shaman is a respected priest(ess) and moral arbiter employed by families to communicate with Dayak spirits and gods in order to make sure that the transition from the liminal period of recent death to the final period of eternal death (i.e., ancestorhood) goes well.

Other types of shamanistic cults are found in different parts of the world. The zar cult in North Africa and similar cults elsewhere in the Middle East still operate among Muslim women. In these cults a woman unhappy with her lot is believed possessed by an irresponsible, alien spirit (*jin*), and the shamaness who is consulted prescribes an expensive treatment, typically to be paid for by the patient's husband. *Jins*, however, lurk in every corner, and can strike at any moment—hence the need for prophylactics or amulets such as the hamsa, or inverted hand-eye symbol. If and when something goes wrong with the person despite having consulted a shamaness, the failure can be explained away as an error in the application of the treatment or the interventions of a malevolent other.

Shamanism has ancient roots in East Asia, as well. In China, shamans believed to be possessed by the minor deities of a village or town participated in all community ceremonies in order to make these events more auspicious. There were even shamanesses who specialized in aiding unhappy girls and subordinate wives who had become despondent. In Japan, the priests of some Shinto and Buddhist sects were shamans licensed by the government to perform certain purification functions or other rites as needed. Among the indigenous Ainu of northern Japan, shamanism has an ancient lineage; shamans were known for their ability to fly, transform into animals, control spirits, and assist in hunting, fishing, and wars.

Healing Magic

In traditional, preindustrial societies, sudden and severe illness was usually ascribed to supernatural powers. Whether invisible gods, upset ancestors, or evil witches, the causes were thought to bring sickness as punishment for neglect or wickedness. In so doing, these inflictions were understood to threaten not only individuals but, potentially, all members of a society. Thus, fear and anxiety were frequent accompaniments to illness.

Supernatural healing went hand in hand with traditional theories of illness. The practices drawn on include divination used for diagnosis along with various curing practices. Among the Azande of Central Africa, divination undertaken by a shaman or "witch doctor" classically involved a variety of different means—mechanical, spiritual, and psychological (trance). Treatment often utilized plant substances based on their homeopathic qualities, meaning that they resembled or reacted in such a way as to look like a patient's condition. For example, the bark of a tree with reddish patches was used to treat skin rashes, because of the resemblances involved. Plant substances used by shamans in some cases contain actual curative properties but are described by the healer in mystical or magical terms. The Yoruba of West Africa, for example, traditionally used a type of *rauvolfia* (dogbane) as a tranquilizer. (It acts as an-antihypertensive.) When collecting the plant material, the healer spoke to the tree (or shrub) from which it was taken, asking for its aid. The Yoruba understood that the substance worked only if the tree cooperated in the healing process. Thus, if the rauvolfia drug worked better on some patients than it did on others, which often was the case, the outcome was explained as being the result of the tree's greater or lesser participation in the cure—or perhaps as the healer's failure to perform the proper interactions with the source.

Traditional healing entails the use of symbolic media including words, images (from myth), and sounds along with invocations of or references to beliefs, feelings, and expectations. It is invariably a social phenomenon that provides the sick and their relatives with emotional reassurance through the use of elaborate rituals.

One widely used form of healing consists of the extraction of a purportedly harmful object from the body of the patient. Typically, the shaman sucks a maleficent substance from the patient's body either directly or using a cup or horn of some kind. (In this, the practice is not unlike the phenomenon of cupping.) The act usually includes a demonstration or proof, in the form of a piece of bone or bit of blood, shown the patient by the shaman who had been concealing it in his mouth.

Other diseases have other causes. "Soul loss" occurs when a person loses his or her soul either deliberately through sorcery or accidentally during sleep. The shaman must locate the lost soul and restore it to the patient. In possession or "spirit intrusion" the patient becomes mentally unbalanced, the result of being targeted by evil persons or forces. In these cases, an exorcism is advised. Finally, with "taboo breaking," the person is believed to suffer as a result of having violated social or moral codes, thus angering the ancestors and/or gods. The resolution in this case might come through confession and a promise henceforth to uphold societal regulations.

The New Shamanism

The spread of modern medicine brought with it an array of complex changes, not the least of which was a general decline in the status of traditional shaman-healers. Yet despite the gains of technologically advanced society in controlling the environment, reducing infectious disease, and establishing effective medical systems, there remain vast areas in the social sphere—that is, in the area of human experience—that are resistant to technological solutions and open to explorations of a more human kind. It is here that one continues to see the expression of religion and magic, of faith and belief.

Although he may not have been the sole force behind the development of "neo-shamanism," or shamanism for the modern world, the anthropologist and educator Michael Harner (1926–2018) is often credited with being its foremost proponent and popularizer. When doing field research among the Jívaro people of the Amazon basin in the 1960s, Harner decided to experiment with a local hallucinogenic concoction called yage or ayahuasca. After writing several academic studies about the Jívaro and shamanism, Harner founded, in 1979 in Norwalk, Connecticut, the Center for Shamanic Studies. He examined shamanic practices worldwide and wrote a guide for contemporary seekers, *The Way of the Shaman: A Guide to Power and Healing* (1980). This book and the work of the center inspired students and New Age health seekers in the United States and elsewhere to incorporate shamanism into their worldview. Suddenly "shamanic journeying," accompanied by drumming, dance, and occasionally hallucinogenics, became widespread. So, too, did reliance on a personal "power animal," or totem said to embody one's essential spirit. A power animal was not assigned but rather discovered during a trance experience. Modern neo-shamans were more about self-discovery or self-realization than about healing others.

That changed in time, however. As the New Age era itself transmuted into the post–New Age era sometime in the mid-to-late 1990s, neo-shamanism became less widely practiced as a personal journey and more commonly found as a specialized form of practice among complementary and alternative medicine (CAM) practitioners. By then, critics had already begun complaining not only that neo-shamanism represented an act of cultural appropriation by (white) New Agers, but also that it was a false system based on picking and choosing from among widely differing indigenous cultures. Moreover, no one could really vouch for the expertise of any given modern shaman or the rate of effectiveness of his or her cures. There were more and more stories about sham spiritual healers appearing in the media, although such troubles afflict many different professions besides the CAM health and wellness field. In any case, today's neo-shamanism is not the hot new thing that it once was. Its practitioners continue to trace the journey, however, as can be discovered in such publications as *Shamanism Annual* and *Sacred Hoop* magazine.

Michael Shally-Jensen

See also: Alternative Diagnostics; Crystals; Cupping; Folk Medicine; Native American Traditional Medicine; Paleo Diet; Psychedelic Drugs; Sweat Lodges and Saunas; Voodoo and Santería; Witch Trials and Exorcisms

Further Reading

DuBois, Thomas A. 2009. *An Introduction to Shamanism.* New York: Cambridge University Press.

Harner, Michael J. 1990. *The Way of the Shaman: A Guide to Power and Healing.* 10th anniversary ed. San Francisco: Harper and Row.

Harvey, Graham. 2003. *Shamanism: A Reader.* New York: Routledge.

SHIATSU

Shiatsu is a "hands-on" therapy from Japan, originally, that involves the use of finger pressure to address conditions both of the body and of the person. It is, in other words, an "integrative" technique that is designed to heal the physical body as well as the mind and even, its proponents say, the spirit.

Shiatsu in fact means "finger pressure." Yet, in employing the technique practitioners use thumbs, fingers, palms, and even elbows sometimes to bring different types and amounts of pressure to bear. Shiatsu points are called *tsubo* in Japanese, and their location and the effect of Shiatsu on them is based on an understanding of traditional "energy" medicine and body systems. Additionally, today's Shiatsu professionals commonly understand about modern anatomy and physiology. The idea behind the technique is to identify trouble areas and adjust the body's physical structure and balance its energy flow. Shiatsu can be a relaxing experience and is generally effective in alleviating stress and promoting a sense of health and well-being. It can also be somewhat painful, depending on the pressure point being utilized and the degree to which the practitioner works it to achieve results.

Thus, Shiatsu is both a diagnostic technique and a corrective measure. The Japanese expression *shindan soku chiryo* means "diagnosis and therapy combined" and conveys this dualism of purpose. The hands of the trained expert are supposed to be sensitive enough to detect, in the first phase of the process, any irregularities in the skin, muscles, or body temperature that might indicate a problem. Not only surface abnormalities but deeper tissues and organs may be "read" in this way. Each condition, its location, and its degree of severity are assessed. Often, at the same time that an abnormality is detected a Shiatsu treatment is applied to it. In other cases, an overview may be obtained first, followed by a series of treatments. The volume of pressure needed and its intensity are worked out as well, as the patient reacts and the practitioner gauges the treatment's effects on an ongoing basis.

Roots and Range of Approaches

Traditional Chinese medicine, including acupuncture, herbalism, and massage, is thought to have been introduced to Japan by a Buddhist monk in the sixth century CE. The Japanese refined and altered many of the traditional practices as well as developed their own, to suit their own needs and preferences. In particular, they cultivated the manual diagnostic and healing arts, such as abdominal diagnosis and treatment, which combined with massage formed the basis of Shiatsu.

The founder of modern Shiatsu therapy, Tokujiro Namikoshi (1905–2000), discovered, while trying to help his mother with her rheumatism as a youth, that he could achieve beneficial results by using his fingers, thumbs, and palms to apply pressure at certain locations on the body. This was the beginning of Shiatsu. Namikoshi's later researches led him to establish an anatomical and physiological basis for Shiatsu, which partially incorporated Western medical conceptions and disciplines such as physiotherapy and chiropractic. He further developed his theories at a school he opened in 1940, Japan Shiatsu College. In 1953, he was invited to present his Shiatsu system at the Palmer Chiropractic School in Davenport, Iowa. There he developed a relationship with the redoubtable D. D. Palmer, founder of chiropractic. In 1964, Japan's Ministry of Health recognized Shiatsu as a uniquely Japanese therapeutic treatment, distinguished from both an older massage method known as *anma* and Western massage.

Another early practitioner, Shizuto Masunaga (1925–1981), incorporated his learning of Shiatsu into his studies of Western psychology and Chinese medicine. He also further developed the existing methods of diagnosis. Masunaga's extended system incorporated special exercises, known as *makko ho*, to stimulate the flow of *qi* (chi) energy, and he developed a set of guiding principles to ensure that his techniques remained effective once transferred to others. He called his system Zen Shiatsu, after the simple and direct approach to spirituality of Zen Buddhist monks in Japan. In Zen Shiatsu, however, practitioners may also use their elbows, knees, and bony parts of the body to apply stronger pressure to the pressure points. (*Qi* can be a stubborn entity.)

Thus, influential Shiatsu practitioners developed their own styles and established their own workshops or schools to help advance their form of Shiatsu as a therapy. Each form has a slightly different theoretical basis and tactical approach. Some focus on acupressure points, *tsubo,* while others emphasize more general work on the body or the classic "meridian" pathways of *qi* that run through it. There are even differences within approaches. In Meridian Shiatsu, for example, some practitioners rely on the "root-branch theory," or the view that an outward condition or abnormality must be traced back to its root elsewhere in the body/energy system, whereas others generally apply pressure to the meridian points closest to the problem area.

In Japan these alternative Shiatsu techniques are referred to as "derivative Shiatsu" to distinguish them from the original Shiatsu taught at the Namikoshi school and sanctioned by the Japanese Ministry of Health. A form known as Tao (Dao) Shiatsu, for example, stresses religious and spiritual elements. A form called Oha Shiatsu, in contrast, employs only light thumb pressure and focuses more on balancing the body through *seitai*, a type of stretching and bodily manipulation. And then there is Macrobiotic Shiatsu. The macrobiotic diet is fairly well known throughout the world. It was developed by Michio Kushi (1926–2014) and based on yin-yang principles. Today, it is often also part of an overall system of complementary medicine founded on diet, acupuncture, meditation, Shiatsu, and Chinese herbal medicine.

Although the term *Shiatsu* was originally Japanese, its meaning has come to be understood today in English-speaking countries and throughout the world as a form of (Japanese-ish) therapeutic "massage" or acupressure. It has been used by millions of clients, including the actors Dan Ackroyd, Juliette Binoche, Anne Hathaway, and Frida Pinto, the musicians Mick Jagger and Madonna, and former British Prime Minster David Cameron's spouse, Samantha Cameron. Many athletes have tried it as well, to treat both movement issues and "imbalances" in their overall sense of health and well-being.

Shiatsu vs. Acupressure

There are some similarities between Shiatsu and acupressure, and some differences as well. Both techniques assess for "imbalances" in the body and use pressure to restore balance and health. Some, but not all, Shiatsu styles use the meridian points associated with acupuncture and acupressure (from Chinese traditional medicine).

Generally, neither Shiatsu nor acupressure use oils or creams during the application of pressure—unlike regular massage. And some of the points pressed are the same. Yet, there are notable differences too. First, Shiatsu is a holistic discipline that approaches treatment by considering the whole body, whereas acupressure, in many cases, involves treatment of a few points only. Second, the pressure used in Shiatsu is always stationary and sustained. In acupressure, in contrast, the pressure applied is often circular or may use a pumping action in which the thumb repeatedly presses and releases pressure quickly. Third, in Shiatsu, the thumb is normally held flat—that is, fully extended—whereas in acupressure it is more commonly used in a bent position. Finally, Shiatsu uses the whole weight of one's body to apply pressure, whereas acupressure uses mostly the strength of one's arms or hands.

Not a great deal of scientific evidence exists for the effectiveness of either Shiatsu or acupressure, but people who use one or the other often return for additional treatments and generally find themselves satisfied upon doing so. One extensive review of the medical literature did find that acupressure could be beneficial for pain, nausea, and sleep irregularities, whereas the evidence for Shiatsu was less consistent (Robinson, Lorenc, and Liau 2011). Shiatsu, in short, has achieved a degree of popularity worldwide but its status is not necessarily backed up by the medical literature. It remains an available resource for those seeking "balance" and "harmony" in their lives.

Michael Shally-Jensen

See also: Acupuncture; Chinese Traditional Medicine; Chiropractic; Craniosacral Therapy; Macrobiotics; Mind–Body Medicine; Reflexology

Further Reading

Cabo, Ferndando, et al. 2018. "Shiatsu and Acupressure: Two Different and Distinct Techniques." *International Journal of Therapeutic Massage and Bodywork* 11(2):4–10. www.ncbi.nlm.nih.gov/pmc/articles/PMC5988345/

Canadian Shiatsu Society of British Columbia. www.shiatsupractor.org/aboutshiatsu.html

Namikoshi, Tōru. 2002. *The Shiatsu Way to Health: Relief and Vitality at a Touch.* New York: Kodansha International.

Robinson, Nicola, Ava Lorenc, and Xing Liao. 2011. "The Evidence for Shiatsu: A Systematic Review of Shiatsu and Acupressure." *BMC Complementary and Alternative Medicine* 11, October. https://bmccomplementalternmed.biomedcentral.com/articles/10.1186/1472-6882-11-88

STRESS AND STRESS MANAGEMENT

The experience of stress, when it occurs in its most extreme form, is regarded as a debilitating psychiatric condition. For example, persons diagnosed with posttraumatic stress disorder (PTSD) or acute stress disorder (ASD), both of which arise from exposure to severe, traumatic events, are subject to flashbacks, dissociation, sleep disturbances, depersonalization, "hypervigilance" regarding anything having to do with the original traumatic event, bursts of anger and hostility, hallucinations, and a sense that the future is nonexistent or bleak. Such persons are, of course, advised to remain under the care of medical or mental health professionals and to seek social support as they try to return to a degree of normalcy in their lives. The number of persons in the population that at any given time can be said to fall under a diagnosis of PTSD or ASD is not known precisely, but, clearly, the figure goes up or down depending on the existence of major stressors such as wars and disasters.

At the same time, there is a much larger pool of individuals who may be regarded as suffering from "ordinary" stress—the kind related to such circumstances or conditions as work, school, family problems, financial difficulties (including poverty and unemployment), marital discord, poor housing or living conditions, or having a medical condition (including a mental disorder). Indeed, for many people even important social events such as weddings and holidays can be sources of stress. Because of its nature and its source in society, this type of "ordinary" stress is sometimes termed *social stress*. As with the more severe, trauma-based forms, social stress can be chronic or acute. It may pass when the situation causing it passes (acute stress), or it may linger and affect an individual's physical and psychological well-being over the long term (chronic stress).

Variable Responses to Stressors

It is a commonly said that some people "thrive on stress." And, indeed, it does seem that certain individuals not only are not bothered by stress but welcome it, within limits, as a way to energize themselves. That is because stress is the body's automatic, protective response to a perceived threat or challenge. It is triggered by those "fight or flight" situations that require a sudden behavioral adjustment. On a physiological level, stress involves changes in many different systems of the body, notably those regulating heart rate, blood pressure, skin sensitivity, and the flow of adrenaline. On a psychological level, stress involves a heightened state of alertness, fear, or anxiety. Although a modest amount of stress is considered harmless, perhaps even beneficial, stress that is excessive or prolonged can take a toll on the individual's physical and mental health.

A stressor is a situation, individual, or environment that causes a state of stress. The stressor need not be present for the stress to be felt, for the individual can think about or worry over the stressor at any time (including during sleep). Moreover, stressors are not necessarily the same for all people. One person, for example, may take an airport delay in stride and use the time to catch up on work, while another may construe it as a personal affront and an example of the ineptitude of the officials in charge. The same stressor is present, but there are two different responses to it.

The body's system for handling stress is designed to remain in a "ready" status most of the time, coming into other difficulties. Regardless of these physiological realities, some people do have an overactive stress response that makes them react strongly to even minor provocations. It is possible, according to some researchers, that a genetic predisposition, or genetic dysfunction, exists in individuals who overreact to stressors in this way. It is possible, too, that an exaggerated response is rooted in prolonged or extreme exposure to stress during early childhood, when critical pathways in the brain are still developing.

Internal conflicts can also be a source of stress. Such conflicts exist, for example, when an individual must decide between two equally compelling but antagonistic options (e.g., take a year off before college or get some prerequisites out of the way?) or between two equally unattractive options (accept a bad job or risk staying unemployed?). Again, some people are better able than others to handle these kinds of situations. Erik Erikson (1980), in his theory of development, notes that often the central internal conflicts revolve around issues of (1) autonomy versus dependence, (2) intimacy versus isolation, or (3) cooperation versus competition. Thought of in that way, it is understandable that some individuals might experience a kind of existential angst in facing important decisions. Most of us, however, experience stress in more prosaic terms and at a more practical level.

Culture, Society, and Stress

Culture and society may shape what stresses will turn us toward assistance. In traditional Indian culture, for example, stress is generally understood to be an integral part of life—a kind of energizing principle—not something that needs to be brought to the attention of a mental health professional or other expert. When stress does become a negative force, there are forms of self-healing available, such as meditation and yoga.

In Latin American cultures the concept of *nervios* ("nerves") is drawn on to account for symptoms such as headaches ("brain aches"), emotionality, irritability, sleeplessness, dizziness, and so on. Nervios is an expression of psychological distress that is more common among women than among men. It is distinguished from a similar disorder, *susto* ("fright," or "soul loss"), in that it is a long-term, or chronic, condition and is more strongly linked to both stress and depression.

Long ago the sociologist Robert Merton (1963) suggested that society can induce stress by promoting values that conflict with the institutions and social structures through with those values are to be realized. Merton argued that the system of values in the United States promotes attainment of monetary success among more people than can possibly be accommodated by the opportunities available. As a consequence, many of those who have internalized these culturally valued goals are doomed to failure.

There are variations in the prevalence of stress among groups in the United States. For instance, U.S. women are far more likely than U.S. men to be diagnosed with anxiety and stress-related disorders, but this may have to do, in part, with a greater willingness among women to seek professional help for these conditions. People who feel marginalized or situated outside the sociocultural mainstream, such as gays and lesbians, people of color, and physically and mentally challenged persons, are also more likely than those from the general population to feel the impact of stress in their lives, a result of discrimination, harassment, economic deprivation, and other factors. Such ongoing adversity can have serious consequences in terms of the individual's neurophysiological health.

Addressing Stress

Stress management can refer to any action that helps prevent or reduce the body's stress response. A variety of strategies are available. One of the most common involves relaxation techniques, such as meditation or progressive muscle relaxation, perhaps aided by calming aural and aromatic stimuli. Education about stress is another standard element of most stress management programs. Participants learn how to identify their personal sources of stress, how to recognize the physiological and psychological signs that they are becoming overly stressed (including through biofeedback), and how to avoid or control stressors to the extent that this is possible. For those who subscribe to them, aromatherapy and/or crystals might be utilized, while a hot tub or whirlpool bath can provide relaxation—both mental and physical. Exercise, likewise, including stretching exercise like yoga, has also been shown to help reduce stress.

Sometimes it is necessary to employ a more serious or comprehensive approach, such as cognitive-behavioral therapy. Under this approach, individuals are taught to monitor and change stressful thoughts, to reorganize their activities and behaviors in such a way as to minimize stress, to actively schedule "time off" or other pleasing activities, to prioritize and manage their workloads, and to generally adopt a healthy lifestyle. Often, too, an antianxiety (anxiolytic) drug may be prescribed.

Michael Shally-Jensen

See also: Anxiety and Its Treatment; Aromatherapy and Essential Oils; Biofeedback; Breathwork; Crystals; Hysteria; Meditation and Mindfulness; Mind–Body Medicine; Neurasthenia, or Nervous Exhaustion; Spas and Mineral Waters; Sweat Lodges and Saunas; Yoga

Further Reading

Erikson, Erik. 1980. *Identity and the Life Cycle*. New York: Norton.

Folkman, Susan. 2011. *The Oxford Handbook of Stress, Health, and Coping*. New York: Oxford University Press.

Marohn, Stephanie. 2003. *The Natural Medicine Guide to Anxiety*. Charlottesville, VA: Hampton Roads.

Merton, Robert K. 1963. *Social Theory and Social Structure.* Rev. ed. Glencoe, IL: Free Press.
Tummers, Nanette. 2013. *Stress Management: A Wellness Approach.* Champaign, IL: Human
    Kinetics.

SWEAT LODGES AND SAUNAS

Originating in North America (sweat lodges) and Europe (saunas), sweat lodges
and saunas are both structures in which people are exposed to high temperatures,
but for different reasons. Sweat lodges were constructed by some Native American
tribes as spaces in which to hold religious ceremonies. The northern European
sauna tradition, on the other hand, which is particularly linked to Finland, was
used for cleansing the body of impurities. Saunas eventually became widespread in
Europe and North America, whereas most Native American leaders have attempted
to keep the sweat lodge tradition limited to members of those who have traditionally used them. They have not been completely successful in doing so, however,
as sweat lodges were also adopted by the New Age movement of the 1980s for the
purposes of health and spiritual enlightenment.

Sweat Lodges

For several tribes of Native Americans who lived on the Great Plains, the sweat
lodge and its associated rituals have been a part of the culture as far back as collective memory goes. Because these tribes were nomadic, having no permanent settlements, the sweat lodge, like other such structures, was built from saplings that
were bent to form a domed structure. Historically, it was then covered with animal
skins, buffalo being the most common. In current usage, however, a wide variety
of materials are employed, including blankets and tarps as well as skins. In the
center of the lodge, a pit is dug in which rocks are placed as part of the ceremony.
The single entrance to the lodge is oriented toward a specific compass direction,
depending upon the tribe and the reason for constructing the lodge.

Because the Native American sweat lodge was, and is, used for religious/cultural
ceremonies, it is built tall enough for a person to sit or kneel in, but not normally
high enough to stand in. For the Northern Plains Indians, only individuals who
have been trained in the sweat lodge ceremonies can lead people in a sweat lodge
gathering. This not only includes having participated in ceremonies for several
years but also fluency in their ancestral language in order to communicate with
the ancestors. Prior to the ceremony, rocks are heated outside the lodge, and then
moved into the lodge at the start of the ceremony and placed in the pit in the center. Just as the rocks can remain hot for several hours, ceremonies can also last an
extended period of time. A variety of spiritual exercises can be conducted by those
gathered in the sweat lodge. Sometimes this is the reason for the gathering, while
at other times the lodge exercises can be a preliminary step in a larger event, such
as the Sun Dance.

Sometimes, in the spirit of Native American unity, the Plains tribes will invite members of other tribes to join with them in sweat lodge ceremonies. However, most stand in opposition to the appropriation of the sweat lodge by New Age practitioners, who typically teach nontraditional beliefs regarding sweat lodges and do so for monetary gain. Native leaders, as well as medical professionals, point to the possible risks of subjecting people to high temperatures for an extended period of time. A noted case occurred in 2009, when three individuals died in a sweat lodge in Arizona run by a New Age teacher; the teacher was subsequently convicted of negligent homicide. The leaders of the sweat lodge tradition among the Plains Indians see those who use sweat lodges for monetary gain or as part of the teaching of other philosophies/religions as pernicious. Some have even filed lawsuits in an unsuccessful attempt to stop outsiders from using the Native American traditions inappropriately. Nonnative users counter that they are not seeking to diminish the culture of any one tribe but are merely drawing on ancient human knowledge regarding the use of physical challenges to engage in spiritual quests. Often, that is, these users employ the sweat lodge as part of a series of challenges that include such things as fasting, sleep deprivation, fire walking, cold exposure, and so on. The goal is to experience a kind of out-of-body vision of the spiritual world, or at least to reconfigure the normal relationship between the mind and the body.

Saunas

Although it is possible that at some point in the distant past saunas were used for religious ceremonies, this has not been part of the sauna tradition in recent centuries. The fact that in Finland there have been sauna rituals for birth, marriage, and death, and that in Finnish tradition each sauna has a guardian gnome/elf associated with it, seems to suggest the role that saunas may have played in the (pre-Christian) religious culture of the Finns. However, in recent times saunas have been primarily a means of personal cleansing, in the manner of a shower. Finland is seen as the home of modern sauna culture, although saunas were present in one form or another in other parts of Europe prior to the present era. While many associate saunas more with Sweden than with Finland, due to the specific type of sauna that found favor outside of Scandinavia and the broader spread of Swedish culture, Finland is the sauna's traditional home and the Finnish language the source of the word *sauna*. In Finland, in fact, the tradition is so strong that virtually every house is built with a sauna as part of its design.

It is traditional in Finland for individuals using saunas to be naked. The user stays in the sauna until it starts to feel too hot, and then may leave to take a cool shower, jump into cold water, or fall into the snow in wintertime. This cycle is typically repeated a few times. A shower is normally taken both before and after using a sauna. After the final cycle, refreshments are taken to replenish the body with liquids.

Over the course of the centuries, technological and architectural changes have affected the design of saunas. Beginning as covered pits, or primitive buildings with dirt floors, saunas later evolved to incorporate wood stoves, chimneys, and, most recently, alternative (nonwood) heat sources. This last step made it possible to have saunas in virtually any building or area. In all of these traditional structures, stones were heated to provide warmth during the time people came to be "cleansed." The key to the sauna experience was the intense heat that caused participants to sweat extensively. The traditional, and for some, current belief was that sweating allowed the body to rid itself of toxins, thus contributing to better health. Other current advocates for saunas, outside northern Europe, point to Finnish studies showing that those who regularly use saunas have better heart health, likely owing to the endurance of heat or the contrast of heat and cold. Whatever long-term health benefits of saunas, they do relax muscles and provide a pleasant overall experience for most people.

There are two main types of saunas, wet and dry. Even though it is common for people in Finland to throw water on the hot rocks, increasing the humidity and the effect of the sauna, they traditionally use less water than do other Scandinavian cultures. Thus, at the same temperature the relatively dry Finnish sauna tends to feel cooler than the so-called Swedish sauna. The higher the humidity, generally the more intense the experience of heat, which some find pleasing and others less so. Many Finns, in fact, prefer the traditional smoke-sauna, wherein stones are heated by means of an unvented wood fire, with the smoke being released just prior to the participants entering the space. The use of smoke is seen to purify the sauna and perhaps the user as well. Sometimes a small, wet birch branch is used to flagellate oneself while in the sauna. The idea is to free the pores and increase circulation at the skin's surface. For the Finns, the sauna is generally a communal experience; depending on the setting, it can be either single-sex or mixed. Perhaps the social setting and the physical and mental relaxation produced have contributed to the Finns' being consistently ranked as one of the "happiest" or most satisfied people on the planet.

Donald A. Watt

See also: Aromatherapy and Essential Oils; Detox Diets; Hydrotherapy; Mind–Body Medicine; Native American Traditional Medicine; Shamanism and Neo-Shamanism; Spas and Mineral Waters; Stress and Stress Management

Further Reading

Bosworth, Mark. 2013. "Why Finland Loves Saunas." *BBC News.* London: The British Broadcasting Corporation. www.bbc.com/news/magazine-24328773

Bucko, Raymond A. 1998. *The Lakota Ritual of the Sweat Lodge: History and Contemporary Practice.* Lincoln: University of Nebraska Press.

Central Finland Sauna. 2018. "Sauna." Jyvaskyla, Finland: Visit Central Finland. saunaregion .fi/sauna/

Edelsward, Lisa-Marlene. 2001. *Sauna as Symbol: Society and Culture in Finland.* American University Studies Book 53. New York: Peter Lang Inc.

Tanahuachi: Native American Church. 2015. "Inipi (The Sweat Lodge)." *Tanahuachi: Native American Kiva.* Georgetown, FL: Tanahuachi American Indian kiva. tanahuachi.org/?p=779

TAI CHI AND QIGONG

Tai Chi

Tai Chi Chuan (taijiquan), usually shortened to Tai Chi (taiji, meaning "grand ultimate"), is a graceful, gentle exercise widely performed by men, women, and children in China, in the Chinese diaspora, and among Westerners. It has become popular in many countries, where it is sometimes practiced in conjunction with body-awareness training and/or meditation. The movements of Tai Chi are related to those of Kung Fu—TaiChi is considered an "internal" martial art—but Tai Chi unfolds in a slow, stylized manner, as opposed to Kung Fu's quick hand-and-foot action. Although not a self-defense activity, Tai Chi can be used for self-development or internal strengthening.

In Chinese philosophy, the term *Tai Chi* refers to the eternal source and cause of all reality. In the *I Ching* (*Book of Changes*), the ancient philosophical text in which the concept is first mentioned, Tai Chi represents the union of the two primary aspects of the cosmos, *yin* (passive) and *yang* (active). Some philosophers associated Tai Chi with *li*, the supreme rational principle of the universe. Li generates *chi* (*ch'i*), or vital matter, which in turn is transformed through the actions of yin and yang into the Five Elements (wood, earth, fire, metal, and water). Thus are produced the basic constituents of the physical universe, which nevertheless carry within them their origins as pure force or energy.

The performance of Tai Chi, therefore, engages the whole body in carefully arranged and rhythmically precise movements that serve to intensify and refine natural vital energy. After the beginning stages, in which the postures and movements seem somewhat artificial, the student becomes proficient in feeling or experiencing the harmony of the universe and integrating the practice of Tai Chi with daily activities. For this reason it is sometimes called (by Westerners) "meditation in motion." Each movement of posture generally flows into the next without pausing. Breath control as well as—obviously—muscle control and balance are essential elements in Tai Chi. It is self-paced and noncompetitive, although it can be performed in a group setting.

Tai Chi became popular in Western countries both as Chinese communities expanded there and as interest in complementary and alternative approaches to health and wellness arose beginning in the 1970s but taking off in the 1980s and 1990s. Besides having an intriguing philosophy behind it, Tai Chi is appealing for its health benefits. It is used as part of a basic exercise program and as a complement to other health care methods. It is particularly popular among older adults, because its movements are low impact and put minimal stress on muscles and joints. It is considered to aid in the reduction of stress, the increasing of flexibility, the improvement of muscle strength and definition, and the optimization of energy, strength, and agility. Research continues as to whether it may play a role, like any physical exercise, in lowering blood pressure, moderating cholesterol levels, and lessening the likelihood of congestive heart failure. Irregularities of mood (anxiety, depression) may also be addressed through the consistent use of Tai Chi.

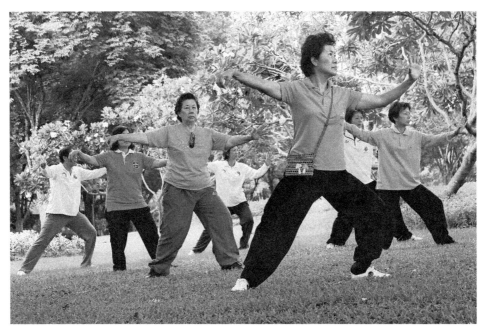

A tai chi group session in a park. (Kanjanee Chaisin/Dreamstime.com)

If there is any critique to be made regarding Tai Chi and its cousin, Qigong (see below), it is only that, from the perspective of Western science, the traditional Chinese concepts of yin and yang and of energy flows from one substance or agent to another substance or agent don't hold water. In the Western view, in the case of living matter, at least, energy is not transferred directly from point A to point B like a continuous wave or like the energy from one billiard ball passing to the next. Rather, "the energy of the response is provided by the respondent," as the naturalist-scientist Gregory Bateson put it (Bateson [1972] 2000, 409). This means, basically, that if one neuron has become excited and fires another, the second neuron fires (or not) by means of its own energy source, not because it has absorbed energy directly from the first. It may receive a charge, or change in charge, but not energy, or "power," as such. Cause and effect in living systems is always *mediated,* not direct. Thus, the notion of energy transfer underlying Chinese traditional medicine, as well as some forms of modern complementary and alternative medicine, is suspect in the eyes of mainstream Western medicine. This is not to say that people cannot benefit from these practices, both physically and mentally. They most definitely can. It is only to restate the philosophical divide separating these two very different systems.

Qigong

There are a variety of different forms of Qigong (or Qi Gong), ranging from a practitioner who uses his or her hands on an individual to forms that use meditation and exercise. It is taught and conducted both on an individual basis and in groups.

The essence of Qigong is the use of gentle, focused exercises for the mind and body designed to restore and increase the flow of *qi* (or *ch'i*, "life force") or, in a health and wellness setting, to accumulate qi with the aim of encouraging the healing process and accelerating its pace.

Qigong means, basically, "qi work," or "working with the energy of qi." Its concepts and techniques are related to ancient traditions associated with Taoism. Qigong, however, is not exclusively Taoist but shares its principles and goals with traditional Chinese medicine, the martial arts, and Tai Chi Chuan. It consists of two main arenas of action, internal and external. The objective is to remove any blockages of qi, thus restoring health and vitality. Internal Qigong is primarily self-directed (albeit sometimes reliant on an experienced guide) and involves the use of meditation and movement. External Qigong is performed by a qualified practitioner using the hands and other parts of the body and is designed to direct qi energy onto the patient. As with Tai Chi, controlled breathing and slow body movements are important elements of Qigong, whether internal or external. The motions and energetics involved are thought to have positive effects on the muscular system and the cardiovascular system as well as benefiting balance, coordination, and mood. There is evidence that Qigong might be effective in people with hypertension.

Qigong, like Tai Chi, is best regarded as a lifelong endeavor the regular practice of which is essential to achieving lasting effects. Individual sessions may differ in length but usually run to 30 minutes. As with Tai Chi, daily practice is the norm for longtime users but, minimally, Qigong should be performed two or three times a week. External Qigong tends to be for beginners who have not yet learned internal Qigong, which is considered superior. But external Qigong may also be requested in cases where a regular user does not seem to be able to get the result that he or she desires.

One variety of Qigong known as Falun Gong became wildly popular in China in the late 1990s and early 2000s. Falun Gong (which means "Dharma wheel practice") combines the slow movements and meditation of traditional Qigong with a moral philosophy centered on the concepts of truthfulness, compassion, and tolerance. Chinese authorities came to suspect Falun Gong practitioners, who often performed their exercises together in public spaces, of belonging to a subversive cult of some kind being operated by charismatic Qigong masters. Any such social movements are strictly prohibited in China on the grounds that they run counter to the idea of total control by the Communist Party. The authorities also felt that Falun Gong contained religious elements, again going against official Communist ideology. Thus, Falun Gong practitioners, whether masters or beginners, were persecuted, and Falun Gong groups were broken up. This is perhaps another reason why Qigong, including Falun Gong, became popular in the West: it could no longer be safely practiced in China—except, maybe, in the confines of one's home.

Michael Shally-Jensen

See also: Acupuncture; Chinese Traditional Medicine; Meditation and Mindfulness; Mind–Body Medicine; Reiki and Therapeutic Touch

Further Reading

Bateson, Gregory. [1972] 2000. *Steps to an Ecology of Mind.* Chicago: University of Chicago Press.

Jarmey, Chris. 2011. *The Theory and Practice of Taiji and Qigong.* 3rd ed. Berkeley, CA: North Atlantic Books.

Kohn, Livia. 2005. *Health and Long Life the Chinese Way.* Cambridge, MA: Three Pines Press.

Wang, Robin R. 2012. *Yinyang: The Way of Heaven and Earth in Chinese Thought and Culture.* Cambridge, UK: Cambridge University Press.

VITAMINS AND MINERALS

Taking a daily multivitamin is part of their morning ritual for millions of Americans. Vitamins are indeed necessary for the conversion of food into energy and the performance of other functions. Although some vitamins are made inside the body, most are not and must be consumed in foods—or as supplements. The question is, "Do we get enough vitamins in the food we eat?" Each person may have a different need, but in most cases the recommended daily allowance (RDA) as determined by nutrition experts is sufficient. And, in most cases too, those who eat a diet of mixed foods need not worry about running up short. The problem is that, whereas nutrition experts generally agree that the RDA is adequate and that most people's routine diets serve the purpose, many health advocates and dietary supplement industry representatives argue that foods do not contain enough vitamins and minerals and that larger quantities of each are needed. The science, however, mostly suggests that multivitamins—and especially "megavitamins" (large quantities)—are not really necessary. The supplement industry and many individual Americans, however, say that that is incorrect and one should always take one's daily vitamins.

Vitamins

Vitamins are the natural components in food—different from proteins, carbohydrates, and fats—which help ensure normal metabolism. They are essential for good health and growth, and when they are deficient or absent, dramatic problems can develop. Vitamins fall into two categories, essential and nonessential. The essential vitamins are needed to sustain life and to maintain good health, yet the body must get them from outside sources. Nonessential vitamins are vital but the body can manufacture them on their own.

A well-balanced diet should satisfy the RDA of each vitamin. RDAs are guidelines first developed by the Food and Nutrition Board and the National Academy of Sciences–National Research Council based on the nutritional needs of the average healthy person. The U.S. government eventually adopted the National Research Council's RDAs. They are expressed in milligrams or international units (IU), and these recommendations differ for adults and children as well as for people who must follow special diets or women who are pregnant or lactating.

The vitamins include vitamin A; the eight vitamin B complex group of B1, or thiamine; B2, or riboflavin; B3, or niacin; B5, or pantothenic acid; B6, or pyridoxine; B7, or biotin; B9, or folic acid; and B12, or cobalamin; vitamin C; vitamin D; vitamin E; and vitamin K.

Vitamin A is fat-soluble and comes from animal foods like liver, egg yolks, cream, or butter or from beta-carotene that occurs in leafy green vegetables and in yellow fruits and vegetables. Vitamin A is important to skeletal growth as well as the health of the skin and mucus membranes. It is often used as a supplement to improve eye function and general longevity—with limited scientific support. A deficiency of this vitamin can cause slowed skeletal growth, skin abnormalities, and susceptibility to serious infection.

Thiamine, B1, is part of the vitamin B complex and plays an important role in the metabolism of carbohydrates. It also helps maintain appetite, normal intestinal function, and the health of the cardiovascular and nervous systems. It is used to treat such disorders as beriberi, a neurological disorder associated with excessive reliance on white (polished) rice as a food. Yeast, legumes, whole grains, thiamine-enriched cereal products, and nuts are all good sources of thiamine.

Riboflavin, also known as B2, is needed by the body to effectively metabolize carbohydrates, fats, and respiratory proteins. It is sometimes used as a supplement to prevent migraines. Good sources of riboflavin include liver, milk, meat, dark green vegetables, whole grain and enriched cereals, and mushrooms. Deficiency can cause skin lesions and sensitivity to light.

Niacin, B3, aids in the release of energy from nutrients. A deficiency of niacin causes pellagra, the symptoms of which include a sunburnlike eruption that breaks out when skin is exposed to sunlight. Other symptoms are a red and swollen tongue, diarrhea, mental confusion, and depression. Large doses of niacin have been used to reduce levels of cholesterol in the blood, but over long periods they can cause liver damage. Good sources of niacin are liver, poultry, meat, tuna and salmon, dried beans and peas, and nuts.

Pantothenic acid, B5 vitamin, plays a role in the metabolism of many substances, including fatty acids, steroids, and carbohydrates. The adrenal gland is an important site of pantothenic acid activity. Deficiencies of vitamin B5 are extremely rare, for pantothenic acid is abundant in many foods, including liver, kidney, eggs, and dairy products. There is virtually no problem with deficiency since it is also manufactured by intestinal bacteria.

Pyridoxine, or vitamin B6, is needed for the absorption and metabolism of amino acids, glucose, and fatty acids. It also plays a role in the formation of red blood cells. The relatively uncommon instances of B6 deficiency involve skin conditions like seborrheic dermatitis. The best sources of pyridoxine are liver and other organ meats, along with spinach, avocados, green beans, bananas, whole grain cereal, and seeds.

Biotin, a B vitamin, also plays a role in the metabolism of carbohydrates, fats, and amino acids. It is synthesized by intestinal bacteria and is widespread in foods, especially egg yolks, tomatoes, yeast, kidney, and liver. Biotin deficiency occurs, infrequently, in breastfeeding mothers. The solution is biotin consumption as a supplement or food.

Folic acid, or vitamin B9, is rich in green leafy vegetables, fruits, dried beans, sunflower seeds, and wheat germ. It works to form body protein and hemoglobin, and deficiencies have been linked to neural tube defects, a type of birth defect that causes serious brain or neurological disorders such as spina bifida. Folic acid is lost in foods stored at room temperature and during cooking, so to increase access to this important vitamin the government has required enrichment of flours, corn-meal, rice, and pasta with folic acid since 1998. Unlike other water-soluble vita-mins, folic acid is stored in the liver and does not need to be eaten daily.

Vitamin B12, cobalamin, is the most complex of all known vitamins and is important in nervous system functioning. It comes only from animal sources—liver, kidneys, meat, fish, eggs, and milk—and vegans or vegetarians, who eat few or no dairy products, are advised to take a supplement to ensure that they have adequate amounts. This vitamin is also necessary for folic acid to fulfill its role, and both are involved in the synthesis of proteins.

Vitamin C is perhaps the best known of the vitamins and is important in the formation and maintenance of collagen, a protein that help form bones and teeth. Vitamin C also enhances the absorption of iron from foods. Deficiency of this vitamin causes scurvy, the symptoms of which include hemorrhages, loosening of teeth, and bone problems, especially in children. The use of large doses of vitamin C in treating common colds, vigorously promoted by the Nobel Prize–winning chemist Linus Pauling (1901–1994), is not as yet scientifically supported, despite ongoing research.

Vitamin D is needed for healthy bones and for the retention of calcium and phosphorus in the body. Called the "sunshine vitamin," it can be manufactured in the body with as little as a half-hour of sunlight. Rickets, from vitamin D defi-ciency, is usually caused by a lack of exposure to sunlight rather than a dietary deficiency. Symptoms include bowlegs, knock knees, and other bone deformities, or, in adults, softening of the bones. However, because this is a fat-soluble vitamin, it is stored in the body. To prevent deficiencies, the government requires milk to be fortified with vitamin D. Infants and breastfeeding women are generally advised to take small doses of supplementary vitamin D. On the other hand, excessive consumption can cause nausea, loss of appetite, and kidney damage. Good food sources of vitamin D include egg yolk, liver, tuna, and vitamin D–fortified milk or juice.

Vitamin E plays a role in forming red blood cells and muscle and other tissues. It is also a potent antioxidant, and studies show that it protects against arterial plaque buildup and, arguably, cancer. On the other hand, excessive amounts of vitamin E can have significant negative consequences, including risks of bleed-ing and other issues. It is found in vegetable oils, wheat germ, green leafy vege-tables, and liver.

Vitamin K is necessary for the clotting of blood and its richest sources are alfalfa and fish livers. Other sources include leafy green vegetables, egg yolks, soybean oil, and liver. The bacterial synthesis of this vitamin usually provides enough for a healthy adult but those suffering from blood diseases can experience some deficiency.

Minerals

A mineral, as understood by nutritionists, is an element needed by the body other than the basic molecular elements of carbon, hydrogen, nitrogen, and oxygen. The main nutritional minerals are calcium, phosphorus, potassium, sodium, and magnesium. A number of others (including chromium, cobalt, copper, iodine, iron, manganese, selenium, and zinc) are needed in trace amounts only.

Minerals are "earth" elements that occur naturally in such foods as whole-grain cereals, fruits, vegetables, dairy foods, meats, and fish. As with vitamins, a healthy, balanced diet usually supplies all the minerals the body needs. Minerals that are absorbed are carried through the body with the help of proteins. Any excessive amounts of minerals are simply evacuated.

Calcium has a central role in many physiological processes, including growth and maintenance of bones along with processes like blood clotting, nervous system activity, and regulation of enzymes and hormones. Women, particularly older women, sometimes consume less calcium than recommended, which can contribute to osteoporosis, or weakened, brittle bones. Excessive calcium, on the other hand, can cause kidney problems and calcification of blood vessels. Fresh milk contains calcium, as do fish, beans, nuts, egg yolk, and cauliflower.

Phosphorus is an important element in metabolism and energy production. Dietary phosphorus is plentiful, and cases of deficiency are uncommon. When they do occur, typical symptoms include fatigue and weakness, among others. Too much phosphorus can harm the kidneys and weaken bone.

Potassium, like sodium, is involved in water balance, heart rhythm, muscle contraction, and nerve-signal conduction. Potassium also affects the metabolism of glucose and lipids. Potassium deficiency is uncommon but can lead to nausea, weakness, and cramps. Excessive potassium can lead to heart irregularities. The main sources of potassium in the diet are dairy products, meats, poultry, fish, vegetables, whole grains, and fruits.

Sodium, or "salt," is involved in balancing the body's water levels, maintaining proper heartbeat, regulating muscle action, and the conduction of nerve impulses. High sodium intake can lead to water retention, hypertension, and heart failure. Sodium deficiencies are rare but can produce adverse mental activity and convulsions. In addition to table salt, sodium is contained in cheeses, breads, and many processed foods.

Magnesium is needed for the proper functioning of the nervous system, the support of cell membranes, and the building of healthy bones. An imbalance of magnesium can lead to blood pressure issues, heart problems, muscle cramps, and even mental conditions like disorientation and depression. The main sources of magnesium are dairy products, seafoods, and green leafy vegetables.

Iron is among the more important trace elements. Iron is necessary for the proper functioning of red blood cells, the immune system, and enzyme production. Anemia is the principal adverse effect of low iron levels, which can produce weakness and tiredness as well as cognitive problems. Women show higher iron-deficiency rates than do men, owing to the loss of iron through menstruation. Meat, poultry, fish, eggs, breads, cereals, potatoes, and green vegetables are the major sources of iron.

Iodine, another mineral, is essential in the synthesis of thyroid hormones. More common in the past than today was the condition known as goiter, caused by an iodine deficiency and characterized by an enlarged thyroid gland. Iodine is present in seafood (including seaweed), dairy products, and eggs, but only if the animals ingested iodine in their diets, based on food sources and iodine levels in the soil. Today, most salt in the United States (and elsewhere) is iodized to help prevent deficiency.

Marjolijn Bijlefeld,
Sharon K. Zoumbaris, and Michael Shally-Jensen

See also: Antioxidants; Bottled Water; Detox Diets; Diet Pills and Metabolism Boosters; Eating Organic; Herbal Remedies; Juice and Juicing; Macrobiotics; Vegetarianism

Further Reading

Bijlefeld, Marjolin, and Sharon K. Zoumbaris. 2014. *The Encyclopedia of Diet Fads.* Santa Barbara, CA: Greenwood.

Hamblin, James. 2016. *If Our Bodies Could Talk: A Guide to Operating and Maintaining a Human Body.* New York: Doubleday.

Schiff, Wendy J. 2017. *Nutrition Essentials: A Personal Approach.* 2nd ed. New York: McGraw-Hill Education.

WALKING AND JOGGING

As far as exercise for human beings goes, walking may be one of the first and best activities we engaged in. We started walking on two legs and began searching for food in new ways. Scientists now believe that our prehistoric Neanderthal cousins existed mostly on plants—nuts, berries, and roots. Foraging for food this way meant moving across regular terrain to ensure that there was enough food for the whole social group.

Jogging is often considered distinct from running, but in terms of physical movement, it is a slow, gentle run. The idea of jogging for fitness began in the 1960s. For many animals, a slow and easy lope is the most energy-efficient way to move over longer distances. When humans needed to move from one area to another, that sort of jog was probably a good way to move.

While walking and jogging were simply ways to get around that served us for eons, working in modern offices and having modern transports like cars, subways,

Walking and Jogging: Does Couch to 5k Work?

If you try to get involved in the running or marathoning world, one of the first programs you might hear about is Couch to 5K, or C25K as many of its fans refer to it. This is a nine-week program that promises to turn the average person from a couch potato into someone who can run three miles (roughly five kilometers).

What's great about the program is that it's based on combining periods of walking and then running to help your body build up endurance and strength. Each session, the running periods are a little longer while the walking periods are a little shorter. Over those nine weeks, the program should build the endurance needed to run those three miles.

Does Couch to 5K work? As with many fitness programs, it depends on the runner. It's a great program for absolute beginners who want to become runners but don't know how to get started. Running also has the benefit of not really needing more equipment than a decent pair of sneakers.

That said, many experts feel that C25K isn't a good program for true beginners. There isn't a strength or stretching component to the program, which leaves beginners prone to injury and doesn't show them how to strengthen their body and make running possible. Many people have a lack of strength in their lower bodies; while they need the endurance to keep running, they also need to be stronger overall.

Like many other workout programs, make sure to do your research if you're going to try out C25K, and be cautious if you're new to running. Injuries can set you back and leave you disappointed.

and elevators left us looking for ways to increase our exercise so as to maintain physical fitness. Jogging developed as a counter to the sedentary lifestyle that came with living in cities and suburbs in modern industrialized society.

From Competitive Sport to Exercise

Marathons became part of the Olympics in 1896, and the Boston Marathon was first run in 1897. While many other races are run in round distances—5 kilometers, for example—marathons are always 26.2 miles (42.2 kilometers). This is a reference to Pheidippides, the Greek soldier who ran from Marathon to Athens to announce that the Persians were defeated. According to the story, he declared the victory, then immediately fell over dead.

Since then, training for marathons has become a much more intense project, and few people try to run a marathon without extensive preparation. Along marathon routes, medical personnel are prepared to deal with emergencies if they arise.

More than 500 marathons are run each year now; marathoners joke that the first 26 miles are easy, and that it's the last quarter of a mile that will kill you. There are even ultramarathons of 100 kilometers (62.1 miles). And of course there is race-walking, which also is strenuous exercise.

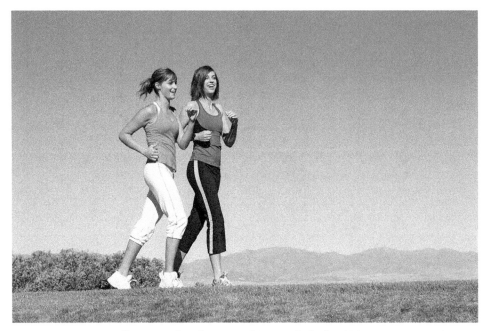

Two women power walking together along a trail in a park. (Yobro10/Dreamstime.com)

Walking certain distances as wagers was popular for hundreds of years in Europe, but walking and running became more popular as exercise options when they became part of the Olympic Games. In 1963, perhaps the first *Joggers Manual* came out, in pamphlet form, in Portland, Oregon; its basic advice was:

"Jogging is a bit more than a walk. . . . Start with a short distance then increase as you improve. Jog until you are puffing, then walk until your breathing is normal again. Repeat until you have covered a mile or two, or three." (quoted in Latham 2015).

In 1964, the first dedicated running shoe was made by the company that would eventually become Nike, also located near Portland (in Beaverton). By the 1990s, walking and jogging were considered the most popular forms of exercise in the United States.

And while we may think of something like meditation as being the complete *opposite* of running or walking, some religious orders have in fact embraced walking meditation. The most well known version of this is kinhin, a practice in Zen Buddhism where practitioners walk in single file, often in time to a clapper or bell. Synchronized breathing and stride may help create mindfulness.

Walking and Health

Both walking and running are considered good exercise for the cardiovascular system—that is, the heart and lungs. The heart has to work hard while one is walking, and since the heart is a muscle, working it makes it stronger. When the heart is strong, one's resting heart rate and blood pressure are lower, both indications of good health.

These activities are also said to provide mental benefits: some evidence suggests that walking, in particular, improves mood, sharpens mental acuity, and can be very beneficial for people with mild anxiety or depression.

One great debate in the exercise community is whether just walking (or jogging) is enough to get healthy. Some fitness experts say that walking at a brisk pace for 30 minutes, six days a week, is enough to lower your weight, improve your heart health, and strengthen your lungs.

But those are not the only measures of fitness. While walking can improve your cardiovascular fitness in certain ways, there are other fitness measures that neither walking nor jogging will really touch without some additional work.

- Cardiovascular or aerobic fitness: this is where walking really shines. Walking raises your heart rate, gets your big muscle groups working, and keeps your blood circulating. Ideally, you should be able to hold a conversation with a walking partner without needing to pause to catch your breath—but it should be work to keep talking.

- Strength training: if you don't walk around much, when you first start walking or jogging, you'll see a difference in your legs as these muscles get stronger. But unfortunately, walking won't do much for the other major muscle groups of your body. In fact, if you have back or shoulder problems, walking can actually make them worse.

- Flexibility: while walking doesn't directly improve flexibility in your joints, it can improve joint health. Research has shown that weight-bearing exercise increases blood flow and nutrition to the joints, which helps to prevent arthritis and other joint problems. If you have really loose joints—hypermobile joints—strengthening the surrounding muscles can help to reduce pain and improve your overall quality of life.

Exercise Options

Should one start with walking or jogging? As with so many other types of exercise, the answer is: it depends. Some people will benefit greatly from starting a walking program; others may need some physical support to get the most out of walking; still others may find a different method of exercise to better support their overall health.

If you are someone who has not regularly exercised and are looking for a slow start to improve overall fitness, walking is a good way to take that first step. The usual advice is to start out slow, keep the pace easy, keep track of your breathing, and gradually increase distances. Jogging is better saved for when one's cardiovascular health has improved and joint health is improving. It is possible to run with ankle, knee, or hip problems, but in that case it is helpful to get the support of an experienced trainer.

If one is moderately fit and looking to take things to the next level, a jogging program might be a way to continue to develop cardiovascular fitness and maintain a healthy weight, but achieving a new level of fitness is probably going to take something different. Once walking is fairly easy, it may be time to either invest in some hand weights at home or get a gym membership. Directly training one's muscles, in conjunction with walking/light jogging, is probably the next step toward physical performance.

If a person is strong but not flexible, walking isn't going to make much of a difference. Instead, consider a program that directly emphasizes flexibility, like yoga or Pilates. A great benefit of these programs is that they emphasize healthy "core" fitness (torso, abdomen, hips), something that not all workouts do. Having a strong, fit core will help you be successful in any exercise program. In fact, core fitness may be one of the best ways to support one's body overall.

As with any other exercise program, before you get started, it's a good idea to speak with your doctor. With walking and jogging, it is particularly important to do so if you have a history of joint problems, asthma, or other concerns. Yet most people can be successful with a walking program, especially if they start slowly and work up gradually to jogging. Overall, running and jogging are incredibly accessible sports. All that is needed is a good pair of shoes and a little willpower.

Kay Tilden Frost

See also: Aging Prevention, or "Successful Aging"; Dance Therapy; Diet and Exercise; Meditation and Mindfulness

Further Reading

Bumgardener, Wendy. 2018. "A Brief History of Walking," *Very Well Fit*. February 10. https://www.verywellfit.com/a-brief-history-of-walking-3436273

Latham, Alan. 2015. "The History of a Habit: Jogging as a Palliative to Sedentariness in 1960s America." *Cultural Geography* (January) 22(1):103–26. https://www.ncbi.nlm.nih.gov/pmc/articles/PMC5897920/

Meyers, Casey. 2007. *Walking: A Complete Guide to the Complete Exercise*. New York: Ballantine Books.

Peterson, Dan. 2010. "Why Are Marathons 26.2 Miles Long?" *Life Science*. April 19. https://www.livescience.com/11011-marathons-26-2-miles-long.html

2000–Present

INTRODUCTION

As the 21st century unfolded, doctors, no longer lording over their patients but working more or less in partnership with them, began opening up to practices once considered alternative but now regarded as part of treating the whole person—mind, body, and spirit. Indeed, the very word *alternative* (along with the phrase *complementary and alternative*) began to fade somewhat in favor of a new term, *integrative*. Integrative medicine, or integrative therapeutics, refers to the practice of using conventional medicine alongside alternative/complementary treatments, particularly those that have some compelling research behind them. Thus, integrative medicine is both a complement to and basically a part of regular treatment. Practices like yoga, progressive muscle relaxation, deep breathing, meditation, and Tai Chi or Qigong have become widely accepted as positively effecting outcomes for a variety of conditions, while maintaining a healthy diet and doing daily exercise, even if only light exercise and of short duration, have become the norm more than the exception for many.

The focus for the past few decades, then, has been *wellness,* or the maintenance of good health and the improvement of the quality of life overall. Even those with serious conditions seek to optimize their health and well-being through the use, most often, of a combination of standard medical treatments and various "natural" or "holistic" methods. At the time of this writing, there were more than 50 institutions in the United States with the word *integrative* in their name, ranging from those linked to universities such as the University of Arizona and the University of Maryland to public-private or nonprofit organizations like the Mayo Clinic and the Cleveland Clinic. Most of them offer treatments like acupuncture, massage, and nutrition counseling along with conventional drugs and surgery. Motion therapies, particularly among older consumers, are enjoying a renaissance.

Whatever treatment is used, the integrative doctors in these centers and clinics hope to make chronic disease more manageable, temporary (or acute) conditions more tolerable, and overall health better in their patients. In doing so, they are researching and monitoring therapies that once were considered secondary, at best, subjecting them to testing and making use of them in much the same way that they would make use of any evidence-based medicine.

The goal is generally to enhance or optimize the body's natural healing functions. A patient, for example, who has high blood pressure, irritable bowel syndrome, and a skin rash is no longer simply given separate medications for each and sent home. Rather, the physician works with the patient to identify how or why these symptoms have appeared and how they might be connected through a common root. Traditional categories of illness and knowledge begin to break down as, again, the whole person is considered and treatment developed accordingly. Perhaps in this example, then, meditation and a natural medicament or two would be prescribed in addition to conventional drug therapy. Another example would be acupuncture prescribed after a surgical procedure to lessen nausea or help control pain and inflammation.

Integrative medicine, moreover, is not just about assigning therapies when the body (or the mind or spirit) is broken; it is about trying to prevent such a breakdown in the first place. It's about health maintenance and wellness. Sometimes, in fact, an experience of illness and an exposure to integrative care leads people to make long-lasting changes to their lifestyle—changes that they might not have made otherwise. One can see this as a kind of ironic twist on Nietzsche's "What doesn't kill you makes you stronger"—or "healthier," in this case.

Integrative care tends to be more personalized than standard care. Under the new model, the physician may order targeted lab workups while also holding lengthy consultations with patients to check on everything from family, school, and work issues to diet and environmental exposures. These are the types of things that can interact at the physiological or even the genetic level to determine the nature and course of an illness. Many patients who enter integrative health centers leave with three- or six-month health plans in hand.

Most integrative approaches explore dietary questions to a degree that goes well beyond ensuring the usual balance of food groups or avoiding excessive salt and trans fats. They consider the prospect of undiagnosed food sensitivities, hormonal imbalances, or autoimmune factors. These problems have increasingly been seen as accounting for many chronic health complaints and may cause more serious underlying damage over time. The topic of intestinal bacteria—the gut microbiome—looms large in current medicine, as researchers have found potential connections between various external symptoms and the internal state of the gastrointestinal tract.

According to a survey by the National Center for Complementary and Integrative Health and the National Center for Health Statistics (2017), greater than one in three adults in the United States uses some form of integrative medicine. The most commonly used form was dietary supplements, that is, products such as fish oil, probiotics, and herbal preparations like ginseng. Other therapies that ranked high on the list included yoga, chiropractic, and massage therapy along with meditation and osteopathic consultation/treatment. Moreover, all these therapies have increased significantly in usage (between 4 and 14 percent) since the last survey was conducted in 2012. Use tended to be higher among women than among men, as it did for those with higher levels of education as against those with less education. The study also found that integrative methods and products were used by people of all backgrounds.

It seems clear, then, that we have arrived at a significant moment in the evolution of complementary and integrative health, and that the trend toward "whole person" health and wellness is likely to continue in the near future. Popular media outlets have picked up on, and led, this trend, with online and cable and network television productions, along with classic print resources, seeing a great spike of interest among the U.S. populace. Alternative/integrative health and healing are now mainstream.

Further Reading

Gritz, Jennie Rothenberg. 2015. "The Evolution of Alternative Medicine." *Atlantic,* June 25. https://www.theatlantic.com/health/archive/2015/06/the-evolution-of-alternative -medicine/396458/

Mayo Clinic. 2017. *The Integrative Guide to Good Health.* New York: Time, Inc.

National Center for Complementary and Integrative Health and National Center for Health Statistics. 2017. National Health Interview Survey. https://nccih.nih.gov/research /statistics/NHIS

BOTTLED WATER

Water, of course, is a basic necessity of life for all organisms on earth, humans included. As humans spread across the continents, the quantity and quality of potable water available varied drastically. However, people did have the ability to create systems (such as the Roman aqueducts) and containers (initially ceramic, later glass) for moving water from one location to another. In Greece, what might be called the first processed bottled water was produced by Hippocrates. After getting water from a stream or well, he advised boiling it and then pouring the water into a clean container through a cloth, thus filtering it. However, that did not become the norm in Greece, or elsewhere. In more recent centuries, bottled water originated as a luxury product assumed to be healthy; it was transformed into a widely used, everyday product only in recent decades.

History

The earliest European records of the commercial bottling and sale of mineral water, in several different locations, occurred in the 16th century. This was mineral water, most of which was sparkling—that is, water with natural carbonation—which was believed to have healing properties. The earliest record of bottled water production in what is now the United States was in Boston in 1767. That same year, the scientist Joseph Priestley invented a way to artificially infuse water with carbon dioxide; he subsequently wrote a paper about it entitled "Impregnating Water with Fixed Air." In 1783, Jacob Schweppes developed a process for manufacturing artificially carbonated water based on Priestley's process. He expanded his sales by introducing fizzy lemonade in 1831, and other companies followed suit. The demand for mineral waters continued until the early 20th century, when many of its health claims were shown to be unfounded.

During the 19th century two factors outside the bottled water industry transformed it. The growth of cities caused an increased demand for safe drinking water, not only because there were more thirsts to quench but because the amount of sewage produced in the cities also increased dramatically, threatening water supplies. Secondly, the glassmaking industry was mechanized, creating a more affordable product, with bottlers in France developing an automated corking machine as an alternative to manually sealing the filled bottles. Although it was not until the middle of the 19th century that certain diseases were clearly understood to be spread by water-borne organisms, the demand for pure spring water, in addition to mineral water, had arisen earlier in the century as a healthy alternative.

By the beginning of the 20th century, clean municipal water supplies had been developed, and these now included the use of chlorine (for bacterial control) and, later, fluoride (for dental health) for city residents. In addition, a better understanding of illness, both its cause and its cure, resulted in a decreased demand for costly mineral water. Public supplies could be utilized as long as the water was certified as safe. Consequently, in the United States the bottled water industry became almost nonexistent. There was a similar trend in Europe, although one not quite as dramatic.

After World War II, bottled water had a revival in eating establishments in Europe. It was a French product, Perrier, that started a revival in the United States. Initially marketing only sparkling water in the United States, which added to its aura of not being for the common person, Perrier was able to convince Americans that the prestige of drinking bottled water made it worth the expense, especially by depicting it as an alcohol replacement at business lunches. Within a decade or so, however, non-sparkling water began to exceed sales of sparkling and soon became the dominant form sold in the United States, as various companies competed for market share. Although Perrier entered the U.S. market using glass bottles, soon, for nonpremium brands, plastic bottles were the cheaper choice in which to market the product.

While generally available in smaller, one- and two-liter "bar" sizes, the most popular variety by the 1970s was the larger five-gallon container used in office water coolers. All told, it was estimated that some 350 million gallons of bottled water were sold annually in the United States when Perrier began its 1977 marketing campaign. By 2017, the American consumer was buying nearly 14 billion gallons of bottled water as part of a $16 billion industry. Globally, the demand for bottled water had increased to about 100 billion gallons. (China was the largest consumer of bottled water, followed by the United States and Mexico.) The United States market has grown every year since 1977, with the exception of two years during the recent recession. Italy has the greatest per capita demand at almost 50 gallons, with American consumption reaching 42 gallons per capita in 2017. By 2016, bottled water had surpassed soda (soft drinks) as the most purchased bottled beverage in the United States.

Part of the recent growth in bottled water sales, and of soda's decline, has been a health emphasis on staying hydrated throughout the day. Although various professional and industry groups, along with many individual companies, push an array of hydrating "sports" drinks and "energy" drinks, medical experts have always asserted any liquid can play a role in hydrating a person, but that water is always the best. Thus, many people's desire to have the optimal level of hydration to maintain their health has come to focus especially on bottled water—both spring-water and purified water—in handy sizes that can be consumed anywhere.

Definitions of Types

The three major classifications of bottled water are purified, spring, and mineral. Obviously, it is possible to create purified water in much greater quantities than either of the other two, as it is simply modified tap water. Mineral water is naturally occurring water that has more than 500 parts per million of dissolved solids (minerals) and can come from artesian wells or springs. Springwater is water that flows out of the ground and, after any necessary filtering, may or may not have sufficient dissolved solids to be classified as mineral water. Sometimes minerals are added, or returned, to springwater after the filtering/treatment process. Purified water can be distilled (condensed steam from boiling), filtered with traditional filters (such as charcoal), or purified by reverse osmosis. Purified water may also have some type of additional treatment, such as ultraviolet light, to insure a safe product.

Bottled Water Issues

Today, in the United States, bottled water can no longer make the claim that it had been able to make in earlier decades, that is safer and healthier than tap water. The International Bottled Water Association's code of conduct states that bottled water companies should not create fear about tap water in order to sell bottled water. However, occasionally headlines in the news do that for them. When locations such as Flint, Michigan, confront catastrophic levels of chemicals entering residents' tap water (in this case, lead), it causes people across the country to rethink drinking tap versus buying bottled water. At the same time, unlike in many other parts of the world, the growth in consumption of bottled water in the United States has not been based solely on the choice between bottled and tap, but also on the choice between bottled water and a sweetened beverage (soda, etc.). The paradigm began to shift as health concerns regarding sweetened beverages began to be raised in the 1990s, and distributors of bottled water made the most of that shift by promoting their product as the healthier choice.

In looking at bottled water versus tap water, there are, in this case too, some concerns about the large-scale consumption of bottled liquid. Questions have been raised about the dental effects, in children and youth, of families relying on bottled water rather than making use of fluoridated public water supplies, where treated water has been shown to help prevent tooth decay. Economically, since most of the water sold in the United States is purified—that is, drawn from the same sources as tap water—it can be asked whether it makes sense to spend hundreds or even thousands of times more than what would spend on tap water in order to access the commercial product. While it may be true that quality concerns have arisen more often for municipal systems than for commercial bottling operations, only in rare instances (such as Flint, Michigan) have there been serious causes for concern regarding the safety of public water systems. The rise of the fracking industry, however, has come with a parallel rise in instances of water contamination in public supplies.

The greatest concern for most regarding bottled water, however, is the container in which it is sold. While a few high-end distributors focusing on upscale restaurants still use glass bottles, the overwhelming majority of bottled water is sold in plastic bottles. In recent years, significant steps have been taken to improve the bottles (the amount of plastic in each bottle has decreased by over 50 percent in recent decades); nevertheless, the fact is that hundreds of tons of plastic water containers make their way into the waste stream every year. Recycling can and does occur in many locations, but that is not universally the case. Moreover, because bottled water is often purchased for its portability, recycling containers are not always available when and where it is consumed, creating landfill and litter problems. Discarded bottles do not biodegrade, and so remain a potential threat to animals and the environment for decades; and when they do break down, they leave vast amounts of tiny flecks known as microplastics, which, tragically, have increasingly shown up in the oceans and in freshwater sources around the world.

For this reason, lately there has been some movement (albeit tiny by comparison) away from bottled water and toward home filtration systems and reusable containers as well as home carbonation devices. Sales of canned "seltzer," another name for carbonated water (often lightly flavored), have also taken off as consumers seek alternatives and rediscover the pleasures of "fizz" as a way to hydrate and refresh.

Donald A. Watt

See also: Antioxidants; Detox Diets; Hydrotherapy; Juice and Juicing; Sanitation Campaigns and Public Health; Spas and Mineral Waters; Vitamins and Minerals

Further Reading

Chapelle, Francis H. 2005. *Wellsprings: A Natural History of Bottled Spring Waters.* Piscataway, NJ: Rutgers University Press.

Dege, Nicholas, ed. 2011. *Technology of Bottled Water.* 3rd ed. Oxford: Blackwell Publishing.

Gleick, Peter H. 2010. *Bottled and Sold: The Story behind Our Obsession with Bottled Water.* Washington, DC: Island Press.

Hawking, Gay, Emily Potter, and Kane Race. 2015. *Plastic Water: The Social and Material Life of Bottled Water.* Cambridge: MIT Press.

International Bottled Water Association. 2018. *IBWA: International Bottled Water Association.* www.bottledwater.org

Moss, Robert. "How Bottled Water Became America's Most Popular Beverage." *Serious Eats.* www.seriouseats.com/2017/07/how-bottled-water-became-americas-most-popular-beverage.html

BREATHWORK

The idea that controlling your breathing can change your state of mind is nothing new; the idea that it can influence the way your body works—or heals—is somewhat newer. After all, modern medicine (compared to medieval or ancient Greek understandings) has a better understanding of how the heart and lungs can influence blood pressure, heart rate, and more.

When people use the term *breathwork* now, they are often referring to a type of breathing that can influence physical, mental, and even spiritual health. Many of the different types of breathing have been taken from Eastern religion, philosophy, and medicine, though not all. Breathing can be directed in different patterns, focusing on different body parts, or with different goals.

Historical Roots

A variety of cultures have a history of using a pattern of breathing to change one's consciousness. The breath is often considered one of the "vital energies" of life—a point that is hard to argue with. Although most of what we understand as breathwork comes from Eastern religions, the Old Testament of Christianity occasionally focuses on breathing, such as the concept of the "breath of life." It also contains the seed of the practice of Hesychia, or The Silence. Learning the practice—focusing only on the tip of the nose as the breath moves in and out of the body—is reported to be what turned a monk named Gregory into Saint Gregory of Sinai.

The Creek (Muscogee) culture hero, Hisagita misa, also known as Breathmaker, taught the people how to fish, dig wells, and cultivate pumpkin; he also made the Milky Way by blowing its stars into the sky. Many cultures similarly associate breath with wind and weather, and see human respiration as a reflection of those larger cosmic forces. No doubt such connections have added to the allure of modern breathwork.

The English word *inspire* has its roots in the concept of being guided by divine or supernatural forces, and ultimately in the Latin term for "to breathe." In the 19th century, a commonly recommended form of therapy was "taking the air" outdoors, especially in mountainous areas where the air was cooler and fresher. This was in fact the *only* treatment available for tuberculosis and a variety of respiratory conditions at the time, with great sanatoriums being created to serve the need. Treks in nature also inspired (!) numerous Romantic-era poets and writers.

Breathwork in Therapy

Breathwork is not generally practiced on its own in the United States, but is often paired with other types of therapy. It can be combined with mindfulness work, couples or group therapy, or trauma therapy, as well as simple stress reduction. Breathwork can also be used with certain types of massage, as well as movement methodologies like Tai Chi or yoga.

Some different types of breathwork include:

- Rebirthing. This might be the most common example of how some people believe that breathing can heal trauma—in this case, specifically trauma that was caused during birth. Leonard Orr, the man who first created this concept, is said to have experienced his own rebirthing in his bathtub at home. Treatments involve either floating in liquid (like a bathtub) or blankets; this is said to simulate being in the womb. Rebirthers then emerge from whatever is containing them while practicing circular breathing—breathing without a pause between the inhale and exhale. While the practice was once popular in certain circles, with people snorkeling in their tubs while they contemplated being in the womb, the practice became much more controversial when a young woman named Candace Newmaker died during a rebirthing treatment in 2000.

- Holotropic Breathwork. Based on the work of Stanislav and Christina Grof, this type of breathwork uses a very rapid breathing pattern to introduce a heightened state of consciousness that practitioners say can be used to aid in trauma healing. Stan Grof, a Czech psychiatrist, was one of the founders of transpersonal psychology in the late 1960s and did extensive research in the area of Shamanism and altered states of consciousness before establishing the practice of holotropic breathwork in the 1990s as an alternative to the use of psychedelics. Unfortunately, the kind of hyperventilation involved in holotropic therapy can also raise the risk of seizures and even psychotic episodes, according to critics.

- Middendorf Breathwork. While Ilse Middendorf created her breathwork method in the 1930s, the concept did not emerge in the United States until 1986. Middendorf's breathing method is the opposite of holotropic; instead of rapid breathing, she pushed practitioners to simply allow their breath to flow in and out without pushing and pulling the air. The goal was to focus on body movements to instill a sense of mindfulness.

- Transformational Breathwork. This type of breathwork draws heavily on practices like Kundalini yoga while also pulling from body-mapping (a kind of art therapy), breath analysis, and other traditions. It was formalized by Dr. Judith Kravitz and is recommended by people like Deepak Chopra and Christine Northrup, both MDs well known for their work in the field of complementary and alternative medicine. Transformational breathwork work focuses on deep, full, relaxed breaths; it is the type of breathing often practiced at the end of general yoga classes.

No matter the type of breathwork, many people report feeling "lighter," more tranquil, and as if their emotional traumas had been eased or healed. They can also discover physical benefits, such as less pain, better sleep, and improved libido. Breathwork may be particularly useful for some people, because it can be done independently. When working with trauma, however, bringing up painful memories without a qualified professional present to guide the experience can be damaging, or even dangerous.

People who can find breathwork beneficial include those with PTSD, generalized anxiety, anger problems, depression, and addiction. Nevertheless, breathwork is not for everyone. There are many situations when breathwork can be risky, as when someone with heart disease, abnormal blood pressure, epilepsy, a history of aneurisms, or severe psychiatric symptoms (psychosis or paranoia in particular) attempts it. People who are pregnant are also advised to stay away from certain forms of breathwork.

Breathwork and the Stars

Like many alternative medicines, breathwork has a number of celebrities and high-profile fans who absolutely swear by its transformative powers. Deepak Chopra and Christine Northrup are both high-profile alternative physicians. Gisele Bündchen, model and wife to the football player Tom Brady, and Christy Turlington, model and filmmaker, both swear by the process in order to relieve anxiety and improve their well-being. Kate Hudson, actress, uses transformational breathing to manage her stress; she learned the practice from her mother, Goldie Hawn.

So, could breathwork ease your anxiety, minimize your depression, help you get a better night of sleep, and generally brighten your outlook on life? The research says that it just may. But will it cure your asthma, relieve your migraines, and reduce or cure your chronic pain? That is probably going to vary from person to person, and may involve other factors besides breathing.

Kay Tilden Frost and
Michael Shally-Jensen

See also: Ayurvedic Medicine; Chinese Traditional Medicine; Faith Healing and Prayer; Health and Wellness Gurus; Mind–Body Medicine; Native American Traditional Medicine; Sanatoriums; Shamanism and Neo-Shamanism

Further Reading

Brule, Dan, and Tony Robbins. 2017. *Just Breathe*. New York: Atria/Enliven Books.
Burke, Abbot George. 2018. "The Christian Tradition." *Breath Meditation*. November 9. https://breathmeditation.org/the-christian-tradition-of-breath-meditation
Serena, Katie. 2018. "The Tragic Tale of Candace Newmaker, The Girl Who Died in a 'Rebirthing' Treatment." *All That's Interesting*. March 14. https://allthatsinteresting.com /candace-newmaker

CUPPING

Cupping is a therapy that involves the application of cups, made of various materials, to the skin. Through different methods, the cupping therapist creates an area of lower pressure inside of the cup. This causes the top layers of the skin and muscle to lift slightly, allowing blood to flow into these spaces. Red marks often form on the skin in the areas where the cups have been applied. The practice dates back thousands of years and has been practiced across several continents. Some modern athletes still use cupping as a way to recover from difficult performances or hard training sessions.

Michael Phelps and Cupping's Olympic Moment

In the 2016 Olympic games, held in Rio de Janeiro, swimming fans noticed that superstar athlete Michael Phelps looked a little different as he got ready for his first swim. He had several circular reddish-purple marks on his shoulders. The Internet went wild with speculation as to what was going on, especially since Phelps wasn't the only swimmer with the marks.

Phelps quickly made sure to ease concerns. He told *The New York Times* on August 8, 2016, that he undergoes cupping before most of his meets and that he'd been doing it for years. "I asked for a little cupping yesterday because I was sore and the trainer hit me pretty hard and left a couple of bruises." He later posted a picture of himself receiving the treatment on Instagram, so his fans could see what it looked like.

Phelps's personal trainer, Keenan Robinson, told *Time* that he didn't turn to cupping specifically to heal his athletes; he believes that while massage works by pressing down to relax muscles, cupping works to relax the fascia—the fibers between and on top of muscles—to reduce soreness and offer more range of motion. When Phelps's workouts are intense and frequent as he works up to a meet, reducing soreness and improving recovery are top priorities.

Phelps is far from being the only famous user of cupping; football player DeMarcus Ware and former Olympian swimmer Natalie Coughlin have shared photos of themselves undergoing the treatment. Actresses Gwyneth Paltrow and Jennifer Aniston have also been seen sporting cupping marks.

History of Cupping

The oldest mention of cupping in surviving writings dates back to ancient Egypt. The Ebers Papyrus is the oldest known medical text; it dates back to 1500 BCE and describes the way both the Egyptians and the Saharan peoples used the practice. Hippocrates wrote about cupping in ancient Greece, around 400 BCE. He believed that cupping would cure internal diseases and fix structural problems.

Muhammad, the founder of Islam, recommended the practice, so Muslim physicians continued to practice and refine the technique. The method then spread into both Asian and European traditions in different ways. Cupping was mentioned by Ge Hong, the Daoist herbalist and alchemist who wrote during 281–341 CE, and by Maimonides, a philosopher within the Eastern European Jewish community, from 1135 to 1204 CE.

During the 14th century, cupping then spread to Italy; from there, the practice found its way into the rest of Europe, lasting well into the Renaissance in the 17th century. During this time, cupping was often used as a treatment for both gout and arthritis.

During the 18th and 19th centuries, cupping was primarily used as a more controlled version of bloodletting. Given the risks of many other methods of bloodletting, cupping must have been almost relieving. Practitioners could nevertheless overuse it, and secondary infections were a possibility, but the risks, overall, were less than those when a vein or artery was nicked. The risk of burning was higher, however: to

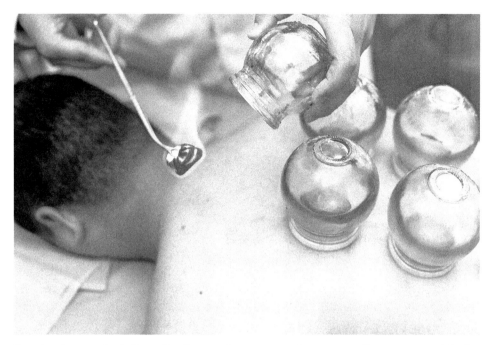

Cupping is an ancient alternative therapy that uses cups to create suction on a person's body. Some believe it helps increase circulation and remove toxins, among other benefits. (7postman/iStockPhoto.com)

create the area of low pressure, a small flame was slipped under the edge of the cup, then rapidly pulled back as the cup was pressed to the skin. If a practitioner's hand slipped, the direct flame could be painful or even result in a serious burn.

Wet cupping and bloodletting fell out of favor around the same time, but dry cupping continued as a treatment for pneumonia and rheumatic conditions through the first half of the 20th century. As modern antibiotics and antiinflammatories became more common, however, it died out too.

How Does Cupping Work?

The goal of cupping is to draw more blood to the skin's surface. The theory behind cupping, to a certain degree, mimics acupuncture. The movement of the blood stimulates pressure points, which allows fluids and energy to be healthfully distributed. The most common area for cupping applications is the back; this is a large surface area with several supposed energy meridians running through it, giving a therapist a number of treatment options.

Why do people use cupping as a therapy?

- By bringing the blood to the surface, the therapy is said to increase circulation.
- Muscle tissue and fascia are relaxed by the treatment, which promotes healing; many modern athletes use cupping to help speed recovery after competition or heavy practice.

- After surgery or injury, scar tissue and adhesions can heal stiffly and cause pain when moving; cupping is believed to gently stretch out the scar tissue, easing pain.
- By moving lymph fluid through the body, treatments can boost the immune system.
- Depression and anxiety can be eased by the gentle relaxation of a cupping treatment.

Types of Cupping

While practitioners have used various methods to complete the actual procedure, the basic theory is always the same. The cup is applied to the chosen area and a seal is created. A pressure change is created within the cup through the application of either cold or hot air, or sometimes using a mechanical pump. The cup is then left in place for as much as fifteen minutes.

Modern practitioners generally use glass cups, but before reliable glass vessels were available, practitioners used horn, clay, or even bamboo. And while cupping practice has spread throughout the world, it is currently most closely associated with traditional Chinese medicine.

The most common type of cupping is called fire cupping. The inside of the cup has rubbing alcohol applied to it; this is then lit before the cup is applied to the skin. When done by an experienced practitioner, the fire extinguishes quickly, having used up the oxygen in the closed environment and creating the necessary change in pressure within the cup. With an inexperienced practitioner, however, fire cupping carries a risk of burning.

Other types of cupping include the following.

- Wet cupping: after the cup has been initially removed, the therapist makes a small incision in the skin, then replaces the cup; this draws out a small amount of blood, which practitioners believe also draws toxins out of the body.
- Dry cupping: instead of using heat to create suction, this treatment uses a special pump to draw out air from the cup and achieve the same lowering of pressure; this gives the therapist more control over the treatment and eliminates the risk of burns.
- Moving cupping: before the chosen cupping method, the practitioner lubricates the skin with oils, often using fragrances that are relaxing and calming; once the cups have been applied, they can be moved over the skin, allowing for different types of treatment.

Most clients report that cupping feels pleasant and relaxing. The sensation is mild, simply a bit of pressure in the area to which the cup has been applied. Those who have experienced moving cupping often compare it to a massage. Some people report that cupping is less painful for deep tissue aches than a regular massage. The mild upward pressure may also be more comfortable than the intense downward pressure of massage, especially when considering the techniques that are often most useful in deep tissue massage.

Modern Resurgence of Cupping

Like many alternative therapies, cupping is often used for those conditions that are not well treated by modern Western medicine. Those who struggle with migraines, asthma, rheumatoid arthritis, or adhesions and scar tissue from surgery, for example, may find some relief from cupping.

Cupping is not entirely safe for some people, however. Those who bleed easily, or whose blood does not clot well, should not have cupping done to them. Practitioners should never place cups directly on veins or arteries, anywhere with varicose veins, or any kind of skin lesion. Open wounds and bone fractures are also unsafe locations for cupping.

A number of modern sports stars have been seen with the marks of cupping on their bodies during competitions. They say that cupping helps them improve recovery times, and that it is better than massage in terms of removing muscle soreness and improving their ability to stay at peak performance during a competition.

Some celebrities have also talked about cupping in terms of its detoxification benefits, massage comfort, and other uses.

There are few dangers of cupping. Scar formation and burns can occur at cupping sites. Abscesses or infections can form. Some people experience anemia after cupping. Many of these adverse effects may come from unskilled practitioners.

There are a few other possible adverse effects from treatment that generally pass quickly. There may be some bruising at the site where the cup was applied. Some people report headaches and dizziness after treatment. In general, the medical community believes the practice to be safe when performed by a trained and skilled practitioner.

Kay Tilden Frost

See also: Acupuncture; Bloodletting and Leeching; Chinese Traditional Medicine; Hydrotherapy; Magnet Therapy; Sweat Lodges and Saunas

Further Reading

Daly, Annie. 2018. "What is Cupping Therapy—And Should You Try It?" *Women's Health Magazine*, October 15. https://www.womenshealthmag.com/health/a19893209/everything-you-need-to-know-about-cupping/

Marcin, Ashley. 2016. "What Is Cupping Therapy?" *Healthline*. April 14. https://www.healthline.com/health/cupping-therapy#conditions

Wu Zhongchao. 2017. *A Practical Guide to Cupping Therapy*. Shanghai: Shanghai Press.

DEEP BRAIN STIMULATION

Treating internal structures of the brain using precisely placed electrode implants as a form of neurological therapy is a fairly recent development in medicine.

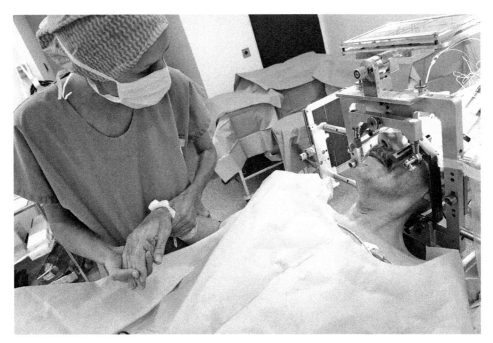

A patient suffering from Parkinson's disease is treated using deep brain stimulation. (BSIP/ UIG Via Getty Images)

Originally developed in the 1990s to address the movement disorders associated with Parkinson's disease, deep brain stimulation (DBS) is now used to address psychiatric problems such as anxiety and depression. Yet, after more than two decades of research and experimentation, DBS remains a viable treatment option only in the most severe cases, where patients have failed to respond to all other treatments. Such caution is perhaps warranted because the use of what is essentially a neural pacemaker does come with some risks. Still, the hope is that in the near future the technique will be refined to the point where it is available as a ready alternative to drug therapy.

Brain Trials . . . and Tribulations

The key to successful brain stimulation is a technique known as stereotactic surgery, or the targeting of specific sites in the brain using precision instruments together with a guidance system—basically a 3-D imaging system—that directs the surgeon toward the site of interest. The first use of this method was in England in the early 1900s, when two surgical researchers targeted an area deep inside a monkey's brain to see what would happen if they altered it. They drilled a hole in the monkey's skull and used a three-dimensional coordinate system built into a fixed metal frame to steady the monkey's head and keep track of the location of the surgical instrument as it proceeded to its target. They found that they could locate any point inside the brain to within a few millimeters using this approach. In this particular case, when they found the spot in the monkey's brain in which they were interested, they used an electrically charged rod to create brain lesions in the area. They could then record the animal's behavior to identify which aspects of behavior the area seemed to control. The experiment was more successful, however, as a pioneering surgical technique than it was as an advance in brain research. In any case, it went largely unheralded until the 1940s.

In 1936, the first lobotomies were performed in Lisbon, Portugal, by the neurologist Egaz Moniz. Moniz borrowed patients from local insane asylums to test his idea about destroying or severing the frontal lobe to make patients less emotionally troubled and aggressive—he had witnessed a similar procedure applied to chimpanzees. Moniz's lobotomy work was later deemed worthy of a Nobel Prize in Medicine, despite indications that it had serious negative consequences for many patients, leaving them rather zombielike, and also causing death in a few cases. In the United States, meanwhile, lobotomies were performed by the thousands in the late 1940s and 1950s. Its proponents claimed that it could cure everything from schizophrenia to homosexuality (which was then thought to be a mental disorder). Only after a decade or more of questionable outcomes did society respond by calling for an end to the practice—about the same time that a new antipsychotic drug, Thorazine, was discovered to take its place. (Thorazine turned out to have its own serious side effects, however.)

Also in the 1950s, a U.S. medical researcher, Robert Heath, began exploring the use of implants as a type of psychiatric treatment. Heath took patients from a mental hospital in New Orleans, cut open their skulls, and slipped electrodes inside their brains. Heath discovered that firing electrodes in certain brain areas (the hippocampus and thalamus) caused patients to react with rage or fear, while firing them in certain other areas (the amygdala and others) caused them to experience pleasure. Heath was a pathbreaking psychiatric researcher at Tulane University School of Medicine who also did work on mental programming for the CIA during the Cold War. Needless to say, some of his experiments would not be considered ethical today (see Frank 2018 for a full account). A 1972 novel by Michael Crichton, *The Terminal Man,* highlighted the dangers of early mind control techniques using implants.

Advances were made in the treatment of Parkinson's around the same time. Initial experiments in the 1950s using stereotactic surgery to disrupt a deep-brain area called the globus pallidus (or pallidum) proved successful in helping to control tremors and other movement problems in Parkinson's patients. Soon, the standard treatment for the condition involved destroying this area by means of electrodes or pure alcohol or else cutting around it with a wire. However, during the 1960s and 1970s, a dopamine compound called L-dopa came to replace psychosurgery for Parkinson's patients, for it was less invasive and seemed to produce excellent results. The use of L-dopa is depicted in the film *Awakenings,* featuring Robin Williams in the role of Oliver Sacks, who worked with people suffering from a serious form of Parkinson's and who wrote the book on which the film is based. As shown in the film, early positive results with L-dopa proved illusory, as over time patients developed severe "dyskinesias," or wild jerking movements, twisted postures, and other disabling side effects. Abandonment of the drug and a return to precision brain surgery was the result.

By the late 1980s, a technique had been developed to avoid surgical destruction of the pallidum and addressing instead a part of the thalamus, another structure deep inside the brain. By electrically stimulating the neurons of this structure at frequencies much higher than their normal rate of firing, they effectively become neutralized and patients could enjoy relief from their movement symptoms. Additional refinements to the method produced the technology we have today: programmed neurostimulators, or "pacemakers," that can be implanted under the skin (in the shoulder or chest area) to continuously control symptoms of Parkinson's and other disorders. This development is a return, in a sense, to *The Terminal Man*—albeit, this time, with better, more targeted goals and outcomes. Implants of this type have been used to treat "phantom limb syndrome," where, after the amputation of a limb, a patient continues to "feel" his or her limb and often experiences severe pain or a sense of dyskinesia regarding the phantom appendage. By artificially firing the neurons connected with pain and motion centers linked to the missing limb, implant technology brings symptom relief for amputees.

From Brain to Mind

One of the unexpected positive benefits of using neural implants for the treatment of Parkinson's disease was that, as patients lost their tremors and muscle discoordination, they also began to show visible signs of an improved *mood*. The change, moreover, did not seem to be linked solely to the pleasure associated with relief of their symptoms; rather, as researchers soon discovered, it appeared to be linked to the use of electrodes in the brain—at least in specific areas of the brain. Although no one knows exactly where in the brain a mood like depression or an experience like anxiety is located—indeed, most experts would agree that there is no single structure or area associated exclusively with either one—an area called Area 25 (in the cingulate region of the cerebral cortex) came to be regarded as crucial in both. Rich in serotonin transporters, Area 25 may be thought of as less a discrete unit having its own function than as a kind of hub for the parts of the brain's neural network that work together to address the effects of negative mood and anxious thoughts and behaviors. Stimulating Area 25 seems to bring joy to its owners.

Thus, today, still on a somewhat experimental basis, persons suffering from obsessive-compulsive disorder (OCD) or depression may receive an electrode implant in Area 25 (and other key areas) to help them with their condition. To qualify, they must first have tried virtually every other available remedy—psychotherapy, drugs of every variety and dosage, electroconvulsive therapy, and so forth—and have their cases reviewed by up to three different medical boards. It is a long, hard journey, but where this form of DBS has been used the results have been "extremely encouraging," according to one expert (quoted in Slater 2018, 320). The hope is that new applications might be found to treat other conditions, such as bipolar disorder, addictions, sleep disorders, and panic attacks. Already, neurostimulation is used in cardiac pacemakers, prosthetic devices, cochlear implants (hearing aids), and for Parkinson's patients. Perhaps a time will come when it is routinely used for mental/emotional conditions too. *The Terminal Man,* updated for the new century, could be in the offing.

Michael Shally-Jensen

See also: Acupuncture; Anxiety and Its Treatment; Biofeedback; Depression and Its Treatment; Electroconvulsive Therapy; Lobotomy and Other "Psychosurgeries"; Mental Hospitals

Further Reading

Aziz, T. Z., and J. F. Stein. 2004. "Brain Stimulation." In *The Oxford Companion to the Mind,* edited by Richard L. Gregory, 129–36. Oxford: Oxford University Press.
Chou, Kelvin L., Susan Grube, and Parag G. Patil. 2011. *Deep Brain Stimulation: A New Life for People with Parkinson's, Dystonia, and Essential Tremor.* New York: Demos Medical Publishing.
Frank, Lone. 2018. *The Pleasure Shock: The Rise of Deep Brain Stimulation and Its Forgotten Inventor.* New York: Dutton.
Slater, Lauren. 2018. *Blue Dreams: The Science and the Story of the Drugs That Changed Our Minds.* New York: Little, Brown.

DRAMA THERAPY

Watching a good movie or play can be a transformative experience, not just for the audience but for the actors as well. The ability to step outside oneself can, paradoxically, reveal profound insights about self-identity for those onstage and in the audience. It is this capacity of drama that psychotherapists sought to apply to mental health treatment starting in the 1950s. Drama therapy (spelled *dramatherapy* outside the U.S.) has its roots in several disciplines, including anthropology, psychology, psychotherapy, sociology, and theater. It uses techniques from theater to facilitate personal growth, the expression of feelings, and help people heal when undergoing times of stress or emotional upheaval. These techniques can include role playing, enaction (scripted or improvised), puppetry, masks, storytelling, and other forms of playacting. It is a type of creative arts therapy that achieves its purposes in the process of the dramatic experience rather than in the final enactment or the standard of the production.

Through the creative medium of drama, clients are encouraged to imagine experiences in inhabiting different roles, express emotions in a safe environment, and explore their own insights in the course of a performance. As an adaptable practice, it can be used to treat individuals, couples, and larger groups in a range of ages. This type of therapy has also been used in a variety of contexts, including schools, hospitals, prisons, and businesses as well as mental health treatment centers.

Drama

The human inclination for role playing and performance can be observed early in children without any exposure to formal theatrical productions. The simple action of a child playacting with a doll is a performance that involves the ability to invent new situations and inhabit roles outside of the self. Anthropologists have traced the roots of drama, from the simple and common action of playing with dolls to flashy theatrical shows with ensemble casts, to the importance of ritual in reinforcing social values and a sense of community. Ritual can take many forms and involves participants constructing a world to explore subjective feelings, as individuals and as members of a group or community. A communal dance to placate the gods allows participants to express fear of events or consequences outside their control, while a shaman's chant can help a subject in his or her desire to cope with illness or loss.

It is speculated that Greek drama evolved from a type of performance (the dithyramb) that involved a group dancing and singing in honor of the god Dionysus. Thespis is usually considered to be the first "actor" to step outside of the chorus and take a speaking role. Over time, the genre evolved to resemble something like the staged performance we recognize today. Stories told in Greek drama often revolved around themes of personal anguish, community values, and coping with an uncertain and unpredictable cosmos. Tragedies from the height of ancient Greek literature about mythical heroes like Oedipus, who killed his father and married his mother, and Orestes, who killed his mother to avenge his father, indelibly influenced Western theater, philosophy, and the development of psychology as a discipline.

It was Aristotle, a Greek philosopher, literary critic, and natural scientist, who first identified the therapeutic qualities of watching a play. In his *Poetics*, Aristotle identified the capability of tragedy to induce catharsis in spectators. In the term *catharsis*, or "cleansing," Aristotle borrowed from medical terminology to describe how tragedy could assist spectators in processing extreme emotions and finding relief. He also noticed in the same work how the most successful dramas have a mimetic quality, that is, they imitate real characters and situations that spectators may recognize from their own lives. These observations influenced later therapists in the incorporation of dramatic structures in their practice.

Psychodrama

Jacob L. Moreno (1889–1974) developed an important bridge between the artistic medium of drama and psychotherapy when he founded psychodrama, a discipline similar to but not the same as drama therapy. A contemporary of Sigmund Freud, Moreno challenged one of the central tenets of psychoanalysis, namely, that the "talking cure" alone was an effective way to achieve psychological change. Instead, Moreno proposed that change occurred for a client through the reenactment of distressing experiences to an audience of peers. After a performance in the practice of psychodrama, discussion ensued between the audience members and the "protagonist," all sharing their experiences. Although Moreno was inspired by his disagreements with psychoanalysis, he applied his ideas about the therapeutic qualities of dramatic performance and creativity not only to mental health treatment but to the operation of social networks.

Drama Therapy

Both psychodrama and drama therapy are forms of action psychotherapy, which means that they encompass more than just discussion between a client and therapist. Whereas psychodrama involves usually one client performing as him- or herself in front of a group, drama therapy encompasses a variety of different techniques and theories. Three people primarily helped the early development of drama therapy as a discipline and developed it as a separate field: Peter Slade, Sue Jennings, and Marion Lindkvist. Slade coined the term *dramatherapy* in England in the early 1950s based on his work with children and educational drama; Jennings next developed the term and expanded the scope of possibilities for using theatrical structures in therapy; and Lindkvist founded one of the first institutes, Sesame, in 1971 to train others in her process for using movement and story for healing.

Drama therapy can include some of the techniques of psychodrama, but in general drama therapy engages protagonists more through fictionalized scenarios, which require protagonists to use more imagination in acting out different roles. Practitioners have often disagreed with each other about the exact nature of their field, leaving the boundaries between psychodrama, drama therapy, and drama per se rather porous.

Principles and Techniques of Drama Therapy

Despite the ambiguities of definition, one of the basic elements in all drama therapy is play, which incorporates spontaneous problem solving and role discovery. Just as children using dolls often use their imagination to create stories and assume identities outside their own lived experiences, adults often distance themselves from thinking in such ways that can paradoxically be crucial in igniting self-awareness. Movement and action also are key elements in all drama therapy. For individuals who find oral expression alone difficult or limited, drama therapy's techniques can offer an alternative to talk therapy. Finally, metaphor is another key tenet, and it also separates drama therapy from the discipline of psychodrama. The ability to reconfigure the world through symbolic means is one way to assist individuals and groups to manage strong emotions and navigate subjective experiences.

Thus, participants can engage in role playing through scripted scenarios, where they must endeavor to understand and relate to the "character" or individual they have been assigned. Improvisation may allow participants to create characters spontaneously. Because they must draw upon their own personality and experiences, participating in improvisational role play often acts as a moment of self-expression or self-revelation.

Rather than being subject to a script or situation, clients can also control the story in another technique of drama therapy. When clients compose their own stories, or take the lead before an audience (either a group or just the therapist), they can often explore hypothetical endings or refocus the event in a way that helps clients cope with their own experiences. Similarly, clients can act out these stories, or act out their own behaviors as a way to consider their past actions. The process of acting out destructive behaviors has often been used for patients seeking treatment for addiction or for other harmful actions, since the distance permits these patients the ability to understand more thoughtfully the effects. Additionally, drama therapists also often use masks, dolls, and other props to assist patients in exploring other roles or in projecting their experiences in a safe, distanced space.

Clients

Owing to its eclectic techniques and origins in a wide range of fields, drama therapy can be and has been beneficial to a wide range of people. Participating in drama exercises has taught children on the autism spectrum how to approach social situations at school and enhance self-confidence. Neurotypical children have also benefited from drama therapy by teaching them how to manage their behavior and effectively manage conflict. Drama workshops in prison have helped reduce tension, improved interpersonal skills, and reduced recidivism. Brian Doerries's Theater of War project has helped veterans process trauma through the performance and discussion of ancient Greek tragedies. The success of Doerries's program and the lasting therapeutic appeal of these ancient dramas proves the great capacity the arts have for maintaining mental health.

Ashleigh Fata

See also: Anger and Anger Management; Anxiety and Its Treatment; Art and Music Therapy; Dance Therapy; Encounter Groups; Milieu Therapy and Therapeutic Community; Primal Therapy and Feeling Therapy; Psychoanalysis; Shamanism and Neo-Shamanism

Further Reading

Anderson-Warren, M., and R. Grainger 2000. *Practical Approaches to Drama Therapy: The Shield of Perseus*. London: Jessica Kingsley Publishers.

Jennings, S., A. Cattanach, S. Mitchel, et al. 1994. *The Handbook of Dramatherapy*. London: Routledge.

Langley, Dorothy. 2006. *An Introduction to Dramatherapy*. Thousand Oaks, CA: Sage Publications.

Malchiodi, Cathy A., ed. 2005. *Expressive Therapies*. New York: Guilford Press.

McFarlane, Penny. 2005. *Dramatherapy: Raising Children's Self-Esteem and Developing Emotional Stability*. London: David Fulton Publishers.

North American Drama Therapy Association. www.nadta.org

EATING ORGANIC

Throughout much of human history, including *all* of prehistory, eating organic was not a matter of choice; it was the only option available. While diets have varied dramatically, based on location and epoch, most food has always been taken directly from nature or cultivated by humans, without any substantial alteration taking place. As hunter-gatherer cultures gave way to agrarian pursuits, humans began to modify the natural world, through irrigation or natural fertilizers, to create more bountiful harvests. However, it has only been in the last few centuries that our knowledge of biology and chemistry, not to mention genetics, has advanced to the point where natural resources can be significantly altered so that new compounds not found in nature can be created for the purpose of producing larger, more resistant crops, "improved" livestock, and many other edible wonders (or disasters) like fast food and Twinkies.

History of the Organic Farming Movement

Early changes in agriculture made use of natural means to increase productivity, such as applying a premodern understanding of heredity to make more productive plants or to selectively breed different types of animals. By the 20th century, advances in chemistry and biology allowed a wide range of products to be made that could affect the growth and health of organisms. In large-scale agriculture, the first major step was developing chemicals that could replace natural fertilizers to ensure productive fields. As early as the 1920s, some critics raised concerns regarding the impact that these chemicals were having, not just on the produce itself but on the surrounding environment. In 1924, in Germany, Dr. Rudolf Steiner gave a series of lectures on soil and crop health, which many see as the first call for a return to organic agriculture. (Steiner is better known as the founder of Anthroposophy.) Nevertheless, the mainstream agricultural industry continued to develop and use new artificial and synthetic products and techniques.

The World War II period (particularly in Europe) created conflicting trends in agriculture. In 1939, DDT was found to be an effective insecticide, with widespread agricultural use beginning in 1942; it became widely available in the United States in 1945. During the same time period, two English nobles, working independently, began researching organic farming. Lord Northbourne, who was the first to use the term *organic farming*, wrote about how a system of organic farming could be sustainable, and profitable. Meanwhile, Lady Eve Balfour performed the first scientific experiment, comparing the productivity of two adjoining farms, one organic and the other utilizing the latest chemical products. Also, in the United States, James Rodale began what is now seen as the modern organic farming movement. He produced his own crops and began publishing *Organic Gardening and Farming Magazine* in 1942. Millions of Britons and Americans became familiar with organic farming techniques through the planting of victory gardens, which were understood to be part of the war effort by making families self-sufficient. At the same time, some chemicals created as part of munitions programs were discovered to have possible agricultural uses (as defoliants, pesticides, and the like). Thus, while the organic food movement was unfolding, so too was modern agribusiness.

Mainstreaming Organic

In 1962, awareness of the harmful effects of some agriculture products was spread through the publication of Rachel Carson's landmark book *Silent Spring*, which documented the harmful effects of DDT. The book helped to create the environmental movement, which of course is related to but not the same as the organic food movement. In addition, during the later 1960s the countercultural revolution got started. As more and more people began to question social norms and seek alternatives, many rejected the usual careers and (conformist) lifestyles. The more enthusiastic youth of the movement looked to back-to-the-land schemes and founded communes, which sought to create a sort of simplified, agrarian self-sufficiency. The 1960s counterculture thus blended with the budding organic movement to create a system that was able to supply organic foodstuffs both at home and to local markets. Both also contributed to a growing awareness of organic foods as healthy alternatives to commercial products.

After a decade of controversy, DDT was outlawed in the United States in 1972 as well as in most other nations. Around this same time, the International Federation of Organic Movements was created, in an effort to support organic farming around the world. Beginning in the 1970s, the organic farming and organic food movement in the United States began a slow but steady growth. By the early 1990s, organic farming passed the $1 billion mark, and at its proponents' request, the federal government began to develop standards for the labeling of products as "organic" for the benefit of consumers. (Up to this time, an "organic" label was based on state standards, or simply on a company's claim.) Based on legislation passed in 1990 (Organic Foods Production Act), in 2001, the U.S. Department of Agriculture (USDA) adopted the final set of regulations to insure integrity in the organic industry and provided a means of enforcement of these regulations. This has assisted the industry to move past $25 billion in annual sales during the second decade of the 21st century.

Current Organic Farming in the United States

Modern organic farming grew out of a movement known as humus farming, which focused on the health of the soil. Thus, a basic outline of organic farming would include taking actions that would increase the quality of the soil and water on a farm. This is the foundation of the effort to reduce pollution, create a more natural and healthier habitat for livestock, and to develop a sustainable cycle of resource development on the farm. Without using synthetic fertilizers or pesticides (or sewage), the organic farmer depends on plant waste, manure, and crop rotation to increase the quality of the soil. Mulch, cover crops, and compost are also used to decrease erosion and increase the soil's quality. Insect traps and predatory insects are used to control some pests. Because of known problems with certain pesticides, an increasing number of home gardeners no longer automatically reach for these. This has increased the demand for alternative solutions. However, these are not always available. In extreme circumstances, crops of commercial growers may be sprayed with some pesticides, under supervision of the USDA, and still be marketed as organic.

Organic animals are supplied with organic feed and graze in natural pastures when available, with living conditions generally being superior to those of modern industrial farms. These animals are allowed to be vaccinated against disease, but they cannot be given any antibiotics or growth hormones.

One area of recent growth—and public concern—is that of genetically modified (GM) plants and animals. While the principal focus of most discussion is on plants, experiments with animals have been ongoing. For example, Canada has allowed the selling of GM salmon, which mature in half the time of natural salmon. Most countries, however, have been resistant to the sale of GM animals. GM plants, on the other hand, have been widely accepted in many countries. By 2010, more than 80 percent of some basic staples in the United States were GM. Corn, cotton, soybeans, and sugar beets fall into this category. Organic farms cannot use any of these items in the production of their crops or as feed for their livestock.

Qualities of Organic Food

The growth in demand for organic food has been based on the idea that this food is better for the consumer and also better for the environment. There have been many nutritional studies conducted in an effort to explore the benefits of organic food. The results are not uniform, with some seeming to reflect the ideals of the organization doing the research. However, some differences in favor of eating organic have been found in some nutrients. Flavonoids (antioxidants) in produce and omega-3 fatty acids (associated with fish oil) in meat, dairy, and eggs are found at higher levels in organic food. Lower levels of toxic metals are found in organic grains, but not other organic products. Less pesticide residue is found on organic produce. The sources of any pesticide are neighboring farms or the organic pesticides allowed under USDA regulations.

In terms of the environment, obviously there is less chance of harmful side effects from organic farming versus agriculture that makes extensive use of chemicals. Organic farming theory generally states that chemicals add stress to the crops, which causes many of the problems seen on conventional farms. By relying on the recycling of agricultural products, more mulching, and cover crops, organic farmers believe that they reduce the stress, resulting in hardier plants and better crops. A major concern directed toward conventional farms is the spraying of chemicals. Organic farming does not have the potential side effect of having harmful compounds drift beyond the borders of the field and cause harm to other plants and animals (including humans).

Donald A. Watt

See also: Anthroposophic Medicine; Antioxidants; Bottled Water; Detox Diets; Diet and Exercise; Juice and Juicing; Macrobiotics; Paleo Diet; Sanatoriums; Spas and Mineral Waters; Vegetarianism

Further Reading

Andrei, Mihai. 2018. "Is Organic Food Actually Better? Here's What the Science Says." *ZME Science.* www.zmescience.com/other/science-abc/organic-food-science02092015/

Carson, Rachel. 2002. *Silent Spring.* 40th anniversary ed. New York: Houghton Mifflin.

Haspel, Tamar. 2018. "The Truth about Organic Produce and Pesticides." *Washington Post.* https://www.washingtonpost.com/lifestyle/food/the-truth-about-organic-produce-and-pesticides/2018/05/18/8294296e-5940-11e8-858f-12becb4d6067_story.html?utm_term=.c788510246a4

Rodale, Maria. 2010. *Organic Manifesto: How Organic Farming Can Heal Our Planet, Feed the World, and Keep Us Safe.* Emmaus, PA: Rodale Books.

Ronald, Pamela C., and Raoul W. Adamchak. 2018. *Tomorrow's Table: Organic Farming, Genetics, and the Future of Food.* 2nd ed. Oxford: Oxford University Press.

USDA National Organic Program. 2012. *2010-2011 Pilot Study: Pesticide Residue Testing of Organic Produce.* www.ams.usda.gov/sites/default/files/media/Pesticide%20Residue%20Testing_Org%20Produce_2010-11PilotStudy.pdf

FAT AND OBESITY SURGERY—AND OTHER WEIGHT-LOSS METHODS

Many people in American struggle with obesity. While some medical professionals and many media figures tout healthy eating and exercise as the keys to losing weight, these strategies simply do not seem to work for some people. No matter what they do, their weight stays high—and high enough to cause problems like joint pain, diabetes, sleep apnea, heart problems, and more.

For those who are somewhat overweight, but aren't necessarily experiencing health problems because of it, a few new treatments have emerged. Cool sculpting, for example, is a noninvasive procedure that uses deep cold to freeze fat cells. The cells die as a result, and are then naturally processed out of the body. As long as a person continues to exercise and eat well, the weight should stay off. Patients most often opt for this treatment when they have selected areas of stubborn fat that are resistant to the person's attempt to lose weight in other ways.

Another procedure, liposuction, also targets specific areas of fat that people are having difficulty losing. The fat is surgically removed in this case, generally through small suction tubes. In some cases, the fat cells are then used to perform plastic surgery procedures, such as filling out the cheeks or cheekbones.

Obesity surgery, a more involved operation, is the modern treatment for those who are morbidly obese and who have tried every other method of weight loss. The first modern weight-loss surgery was developed in the 1950s, and the techniques—which include bariatric and metabolic surgery—have improved since.

Before the arrival of surgery that could help people with serious health problems drop the weight that was killing them, however, there were hundreds of other methods that people used in attempting to lose weight—at any cost, it would seem. Below are a few of the more incredible.

Live Tapeworms

In the Victorian age, a slim figure was popular for both men and women; being overweight was considered a sign of gluttony, and ran counter to the prim Victorian understanding of morality. In order to try and lose weight, some Victorians would swallow live tapeworms.

Now, one sign that a person is infected with a tapeworm is weight loss; after all, tapeworms absorb nutrients before you can. But the tapeworms did eventually need to be killed, which meant taking dangerous antiparasitics or having a doctor remove the tapeworm in a risky procedure. And, while were infected, the patient would experience stomach pain, rectal problems, metabolism issues, and even episodes of epilepsy.

Doctors, even though working with a premodern understanding of the body, likely did not endorse this remedy for weight loss; tapeworms were known to be a dangerous affliction during this time. The practice is made evident, though, in consumer-oriented medical advertisements of the time; people could purchase tapeworms if they wished to. (More recently, Khloe Kardashian has commented that she would happily ingest a tapeworm if it meant losing weight—but you should not try this experiment at home!)

Arsenic

Along with tapeworms, the rigid Victorian society had another suggestion for losing weight: eating arsenic. Arsenic has many uses in modern society—electronics, batteries, and pesticides all use the metallic compound. But according to the U.S. Environmental Protection Agency, all forms of arsenic are dangerous poisons and should not be ingested in any way, or even handled without special tools and methods.

Many Victorian weight loss "remedies," however, did contain arsenic—enough, in fact, to give people severe poisoning. Worse, many of the remedies didn't even list the arsenic they contained as an ingredient; there were no regulations forcing them to do so. People could readily poison themselves without even knowing that they were doing so. Here too, it is unlikely that doctors suggested the use of arsenic as a dieting measure; our knowledge of the method comes mostly from popular advertisements. (In this era advertisements, like the labels on the products, could make any claims they wished to; it was up to the buyer to beware of falsehoods and exaggerations.)

The Great Masticator

The idea of simply not eating has been a concept floating around in the weight-loss field for a long time. Nowadays, of course, those who systematically starve themselves and lose a certain percentage of their weight because of it are often diagnosed with an eating disorder (anorexia or bulimia). In the early 1900s, however,

Horace Fletcher came up with an idea that he thought was a compromise to starving oneself. Instead of simply not eating, Fletcher advised chewing food so that one could enjoy the taste, and perhaps swallowing some of the juices, but then spitting the rest out to avoid taking in the calories.

Of course, chewing one's food but barely swallowing any of it is another name for starvation; it carries much the same risks as simply not eating, and is intensely unsatisfying as well. A person could lose weight this way, but his or her metabolism would likely be thrown off and they probably would immediately gain weight again upon going off the mastication diet.

Cigarette Smoking

One of the early and frequently touted "benefits" of smoking cigarettes was its ability to help people lose weight. This may have worked in a few different ways; nicotine, the addictive chemical in cigarettes, does function as an appetite suppressant. Also, people who tend to be "nervous eaters," or those who eat (and overeat) to calm down or have something to do, could, by smoking, have an alternative to hovering around food, keeping their hands and mouths busy without ingesting extra calories. In fact, when people try to quit smoking, they often discover that they end up gaining a few extra pounds.

While nicotine may be useful in this way, cigarette smoking causes many different additional health risks, particularly an increased risk of cancer in the mouth, throat, and lungs. Vaping nicotine may be a less risky way to take in nicotine, but science has not yet determined its medical safety.

Sauna Pants

Exercise instructors often say that sweating is evidence that a workout is achieving its goal. In the 1970s, therefore, inflatable sauna pants were developed to make users sweat –while exercising or simply while walking around. These pants looked a little like the water wings that kids used to wear to help them learn to swim, only they extended down the full length of the lower limbs and around the waist. Even today there are still items available that can be worn to increase sweating while working out, and theoretically boost one's weight loss, but they are no longer inflatable. And, unfortunately, they still have the same problem as the inflatable type: they do not do anything to influence how much weight you lose in a permanent way. They can increase the amount of water weight you lose during the workout itself, because of the excessive sweating, but that cannot really affect your weight over the long term. Plus, if you feel dehydrated after a workout, the best solution is to drink water—bringing you back to square one.

Creams and Soaps

For those who wanted to avoid tapeworms or starving themselves, a simpler solution was using various creams and soaps. In the late 19th and early 20th centuries, these were sold as "patent" remedies—that is, commercial products with little or no regulation. The user was advised to rub then on any part of the body that was deemed unsightly, and the fat, supposedly, would just melt away. Naturally, there was no such magic ointment, and these products did nothing but waste people's money.

In the modern day, this method survives in the form of collagen creams and chemicals whose makers swear that they will break down cellulite (fatty deposits) from the outside. Yet, even if these creams do sometimes offer a temporary change to the appearance of the skin, they do nothing to actually attack fat or reduce a person's weight.

Weight-Reducing Girdles

Corsets came into fashion hundreds of years ago, and are still occasionally seen today, either as fashion items, as tight spandex products designed to smooth out the figure, or as "waist trainers" designed to slim the waistline to an hourglass shape. The last of these products appears to have gotten its start in the early 20th century; it was marketed primarily to men, and was guaranteed to help reduce the appearance of an unsightly figure.

In a strange way, waist trainers and flex girdles might actually help a person to lose weight by preventing him or her from overeating. If you have ever needed to unbutton your pants after Thanksgiving dinner, then you know how the abdomen extends when you eat heavily. With stiff corsets, overeating would become uncomfortable even more quickly, discouraging the diner from continuing to eat. If weight gain is caused by overeating, such devices could help a person change his or her eating habits without resorting to a dangerous starvation diet.

Many people suggest that modern Americans who choose weight-loss surgery in order to get their weight under control are wasting their time and money while putting their health at risk. But when compared to such things as arsenic, tapeworms, useless creams, and the like, the procedure can begin to seem less bizarre and more medically precise.

Kay Tilden Frost

See also: Detox Diets; Diet and Exercise; Diet Pills and Metabolism Boosters; Juice and Juicing; Macrobiotics; Paleo Diet; Patent Medicines; Purgatives and Emetics; Sweat Lodges and Saunas; Vegetarianism

Further Reading

Fitzharris, Lindsey. 2017. *The Butchering Art: Joseph Lister's Quest to Transform the Grisly World of Victorian Medicine*. New York: Farrar, Straus, and Giroux.

Stolz, Jonathan L, M.D. 2018. *Medicine from Cave Dwellers to Millennials*. Longboat Key, FL: Telemachus Press.

"Story of Obesity Surgery." 2014. American Society for Metabolic and Bariatric Surgery. https://asmbs.org/resources/story-of-obesity-surgery

NARRATIVE THERAPY AND WRITING THERAPY

Narrative therapy and writing therapy sound as if they should be very similar, and in some ways they are. After all, narratives are stories, and stories are very often written down. There are indeed some similarities between the two approaches, but there are notable differences as well.

Narrative therapy began in the 1970s and 1980s through the work of Michael White and David Epstein (both of New Zealand), becoming more widely recognized in subsequent decades. Writing therapy, as a formalized treatment, goes back to the late 1980s and gained wider interest in the 1990s through the work of James Pennebaker (of the University of Texas at Austin) and others.

What Is Writing Therapy?

Writing therapy is somewhat self-explanatory; the patient writes down her thoughts and experiences. This is often done as part of trauma work. The patient may be given little direction or a great deal of direction; either way, she is usually asked to write for a certain period of time. Expressive writing usually involves simply writing about feelings and reactions to events or thoughts. In other situations, a patient might be directed to write an (unsent) letter to a living or deceased person about a particular event, sometimes with imagined replies. Sometimes these letters can even be addressed to inanimate objects: a recovering alcoholic, say, might write a letter to a bottle of liquor.

For many people, the act of writing down expressions of their traumas, feelings, and reactions helps to improve mood, to decrease symptoms of mental illness, and to release some of the negative emotions that are tied to their conditions. Scientists can measure the physical changes in the body that take place after such writing sessions take place, finding that lowered stress levels and, in some cases, improved immune system responses are among the positive benefits of writing therapy.

What is interesting, though, is that these results tend to be specific: they work best when someone is writing about a trauma, loss, or grief they have already disclosed to another person. Yet, oddly, scientists have also found that when someone writes about a trauma they have *not* experienced, similar decreases in stress and anxiety can be found. They are not entirely sure why this is so, but they are sure that the healthy result can occur—at least for most patients.

With the availability of the Internet, many people have found writing therapy to be particularly accessible. There are simply not enough therapists, especially in rural areas, for the number of people who need them. Many people find that communicating with a therapist by email can still get them the perspective they need in order to begin to heal and improve their quality of life.

However it is done, writing can serve as a kind of meditation or personal reflection. It can function as a private confession, of sorts, where thoughts, feelings, or perceptions that may be difficult to convey in direct conversation can be expressed nonetheless. It can be "creative, cathartic, and curative" all at the same time (quote in Lewis 2011, 231). And it need not be only about the writing of personal stories, or about past (traumatic) events. It can also be in the form of a diary or journal, where the person records his or her thoughts or reactions on a daily (or twice-weekly) basis. This kind of journaling can allow patients to identify issues, see patterns in their lives, and begin to problem-solve on their own. It can provide them with a sense of control over their thoughts, and even give them a new direction in their lives. Poetry, too, along with journals and stories, has helped many to get at experiences they otherwise might not disclose. Veterans of foreign wars have long made use of poetry and storytelling in this way.

What about Narrative Therapy?

Narrative therapy is somewhat different, though underlying it, again, is the concept of story. One of the primary features of narrative therapy is that it views people as separate from their problems. This can be particularly helpful when a person tends to say "I am a depressed person," or "I am an anxious person," for example. Reframing such language to present the situation as someone struggling with depression or working through anxiety can prove very useful in helping people to move through the difficulties facing them.

Narrative therapists often focus on helping people look at what they are facing and determining whether it protects them, harms them, or helps them. For example, a wife might say that she is constantly anxious. When digging into why she is feeling such anxiety, a therapist might discover that her husband is abusive. The wife's anxiety, therefore, is protective—she is on alert toward threats and danger because she needs to be. Instead of addressing the anxiety, the therapist would then move toward helping the woman find a safe way to exit the relationship, and heal the damage done in the process.

During narrative therapy, the therapist often tries to look at stories from a person's past, where they were happy or successful. They can use those moments to point out the ways in which a person succeeded in the past. This can help the person find the tools to succeed in the present.

Ultimately, narrative therapists view our lives as the stories we tell ourselves. Someone might tell him- or herself that he or she is disorganized or unhappy, for example. Identifying the stories that we tell ourselves and then studying them to see if they are true to our hopes and dreams is another way to find out if these stories are helpful or harmful. Once that is known, the therapist and the patient can work together on strengthening helpful, positive stories, and reframing harmful or unhelpful stories.

Narrative therapy can be used in individual or couples counseling, with adults or with children. It can be used to treat many different mental health concerns, but it is most often helpful with people who tend to view themselves and their problems as inseparable.

In a way, it is hardly surprising that narrative should be such a powerful tool in mental health. After all, psychotherapists have, from the beginning, found it useful to ask why someone has come to see them, and then listen to their stories about it and whatever else may be bothering them. Modern psychiatry, in fact, was founded on the case history, or patient stories augmented with the psychiatrist's interpretations and analyses. Such cases have been the foundation for the diagnosis and treatment of patients for over a century. Narrative therapy, then, draws from this rich history and focuses more closely on the intrinsic value of patient stories, making them the centerpiece of the work. It looks at "plot," metaphor, meaning, character, point of view, and other factors in making assessments about the nature of people's stories and determining the best strategies for helping them to navigate the world. (Narrative psychiatry does not necessarily eschew psychiatric drugs in applying treatments, though some individual practitioners might.)

How Are the Two Therapies Related?

While we cannot be absolutely certain why writing therapy seems to be helpful, apart from the fact that it allows a person to formulate and express his or her ideas and emotions, the concept of narrative may be part of why it helps. Humans have been telling stories throughout time. People who have been through trauma often get stuck reliving brief moments of the traumatic event without bringing any real cohesion to what is happening inside their heads. By writing it all down, they may be able to create a reliable narrative of what happened to them and feel more in control of the experience.

There is a theory that relates specifically to posttraumatic stress disorder, or PTSD. This theory says that PTSD occurs when a traumatic memory gets lodged (or "stuck") in the emotional centers of the brain, and is not properly processed out of emotional memories and into long-term memories, as would normally be the case. One can then reexperience the trauma whenever it is "triggered" by an event that directly or indirectly reminds one of the original event.

Writing therapy may work in a similar way. By allowing the person to organize his or her thoughts and exercise the "writing" centers of the brain (both linguistic/ cognitive and mobile/tactile centers) we may help such thoughts and memories to move out of short-term memory and into long-term memory, thereby removing some of their raw emotional power. Professional poets and writers have long understood the impetus behind this, and now many "amateur" writers have discovered its value as well. Some of these amateur writers, in fact, have gone on to write powerful works that turn out to be bestsellers.

Underlying both of these therapies is the idea that our stories are powerful, and that the way we create and relate them has a great impact on our own, and perhaps others', lives.

Kay Tilden Frost and
Michael Shally-Jensen

See also: Anxiety and Its Treatment; Art and Music Therapy; Client-Centered Therapy; Drama Therapy; Existential Psychotherapy; Guided Imagery, or Visualization; Primal Therapy and Feeling Therapy; Psychoanalysis; Recovered Memory Therapy, "Split Personality," and Satanism

Further Reading

Denborough, David. 2014. *Retelling the Stories of Our Lives: Everyday Narrative Therapy to Draw Inspiration and Transform Experience*. New York: W. W. Norton.

Lewis, Bradley. 2011. *Narrative Psychiatry: How Stories Can Shape Clinical Practice*. Baltimore: Johns Hopkins University Press.

Marinella, Stella. 2017. *The Story You Need to Tell: Writing to Heal A Trauma, Illness, or Loss*. Novato, CA: New World Library.

"What Is Narrative Therapy?" *Psychology Today*. November 21, 2018. https://www.psychologytoday.com/us/therapy-types/narrative-therapy.

NEURODIVERSITY

Although it has a number of meanings, the term *neurodiversity* mainly refers to a political and social movement dedicated to advancing the human and civil rights of individuals with neurological differences. The movement has been led primarily by autistic self-advocates, but in recent years other groups, such as those in the "hearing voices" community, have become aware of it and aligned themselves with some of its goals.

Neurodiversity, then, is a natural condition of humanity related to, but nevertheless distinct from, neurological difference. Whereas neurological difference originates in the biological reality that no two brains are identical, neurodiversity involves a choice to recognize differences as a fundamental component of identity and, often, to deliberately identify with a particular neurodiverse group or community (Baker 2006).

Although a neurotypical (or "normal") brain is as much a social construction as s a neurologically different one, differences recognized as sufficiently distinct from the accepted norm tend to come with certain difficulties in the context of society. Most of these difficulties result from factors external to the individual, particularly social, economic, cultural, and political factors. Moreover, some neurological differences constitute a threat to individual comfort or survival. As a result, each individual, in recognizing neurological difference as part of his or her identity, has the right to consider it personally undesirable or not, and to pursue palliative care or a cure, or not. Although objections to the use of "people first" language (e.g., in defense of individuals with disabilities) are sometimes raised by those embracing neurological difference as a core, positive element of their identity, use of such language in law and policy is best considered a means to include the expressed interests of all people with neurological differences.

At the group level, neurodiversity describes an inherently positive characteristic and a natural experience. Traditional classifications drawn from the fields of medicine and education are employed to describe neurodiverse groups. For example, categories and conditions defined in the American Psychiatric Association's *Diagnostic and Statistical Manual of Mental Disorders* (DSM) and in the World Health Organization's International Classification of Functioning, Disability and Health (ICF) are routinely employed in discussions of neurodiversity. Similar to discussions about other forms of diversity, much of the discourse on neurodiversity focuses on conditions understood as connected with minority groups that have historically been excluded, ignored, oppressed, or otherwise systematically disempowered. Examples of such conditions include autism, attention deficit hyperactivity disorder (ADHD), bipolar disorder, dyslexia, schizophrenia, and the hearing of voices. Political activity surrounding neurodiversity involves efforts to restore basic human rights, promote acceptance of neurological difference, and reduce the effects of neurotypical privilege wherever possible. A number of groups have their own organizations centered on specific conditions in addition to the neurodiversity movement.

Origins and Development of the Concept

The history of discrimination against those with disabilities is less well known than the histories of oppression toward other groups. While members of the general public are exposed to information about discrimination against racial and ethnic minorities, religious groups, and women, for example, information about disability is largely absent from public education programs and general public discourse, though some improvement has occurred in recent years. Justification of discrimination against individuals with disabilities is, unfortunately, not yet fully taboo.

The disability rights movement grew steadily over the course of the 20th century, resulting in significant changes in public policy such as deinstitutionalization, or the move away from hospitals for the mentally ill and toward community mental health systems, and the creation of rights-based, inclusionary special education. The neurodiversity movement is part of the larger disability rights movement. For example, the mission statement of the Autistic Self-Advocacy Network (ASAN) ends with one of the main disability rights mantras, "Nothing about Us, without Us!" (http://www.autisticadvocacy.org/).

The term *neurodiversity* began appearing in the media, on the Internet, and in gray literature (i.e., technical reports, working papers, policy statements) in the late 1990s, usually with reference to autistics. By the latter half of the first decade of the 21st century, the concept was being examined and articulated in the academic literature. Though use of the term in law and political discourse remains sparse, by 2011 it had appeared in legislative testimony and court proceedings in several countries, including Australia, Canada, France, Great Britain, and the United States. In the United States, one of the catalytic events of the neurodiversity movement was the so-called ransom notes campaign of 2007, in which poorly conceived advertisements seeking to raise awareness of childhood neurological and behavioral health issues represented autism, Asperger's syndrome, and other conditions as roughly equivalent to being kidnapped by an outsider. A protest led by Ari Ne'eman, the president of ASAN, led to a cessation of the campaign and expanded awareness of questions of rights associated with neurological difference (see Kaufmann 2007; Kras 2009). A key concern of this campaign was the unapologetic portrayal of autism and Asperger's as "totally debilitating.". By mid-2011, "neurodiversity" had been used in a cover story in the *New York Times*, lost its designation as a neologism on Wikipedia, been taught as a college course at a research university, and served as a theme for an academic symposium.

Debate remains as to whether or not neurodiversity can be attributed to differences in neurology or to psychological differences (Ortega 2009). Despite stunning recent progress, our understanding of human neurology is still in its infancy. Even whether or not a human brain should be considered a single entity or a kind of "team of rivals" remains unknown (Eagleman 2011, 109). Many neurological differences continue to rely on behavior-based diagnoses rather than on actual knowledge of underlying physiology. While such fundamental gaps in understanding are likely to continue for the foreseeable future, more relevant from the perspective of the politics of neurodiversity are the implications of this form of diversity as a characteristic of community.

Accommodations, Services, and Infrastructures

Some controversy surrounds the question of services and accommodations in the context of neurodiversity and neurological difference. For many observers, the assertion of disability rights accompanied by a demand for disability services appears contradictory at first glance. Typically, such impressions fail to take into account the existence of exclusionary infrastructures (such as access points, functionality of utilities, etc.). In any case, the denial of some individuals' needs above and beyond the making of infrastructure changes can be harmful to those incapable of self-care or in need of targeted services in order to participate in society even under conditions of full inclusion.

Neurotypical privilege continues to be broadly accepted. If, for example, a noise commonly irritating to those considered neurologically typical is present in an enclosed space (such as the sound of fingernails run down a blackboard), then a level of urgency around removing the source of the noise almost always develops. Stopping a noise similarly irritating to an individual identified as having a neurological difference would often be considered a low-level priority, with greater attention commonly paid either to removal of the individual or toward encouraging him or her to develop greater tolerance of the sound. Social norms and standards are, of course, a necessary condition of society. In fact, as Ann Jurecic (2007) has noted, one disabling but presumably well-intentioned response to the awareness of neurodiversity would be to relieve those with neurological difference of the expectation of conformity to social norms or standards of achievement expected of those considered neurologically typical (Jurecic 2007). However, much in the area of neurological privilege remains unexamined. Considerable deliberation will be required to distinguish between such privilege and expectations surrounding social norms and standards necessary for the functioning of society.

Stakeholders

Because diversity implies a level of interdependence, the direct effects of neurological difference on family members and other intimates of individuals with neurological differences also present dilemmas. The negative effects often experienced by parents of children with autism, for example, include financial suffering, social stigma, disempowerment, unfounded suspicion of deviancy, and marital strain. Significant improvement in this area could reasonably be expected as a result of substantial changes to exclusionary infrastructures and discriminatory attitudes. Nevertheless, the desire for a normal life achieved through a separate peace with society appears to be a common one among families living with neurological differences. A related issue is that of decline or suffering experienced as a result of living with neurological differences—especially when associated with increased risk of suicide, violence, homelessness, or incarceration. Many observers argue for limits to the tolerance of expressions of neurodiversity. In other words, the question of at what point behavior becomes dangerous or risky is a difficult one but one that must be discussed all the same.

There is also the issue of posttraumatic growth and increased sense of meaning that family members and intimates with neurological difference routinely experience. Part of this controversy surrounds the question of who gets to speak for people with neurological differences. This is a core identity-politics issue, common to all forms of diversity. On the one hand, there may be little reason to expect that an individual with a neurological difference is better equipped to speak for others, particularly those with different neurological conditions, simply by virtue of being considered neurologically atypical (Ortega 2009). On the other hand, any individual who has taken the time to learn about the implications of neurological difference has a level of expertise that is potentially relevant to political discourse surrounding neurodiversity, regardless of that individual's own neurological status. Thus the matter of who can speak for whom remains a work in progress.

Conclusion

It now appears that if human neurology were somehow simple enough for human beings to understand it, we would, paradoxically, not be intelligent enough to understand it (Eagleman 2011). Full recognition of neurodiversity, in both senses of the word, originates in a more mature understanding of the human brain than now exists or has existed in the past. Substantial use of that very same human brain, however, will be necessary in order to manage the opportunities and challenges posed by neurodiversity in coming years.

Dana Lee Baker

See also: Electroconvulsive Therapy; Mental Hospitals; Milieu Therapy and Therapeutic Community; Moral Treatment; Neurasthenia, or Nervous Exhaustion; Recovery Movement; Witch Trials and Exorcisms

Further Reading

Armstrong, Thomas. 2010. *Neurodiversity: Discovering the Extraordinary Gifts of Autism, ADHD, Dyslexia and Other Brain Differences.* New York: Da Capo Lifelong Books.

Autistic Self-Advocacy Network (ASAN). http://www.autisticadvocacy.org/.

Baker, Dana Lee. 2011. *The Politics of Neurodiversity: Why Public Policy Matters.* Boulder, CO: Lynne Rienner.

Eagleman, David. 2011. *Incognito: The Secret Lives of the Brain.* New York: Pantheon.

Grinkler, Roy Richard. 2008. *Unstrange Minds: Remapping the World of Autism.* Philadelphia: Basic Books.

Jurecic, Ann. 2007. "Neurodiversity." *College English* 69:421–42.

Kaufmann, Joanne. 2007. "Ransom-Notes Ads about Children's Health Are Canceled." *New York Times*, December 20, 2007.

Kras, Joseph F. 2009. "The 'Ransom Notes' Affair: When the Neurodiversity Movement Came of Age." *Disability Studies Quarterly* 30(1). http://dsq-sds .org/article/view/1065/1254

Neurodiversity: A Symposium. http://neurodiversitysymposium.wordpress .com/

Ortega, Francisco. 2009. "The Cerebral Subject and the Challenge of Neurodiversity." *BioSocieties* 4:425–45.

PALEO DIET

The Paleo diet offers a plan to lose weight and regain health by eating like the early cave dwellers or Neanderthals and lays the blame for many chronic health problems at the feet of what Americans do and do not eat. The Paleo Diet was written by Loren Cordain, PhD, and has become popular with dieters, athletes, and many Americans looking to solve autoimmune disorders and other chronic health issues.

While not the first to look at how cave dwellers ate, Cordain brought the concept to a large audience by writing his diet book supporting the idea of a Paleolithic diet. S. Boyd Eaton was among the earliest supporters of eating like our ancient ancestors and the first to offer a scientific principle based on what he termed *Paleolithic nutrition*. He published his theory in a 1985 *New England Journal of Medicine* article in which he outlined the evolution of human genes and how he thought they interacted with their nutritional environment. He suggested that early man became used to the nutrients in his foods, while modern man finds the convenience foods of today incompatible with his genetic makeup. Eaton and later Cordain publicly blame sugar and carbohydrate-filled foods for the current epidemic of obesity and diabetes in the United States.

Cordain took the idea of eating like our ancestors a step further and published his diet book in 2001 to moderate success. However, upon release of his revised edition in 2010, the word *paleo* had entered the national conversation, thanks to social media and the Internet, where bloggers and others shared their own personal successes with Paleo-style eating plans. An Internet search can deliver testimonials from thousands of people who have written about their stories of weight loss and improved health once they ate like cave dwellers and removed most carbohydrates from their daily menu.

In fact, the Internet continues to provide a forum for others with similar eating plans including Robb Wolf, Sarah Fragoso, Dr. Kurt Harris, and Chris Masterjohn. Wolf, author of *The Paleo Solution*, is a biochemist and offers information as well as podcasts about his unique paleo-eating plan. Fragoso was introduced to paleo-style eating by Wolf, and she also blogs and creates podcasts about her diet, which she calls everyday paleo. Dr. Kurt Harris calls himself an archevore and describes his diet as being based on essential principals. He is in private practice as a board-certified radiologist but blogs about nutrition with a focus on evolutionary biology. Masterjohn was influenced by Weston A. Price, and with a PhD in nutritional science, he has created a website that encourages a diet of quality animal foods based on his research that cholesterol is not the cause of heart disease in America.

In his book, Cordain made clear there are differences between his paleo diet and other similar eating plans as well as low-carbohydrate fad diets. For example, Cordain's paleo diet contains almost no carbohydrates when compared to the typical U.S. diet and includes more protein and more vegetables than the popular high-protein, low-carbohydrate diets like the Atkins plan. Cordain based his eating plan on studies he conducted as a researcher and professor of exercise physiology at Colorado State University.

Specifics of the Paleo Diet

Cordain laid out seven fundamental characteristics of his paleo program that he said sets it apart from any other diet. They include a higher protein intake, a higher fiber intake from a bigger selection of fruits and vegetables, a smaller number of carbohydrate foods, especially grains, and the drop in the glycemic index of foods eaten due to this lack of carbs an increase in consumption of monounsaturated and polyunsaturated fats but not vegetable oils, and an improved balance of Omega-3 and Omega-6 fat levels, higher potassium and lower sodium levels, an increase in vitamins, minerals, antioxidants, and plant phytochemicals and a change to the alkaline-acid load to the kidneys. Cordain reasoned that plant foods provide an alkaline balance rather than an acidic balance in the body. He suggested any increase in acidity is caused by other foods, especially processed foods or refined carbohydrate foods. An increase in acidity has been shown to increase bone and muscle loss along with encouraging high blood pressure. High acidity is also considered a factor in a number of kidney diseases including kidney stones.

So, what exactly are paleo dieters eating? Most fruits are allowed along with nuts and seeds like almonds, chestnuts, pecans, and walnuts. Cordain is very specific about which oils he recommends and has narrowed the acceptable choices to olive oil, walnut oil, flaxseed oil, and avocado oil. He strongly recommends against eating any canola oil and suggests the only oil for cooking should be olive. Other paleo-style diets allow coconut oil or palm oils, even though they are high in saturated fats.

Forbidden foods include all dairy products; all sugars, especially sucrose, fructose, and molasses; all grains from cereals, breads, pastas and other wheat products as well as oats, rice, and even increasingly popular ancient grains like quinoa and amaranth; all legumes such as beans, lentils, coffee, soybeans, and peanuts; all starchy foods including potatoes and sweet potatoes. The diet also recommends that people avoid fatty, salty, processed meats such as bacon, sausage, hot dogs, and lunch meats although in the updated version of Cordain's book he reassures those faithful to the basic principles of his paleo diet that they can eat those meats occasionally with no ill effects on their health. However, he strongly recommends that paleo followers seek out meats from animals that were not produced in a feedlot because they were raised on a grain-based diet. Instead, he recommends eating meat from wild animals or grass-fed animals.

A daily menu for the paleo diet is supposed to resemble what ancient people ate, only the choices are more contemporary. For example, foods like grass-fed meats, eggs, fish or other seafood, fresh vegetables and fruits along with olive, walnut, flaxseed, and avocado oils are all mainstays of the paleo menu. Cordain created three levels in his diet plan: Level I for those who want to move slowly into the diet and ease the feelings of deprivation that often go along with starting any diet, Level II for those willing to make a few more changes to their food choices, and Level III for those who want to make long-term behavioral changes quickly and who want to see immediate weight loss or health benefits.

Breakfast in Level I might include a bowl of diced fruits and vegetables like apples, carrots, and raisins, plus poached eggs, or some leftover protein, like chicken breast. Lunch would be a vegetable-laden salad, maybe with tuna or some other seafood, and a sample dinner might be veal or halibut, a green or spinach salad with some other steamed or fresh vegetable or fruit plus nuts and berries for dessert.

Level II might start with something like an omelet with avocado or a breakfast steak and some fresh fruit slices, lunch would be a spinach salad with crabmeat or leftover chicken and vegetables from the previous dinner. Dinner might include fish, chicken, or beef, with squash or vegetable soup, and some fresh fruit for dessert.

A Level III sample menu would include melon and berries plus a broiled pork chop or beefsteak for breakfast, and lunch might include baked cod, salmon steak or some other fish, and a vegetable salad. Dinner would have a serving of fish and perhaps also some game meat like venison, buffalo, or pheasant along with a green salad, steamed asparagus, or other nonstarchy vegetables and baked apples or other fresh fruits like dates or figs. For those who still feel hungry after eating a paleo meal, Cordain recommends eating additional lean protein, chicken or turkey breasts, fish, lean beef, shrimp or crab, and more crisp vegetables or fresh fruit.

Critics of the diet point to the possible effects on the heart from the high amounts of meat and fats and suggest the increased intake of protein might also create kidney problems. Scientists question whether Paleolithic peoples would have exhibited many of our modern health problems if they had longer life spans. According to fossil remains, it is clear that most people of that time period did not live long enough to reach middle age, which is when chronic diseases like diabetes, heart disease, cancer, and osteoporosis frequently develop in adults.

The lack of whole food groups is also a concern for nutritionists when it comes to high-protein diets, and that is a worry voiced by critics of the paleo diet. Health experts agree that growing obesity rates and rising numbers of diabetics can be linked to our dependence on processed foods filled with fats and sugar, as well as an overall lack of exercise. They admit any diet that focuses on whole foods and increases daily fruit and vegetable intake can't be totally negative. However, the cost of eating a steady diet of specialty meats, fresh fruits, and vegetables can be extremely expensive for the average family.

Marjolijn Bijlefeld and
Sharon K. Zoumbaris

See also: Aging Prevention, or "Successful Aging"; Antioxidants; Detox Diets; Diet and Exercise; Eating Organic; Juice and Juicing; Macrobiotics; Vegetarianism; Vitamins and Minerals

Further Reading

Audette, Ray. 1999. *Neanderthin: Eat Like a Caveman to Achieve a Lean, Strong, Healthy Body.* New York: St. Martin's.

Challem, Jack. 2013. "Is the Paleo Diet for You? The Healthiest Diet for Today and Tomorrow May Very Well Be the Eating Habits of the Past." *Better Nutrition* (April) 75(4):48.

Cordain, Loren. 2001. *The Paleo Diet: Lose Weight and Get Healthy by Eating the Food You Were Designed to Eat.* Hoboken, NJ: John Wiley and Sons.

Cordain, Loren, and Joe Friel. 2005. *The Paleo Diet for Athletes: A Nutritional Formula for Peak Athletic Performance.* Emmaus, PA: Rodale Books.

Sanfilippo, Diane. 2012. *Practical Paleo: A Customized Approach to Health and a Whole-Foods Lifestyle.* Las Vegas, NV: Victory Belt Publishing.

Zuk, Marlene. 2013. "Pondering Paleo: Channeling Your Inner Caveperson." *Nutrition Action Healthletter* (April) 40(3):9–11.

PET THERAPY

Pet therapy, also known as animal-assisted therapy, involves the use of common companion animals like dogs, cats, and horses to help people cope with mental and physical health issues. Animals require care from humans that increases our own mental and physical well-being, according to scientific research; the social bond between animals and humans can also reveal new insights and encourage us to approach our own emotions and experiences in a new light. Animal-assisted therapy can help in a variety of different situations: children struggling to read, patients undergoing difficult surgery, prisoners examining past behaviors, and soldiers struggling with PTSD, to name a few. The popularity and efficacy of animal-assisted therapy continues to prove the extent of the bond between humans and domesticated animals, which can affect the biological foundations of human well-being all the way to complex social functioning.

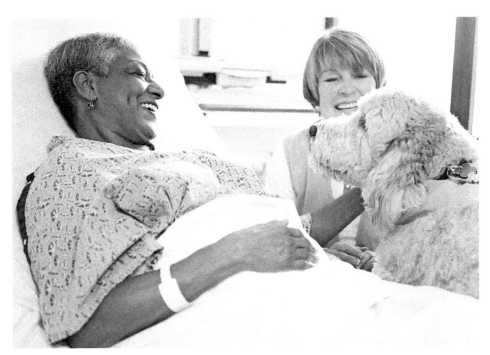

A therapy dog visits with a hospital patient during her recovery. (Monkey Business Images/ Dreamstime.com)

History of Development

A mutually beneficial relationship between humans and certain animals has existed almost as long as human history. Animal domestication follows closely the development of human civilization into complex agrarian societies. Humans in Mesopotamia perhaps first domesticated goats and cattle around 10,000 years ago. These tamed animals provided meat, milk, and hides for their human masters, and also could assist as beasts of burden in large-scale planting and harvesting of domesticated plants. The development of dogs from domesticated wolves is more uncertain. Scientists speculate that hunter-gatherer people anywhere from 20,000 to 40,000 years ago may have captured and raised wolf pups, or friendlier wolves may have incorporated themselves into human camps at the prospect of easy food scraps. Nonetheless, humans fostered this connection with these canines for hunting purposes and eventually companionship, as seen in the modern breeds of dog. The domestication of cats may have followed a similar trajectory: ancient felines found easy sources of food and safety in human homes, and humans found companions who were helpful at driving away disease-bearing or food-spoiling pests.

Some early evidence exists of animals assisting in therapeutic care. The healing cult of Asclepius in ancient Greek and Rome often used snakes and dogs in their practice. Suppliants, who would sleep at shrines of Asclepius, hoped that the physician god Asclepius would appear to them in the guise of a snake or a dog and lick their affected body parts or wounds. This association between dogs and healing continued into the Christian era. For example, Saint Rocco (Saint Roch) is often depicted in icons with his dog, who healed his companion's sores by licking them. Other saints attested as healers were often depicted with animals, such as Saint Christopher and Saint Bernard.

Around the time of the Enlightenment, people began to recognize that interacting with animals had a useful socializing influence too. One of the first recorded modern instances of using animals for therapeutic purposes comes from England at the York Retreat, founded by Quakers in 1792. The care of and interaction with animals like rabbits and birds on the grounds helped soothe patients and foster positive social skills. Around the same time, dogs were becoming more popular as companion pets, rather than seen only as tools for hunting and sport.

Mental and physical health treatment centers throughout the 19th century incorporated the care of animals to help patients suffering from a number of issues. Even Florence Nightingale, the founder of nursing, observed in 1860 that small pets often helped the sick in recovery. Later stories exist of animal-assisted care occurring for people coping with trauma from war, such as at the Pawling Army Air Force Convalescent Hospital in New York in the waning years of World War II. Soldiers recovering from injuries or dealing with psychological trauma worked with farm animals from 1944to 1945, but no data was kept or investigated scientifically that could have allowed researchers to assess the impact.

In 1964, Boris Levinson, a child psychiatrist, coined the term "pet therapy" to describe the effects canine companionship had on children residing at a treatment center. He discovered the usefulness in encouraging children to open up in his presence when he once had his dog Jingles in a room with an uncommunicative and withdrawn child. Levinson expanded on his findings in two later books and proposed that pets worked as "transitional objects": children could relate first to the animal, then to the therapist, and finally to other people in different spaces.

Other studies in psychiatric wards and prisons in the 1970s upheld Levinson's claims. The first professional organization for pet therapy was founded in 1977 and known then as the Delta Foundation (currently named Pet Partners). This group pioneered some of the first scientific studies on the therapeutic effects of animals on humans. Together with veterinarians, this group published the first guidelines for incorporating animals into mental and physical therapy.

Terminology and Techniques

Animal-assisted intervention is the umbrella term used to describe the variety of ways that animals are used to assist people in mental and physical therapy. Animal-assisted therapy (AAT) usually means a goal-directed intervention in a patient's treatment process. Specialized professionals direct this treatment, record the data scientifically, and evaluate the effects at the end. Animal-assisted activities (AAA) cover a broader scope of practice and in many cases do not require specialized professionals to manage the interaction. There are no specific goals in AAA, and the interaction with a therapy animal can occur spontaneously, rather than as part of a predetermined treatment plan.

Not just any pet can become a therapy animal. Prospective pets must pass certain guidelines in order to become certified. Some of the basic requirements include: good health, friendly disposition, good obedience skills, and comfort in new situations. Certain programs will have different rules or required courses for qualifying certain animals, and interested individuals should consult with particular programs themselves to understand these requirements.

Benefits and Questions

Social animals, like horses and dogs, make excellent therapy animals because of their biological instincts and history of breeding. These animals both desire and depend on positive social interactions, because they themselves come from pack or herd systems; these animals can also recognize signs of distress in their human counterparts and actively seek to calm them. Interventions with these types of animals can be transitional for patients who struggle to relate in human social interactions or provide relief by refocusing a person's attention away from a source of distress.

Science shows that engaging with an animal has many health benefits, from the immediate to long term. A brief interaction with an animal can release oxytocin, a hormone that makes people feel happier and strengthens social connections. The relaxation that animals induce can alleviate a patient's physical pain or reduce the amount of medication a person requires for pain management. Interacting with animals can also lower blood pressure, and activity with them can improve cardiovascular health.

Pet therapy has faced some detractors since the beginning of the field, when one heckler asked Dr. Levinson at a speaking engagement if he shared his pay with his dog. As a relatively recent field, pet therapy also suffers from the lack of long-term studies about the efficacy of this treatment. Those who question the efficacy of animal-assisted interventions cite inadequate or anecdotal evidence in studies on the use of animals in therapy and the influence of personal bias from the researchers. After research showed that there were direct physiological changes in humans after interacting with friendly animals, the inclination to disbelieve the effects of pet therapy lessened. The radical increase in pet therapy programs after this research into the physiological effects in 2002 seems to prove the growing acceptance of AAT as valid.

Ashleigh Fata

See also: Anxiety and Its Treatment; Art and Music Therapy; Depression and Its Treatment; Mind–Body Medicine; Stress and Stress Management

Further Reading
Altschiller, Donald. 2011. *Animal-Assisted Therapy*. Santa Barbara, CA: Greenwood.
Chandler, Cynthia K. 2017. *Animal-Assisted Therapy in Counseling*. New York: Routledge.

Fine, Aubrey H., ed. 2010. *Handbook on Animal-Assisted Therapy: Theoretical Foundations and Guidelines for Practices.* 3rd ed. San Diego, CA: Academic Press.

Levinson, Boris M. [1969] 1997. *Pet-Oriented Child Psychotherapy.* Revised by Gerald B. Mallon. Springfield, IL: Charles C. Thomas.

PAWS for People. www.pawsforpeople.org

Pet Partners. https://petpartners.org

PSYCHEDELIC DRUGS

Indigenous healers in the Amazon Basin and the deserts of Mexico, among other places, have known for millennia that plant hallucinogens like ayahuasca and peyote can be used for medical purposes. These botanicals can serve, in particular, to loosen patients' defenses and make them pliable and suggestible, allowing healers to lead them on a spiritual journey with the aid of chants, words, music, power objects, smoke, and other devices. The healers know that the human mind, when in the throes of an altered state of consciousness, can be manipulated, or directed, in such a way as to break down barriers to healing such as conventional worries and habitual patterns of thought. Through the use of hallucinogens, patients can gain a new perspective and, as guided by the shaman, find their way to feeling better.

Here are the words of one such healer:

> Seek and see all the marvels around you. You will get tired of looking at yourself alone, [as] that fatigue will make you deaf and blind to everything else. . . .
>
> You must always keep in mind that a path is only a path; if you feel you should not follow it, you must not stay with it under any conditions. . . . Does this path have a heart? If it does, the path is good; if it doesn't, it is of no use. Both paths lead nowhere; but one has a heart, the other doesn't. One makes for a joyful journey; as long as you follow it, you are one with it. The other will make you curse your life. One makes you strong; the other weakens you. (Quoted in Castaneda 1968, 31–32, 76, 118)

Although these words may not represent a verbatim recording (and were likely embellished or even created by the interlocutor), they serve to show how a person debilitated by negative thoughts or stuck in a psychological or emotional rut might benefit from being jarred awake by a dose of, say, psilocybin mushrooms and, with the benefit of an experienced guide, moved to reconsider his or her perception of reality.

In the case illustrated here, Carlos Castaneda, the person working with the wise man/shaman (Don Juan) quoted above, has taken psilocybin and other substances, and writes later about his own changing worldview:

> I had been experiencing brief flashes of disassociation, or shallow states of nonordinary reality. . . . In going over the images I recalled from my hallucinogenic experience, I had come to the unavoidable conclusion that I had seen the world in a way that was structurally different from ordinary vision. In other states of nonordinary reality I had undergone, the forms and the patterns I had visualized were always within the confines of my visual conception of the world. But the sensation of seeing

under the influence of the hallucinogenic . . . mixture was not the same. . . . After probing and exerting myself to remember, I was forced to make a series of analogies or similes in order to "understand" what I had "seen." (Ibid., 127–28)

More broadly, it was just such a quest for "enlightenment," or new experiences, that fueled the psychedelic drug craze of the 1960s, when millions of young people followed the controversial drug researcher Timothy Leary's advice to "turn on, tune in, and drop out." Indeed, Castaneda's book *The Teachings of Don Juan: A Yaqui Way of Knowledge* (1968), itself played a role in fueling that craze, spreading the word that psychedelic drugs were something to behold and becoming a cult classic in the process.

At the time of the book's publication, psychedelics were not only legal in the United States but, in the case of LSD (lysergic acid diethylamide), used by psychiatrists in selected therapeutic applications (depression, psychotherapy, alcoholism). Hundreds of studies showed their value in mental health settings. A number of celebrity users, like the actor Cary Grant and the writer Aldous Huxley, proclaimed their benefits. LSD has also been used by the CIA in experiments involving brainwashing, which tended only to reinforce its negative characterizations. By 1971, when President Richard Nixon labeled Timothy Leary "the most dangerous man in America," LSD and other such drugs were outlawed in the United States, except for limited academic research purposes. Since then, their use as either recreational drugs or psychiatric pharmaceuticals has taken place only "underground," their users subject to arrest and stiff penalties. That, however, has not stopped advocates from pressing the case for their acceptance as legitimate compounds that should be made available to professionals in the mental health community.

Psychedelic Therapy

Beginning in the 1990s, a second generation of academic researchers began exploring the use of psychedelics. This time, besides mental health applications, the focus was on other uses such as end-stage cancer treatment or remediation. Test trials using psilocybin were undertaken at Johns Hopkins University, New York University, the University of California–Los Angeles, and elsewhere. Cancer patients received relatively high doses of psilocybin and were guided by professional therapists. As recounted by author Michael Pollan, who had tried the drug himself on an unauthorized basis, under the supervision of a trained guide, "patients described going into their body and confronting their cancer or their fear of death; many had mystical experiences that gave them a glimpse of an afterlife or made them feel connected to nature or the universe in a way they found comforting" (Pollan 2018, 35). At the end of a second round of studies, some 80 percent of test subjects showed significant reductions in depression, anxiety, and other symptoms (ibid). Similar results have been reported in other studies focusing on reducing substance abuse and addiction; the working hypothesis in these studies is that psychedelic experiences give subjects a new perspective on their lives, allowing them to distance themselves from old ways of thinking and destructive coping mechanisms (Slater 2018, 269–70).

The Czech psychologist Stanislav Grof (1931–) developed what eventually became the standard model of psychedelic therapy in the late 1960s, although it parallels, in some ways, traditional shamanistic forms. It consists of three stages. The first stage is preparation, that is, working with the patient to identify the focus of the treatment and providing a set of guidelines for what it is to be expected during the psychedelic experience. The key here is developing trust and an openness on the part of the patient to encountering a loss of ego control, even a dissolution of the self, but under conditions that should make the person feel safe. The second stage is the psychedelic session or "journey," guided by an expert. Here, a comforting ambience is created through music and visual aids. Eyeshades and headphones might be used to encourage relaxation and the forgetting of daily concerns. The guide is trained not to intervene but to support and encourage exploration. The final stage (which typically takes place the next day) is that of integration, in which the patient, with the aid of the guide, processes the material that emerged during the psychedelic experience—Castaneda's "making sense" of what happened and figuring out how to explain it to oneself. This stage is often just as important as the central event, in that patients gain additional insight and illumination. They can begin to generalize in constructive ways about self and situation, person and myth, individual and universe. Those who have gone through psychedelic therapy say that it can be a mystical experience with substantial personal meaning and spiritual significance. In the least it has been demonstrated to be helpful in many cases.

Another psychoactive drug that has shown promise in experimental settings is the one-time "date rape" drug known as Ecstasy, or MDMA (methylenedioxymethamphetamine). Ecstasy is considered an empathogen, which means it increases feelings of empathy, connectedness, and sensual experience. Experiments with MDMA have shown that it can be valuable in addressing conditions as diverse as trauma, social anxiety (extreme shyness), autism, and marital discord. The drug seems to help build ego strength in victims of trauma, allowing them to revisit frightening memories in order to discuss them calmly and avoid blaming themselves (a common reaction). At the same time, MDMA boosts one's receptivity to social signals, thus permitting pathologically shy persons or those on the autism spectrum to pick up valuable communication clues and engage better with others. Similarly, partners who can no longer tolerate each other are enabled via MDMA to feel compassion and to begin communicating in healthy ways. The drug does so by stimulating the production of oxytocin in the brain, a molecule associated with social bonding and prosocial behaviors (Slater 2018, 273).

Other willing parties have quietly used microdoses of LSD to control symptoms of such ailments as depression and bipolar disorder. They ingest as little as 10 micrograms of the drug in order to improve their daily functioning, without undergoing all the ritual that surrounds taking a full-scale "trip" with a formal guide (Waldman 2017). Needless to say, this type of activity takes place strictly "underground" and is not well researched; users, therefore, should beware. Micro-dosing could be risky or even dangerous.

Critics of psychedelic therapy argue that it provides a chemical shortcut to a false sense of mystic satisfaction, not real enlightenment or the type of personal healing that might occur, for example, through fasting, meditation, or prayer. Those healers who hew to these other methods take umbrage at the idea that one can swallow a drug and reach nirvana, whereas truly touching divinity, or the secular equivalent of it, takes serious commitment, devotion, righteous behavior, and a progressive uncovering of deep moral truths (Slater 2018, 257). Scientists, for their part, have in some cases questioned the validity of using mystical experience as a measure in a therapeutic context. Such a notion, they say, borders on theology or shamanism, not psychological science. In response, researchers in the field continue to refine their procedures and expand their studies in the interest of advancing the science and demonstrating the value of psychedelic drugs for therapeutic uses (Sassa 2012).

Michael Shally-Jensen

See also: Anger and Anger Management; Anxiety and Its Treatment; Depression and Its Treatment; Shamanism and Neo-Shamanism

Further Reading

Castaneda, Carlos. 1968. *The Teachings of Don Juan: A Yaqui Way of Knowledge.* Berkeley: University of California Press.

Pollan, Michael. 2018. "Guided Explorations: My Adventures with the Researchers and Renegades Bringing Psychedelics into the Mental Health Mainstream." *New York Times Magazine,* May 20, 32–38; 61–65.

Sassa, Ben. 2012. *The Psychedelic Renaissance: Reassessing the Role of Psychedelic Drugs in 21st-Century Psychiatry and Society.* London: Muswell Press.

Shroder, Tom. 2014. *Acid Test: LSD, Ecstasy, and the Power to Heal.* New York: Blue Rider Press.

Slater, Lauren. 2018. *Blue Dreams: The Science and the Story of the Drugs that Changed Our Lives.* New York: Little, Brown.

Waldman, Ayelet. 2017. *A Really Good Day: How Microdosing Made a Mega Difference in My Mood, My Marriage, and My Life.* New York: Knopf.

About the Author and Contributors

Author

Michael Shally-Jensen is an independent editor and author specializing in reference works in history, American studies, the culture of health and wellness, and other subjects. Among his previous edited volumes is ABC-CLIO's *Mental Health Care Issues in America: An Encyclopedia*. He received his doctorate in cultural anthropology from Princeton University.

Contributors

Nicole A. Adamson is on the faculty of the Department of Educational Leadership and Counseling at the University of North Carolina at Pembroke, where she specializes in counseling and behavior therapy.

Dana Lee Baker is an associate professor at the School of Politics, Philosophy, and Public Affairs at Washington State University, where she specializes in public policy and comparative disability policy. Among her recent publications is *The Politics of Neurodiversity: Why Public Policy Matters*.

Charles Barber is a writer in residence at Wesleyan University and a lecturer in psychiatry at Yale. He has written widely on mental health and criminal justice issues, both in popular and scholarly publications.

Marjolijn Bijlefeld is a reporter and editor in Fredericksburg, Virginia. She is the coauthor of several Greenwood books, including *Food and You: A Guide to Healthy Habits for Teens* and *Encyclopedia of Diet Fads*.

Kathleen E. Darbor studies psychology in Texas A&M University's graduate program, focusing on the impact of emotions on cognitive processes.

Ashleigh Fata holds a master's degree in classics and teaches and writes in a variety of subjects as she pursues her doctorate at the University of California, Los Angeles.

Kay Tilden Frost is a historian who writes about health topics and other subjects online. Her work has appeared in such publications as *GeekMom*, *Grok Nation*, and *War History Online*, among others.

Leah Gongola is an assistant professor in the special education department at Youngstown State University and an educator and consultant in the area of autism and behavioral services.

Donna R. Kemp is professor emeritus of public administration in the Department of Political Science, California State University at Chico. Her previous work includes *Mental Health in America: A Reference Guide* (ABC-CLIO, 2007).

Julie Kipp is a practicing mental health social worker in New York City, specializing in schizophrenia and therapeutic communities. She received her PhD from New York University.

Timothy Kneeland is professor (and chair) of history and political science at Nazareth College, Pittsford, New York. He has published extensively on the history of science and medicine, among other subjects. Among his recent publications is an updated version of his *Pushbutton Psychiatry: A Cultural History of Electroshock Treatment in America*.

Victoria E. Kress is the director of the clinical mental health and addictions counseling program at Youngstown State University. Her most recent work, coauthored with Matthew J. Paylo, is *Treating Those with Mental Disorders*.

Heather C. Lench is professor of psychology, and department head, at Texas A&M University. Her work focuses on the interactions among cognitive and emotional processes.

Matthew J. Paylo is an associate professor and coordinator of the student affairs and college counseling program, as well as director of the counseling program, at Youngstown State University. His most recent work, coauthored with Victoria E. Kress, is *Treating Those with Mental Disorders*.

Sarah Raven is a research associate for The Connection Inc., Middletown, Connecticut, where she is working on a study examining the life stories of residents of a halfway house for ex-offenders.

Gretchen Reevy teaches in the Department of Psychology at California State University at East Bay, specializing in personality, stress and coping, and other subjects. Among her works is the *Encyclopedia of Emotion* (with the assistance of Y. M. Ozer and Y. Ito, Greenwood Press).

Dave Sells is an associate research scientist in the Program for Recovery and Community Health in the Department of Psychiatry at Yale University.

Sarah C. Sitton is an associate professor of psychology at St. Edward's University, Austin, Texas. Among her publications is *Life at the Texas State Lunatic Asylum, 1857–1997*.

Robert Surbrug is an assistant professor of history and director of the honors program at Bay Path University's School of Liberal Studies. His scholarly focus is on the social and political movements of the 1960s and 1970s. Among his publications is *Beyond Vietnam: The Politics of Protest in Massachusetts, 1974–1990*.

Richard Van Voorhis is an associate professor in the school psychology program at Youngstown State University.

Donald A. Watt retired to Idaho to write and pursue various educational interests after having served as dean of liberal arts, professor of political science and geography, vice president of academic affairs, and in other professional capacities.

Melinda Wolford is a specialist in neurological disorders of children and a practicing school psychologist. She also serves as an assistant professor in the counseling and special education department at Youngstown State University.

Sharon K. Zoumbaris is a professional librarian and freelance writer/editor. Her published works include ABC-CLIO's *Nutrition: Health and Medical Issues Today*; *Food and You: A Guide to Healthy Habits for Teens*, and *Encyclopedia of Diet Fads*.

Index

Page numbers in **bold** indicate the location of main entries.

Vitamins (*cont.*)
   in vegetarianism, 240
   See also Minerals
Voices, 70–71, 143, 371–372
Voodoo, **241–244**

Walking, 21, 59, 253, 276, 295, **336–340**
Water cure, 2, 14, 20–23, 43, 53, 68. *See also*
   Hydrotherapy
Watson, John, 95
Watts, Alan, 200, 202
Weight-loss methods, 116, 276, 286, 364
Weil, Andrew, 211, 214–215, 237, 251,
   280–281, 314
Weiss, Brian, 299
Wellness promotion, 30, 49, 116, **283–284**
Wertheimer, Max, 132
Western culture, 73, 106, 174, 257, 290
Wheat, 194, 286, 334, 376
Whitehouse, Mary Starks, 198–199
Whole grains, 1, 114, 116, 215, 216, 262, 333,
   335
Wilmer, Harry, 225–226
Witch trials, **71–76**
Witchcraft, 13, 24, 73–75, 176, 242
Wolfe, Tom, 200, 203
Women
   and anger, 256
   and antioxidants, 261
   and anxiety, 86
   and bloodletting, 7
   and depression, 106
   dreams and, 119
   exercises for, 115, 286
   as folk practitioners, 13
   and hydrotherapy, 21–22
   and hysteria, 24, 25
   idealized images of, 273
   in medicine shows, 28

   in mental hospitals, 146–147
   and mesmerism, 32
   and multiple personality disorder, 301–302
   and *nervios,* 324
   neurasthenia and, 43
   reformers, 37, 52
   and sedatives, 170
   spiritualism and, 70
   and sexuality, 161–162
   and witchcraft, 71–75
   and women's health, 172
   and stress, 325
   and vitamins, 334, 335, 336
   and yoga, 342
   zar cult and, 317
Women's health, 21, 86, 106, 170–172, 261,
   334–336
Writing therapy, **368–371**

Yalom, Irvin, 207
Yamas, 245
Yeast, 281, 333
Yin and yang, 10–12, 15, 173–174, 217, 321,
   329–330
Yoga, **245–248**
   in Ayurveda, 188
   breathwork and, 347–348
   in macrobiotic lifestyle, 217
   and meditation, 221
   in mind-body medicine, 290–291
   and reincarnation, 298
   for seniors, 253
   in spas, 67
   for stress, 324–325
   in U.S. population, 341–342
Yogi, Maharishi Mahesh, 223–225

Zodiac, 184, 186
Zombies, 241–243